Teaching Nursing: The Art and Science

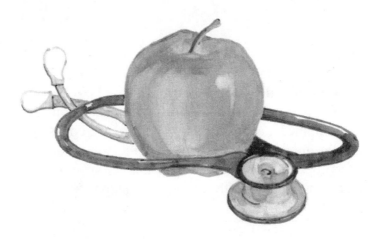

Linda Caputi, MSN, EdD, RN
Professor of Nursing
College of DuPage
Glen Ellyn, Illinois

Volume 3

College of DuPage Press

College of DuPage Press
425 Fawell Blvd.
Glen Ellyn, Illinois 60137

Project Manager: Joseph Barillari
Designer: Janice Walker
Typesetter: Janice Walker
CD Designer: Kevin Dudey
Production Coordinator: Janice Walker
Editor: Sean Brenner

About College of DuPage: For more than 15 years College of DuPage has been a leader in publishing educational materials for nursing education including multimedia computer programs, videos, books, and other print materials. We are committed to providing the highest quality products in the most appropriate format for our colleagues. Visit the College of DuPage website at www.cod.edu/software for information on all our products.

Acknowledgements

After attending the National League for Nursing's Education Summit last September, I was excited and energized! I became acutely aware that the scope of nursing education was even broader than I had realized. Volumes 1 and 2 of *Teaching Nursing: The Art and Science* were not even off the presses and I was eager to start Volume 3. I approached Joseph Barillari about assembling a cadre of experts to write this third volume. As usual, his faith in my work and his support of nursing education were ever present. So, the work began.

The group of chapter authors in Volume 3 are as stellar as those who wrote in Volumes 1 and 2. It always amazes me how dedicated these professionals are. Writing a book chapter is no easy task, and I appreciate all their time and effort. I would also like to acknowledge the three reviewers of this text for their timely and thoughtful comments: Ken Edmisson, Marilyn Frank-Stromborg, and Nancy Kron.

It would be impossible to list all the people at College of DuPage who made this volume possible. I would like to thank the college leadership and my colleagues for their support. I would especially like to acknowledge Joseph Barillari, Director of Information Technology, Special Services, for his support; it is a privilege to work with such an administrator. As always, I appreciate the work of the support staff in information technology who helped maintain a smooth, efficient production process: Gail McPike, Cathy Russo, and Patricia Kaira. I am also grateful for the hard work of my editor Sean Brenner, book designer Janice Walker, and CD developer Kevin Dudey.

Finally, I would like to thank my family for their endless support and patience: my husband Victor, son Vincent, and daughter Linnea.

- Linda Caputi

Preface

Nursing practice is a demanding profession—the serious nature of the work, an exhausting work schedule, the need to juggle many tasks simultaneously, and the breadth of knowledge and cognitive abilities necessary for safe practice.

Teaching nursing mirrors the practice field, requiring skills that all teachers have, plus a lot more! Nursing faculty must deal with college and hospital administration, legal challenges, funding deficits, and numerous other hurdles. Entering the world of nursing education is a complex, multifaceted journey. This book was written to help you on this journey, whether you're at the beginning or nearing its end.

Because of the complex nature of nursing education, I have drawn upon the knowledge of more than 25 experts to help write this volume, bringing their personalities and expertise to the subject at hand. I am proud of the many experts who graciously contributed chapters. These authors bring a wealth of information and a wide diversity of backgrounds and styles. To maintain each author's unique voice, I have made every effort to preserve individuality in writing style, allowing each author to set the tone for his or her chapter. With this approach, the reader can experience the true spirit of the author's personal expertise. My three reviewers also represent diverse backgrounds, and they provided their own unique perspectives as they reviewed each chapter.

The overall character of *Teaching Nursing: The Art and Science* is friendly but professional, so sit back and enjoy!

Foreward

As you read this book, you will no doubt be thinking about how the content might apply to you, your students, and your teaching philosophy. To take full advantage of the varied backgrounds and expertise of the chapter authors, I have asked them to share their teaching philosophies with you. Each author's philosophy appears below the apple icons on the first page of each chapter—providing an array of teaching perspectives for you to ponder.

Teaching Nursing: The Art and Science, Volume 3, is a book whose value lies in both its practical and theoretical applications. To that end, I have created a CD-ROM that holds valuable supplemental material the authors have designed.

Where you see this symbol:

you may refer to the CD-ROM to explore these additional materials. Please feel free to use these tools in your role as a nurse educator. You may wish to use these materials as a springboard to develop your own educational materials. These items are copyrighted as noted.

Editor

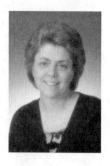

Linda Caputi, MSN, EdD, RN
Linda was awarded a BSN from Northern Illinois University, an MSN from Loyola University, and an EdD in instructional technology from Northern Illinois University.

Dr. Caputi has authored and co-authored more than 25 educational software programs, three books for nursing educators, and several journal articles. She won a 2004 Pinnacle award from Sigma Theta Tau for the software program *PhysWhiz II: Labor and Delivery,* and has won six awards from Sigma Theta Tau, two from American Journal of Nursing Company, and one from the Association for Educational Communications and Technology. Dr. Caputi was acknowledged for teaching excellence in the 1998 and 2002 editions of *Who's Who Among America's Teachers.* Dr. Caputi is a professor of nursing at College of DuPage, Glen Ellyn, Illinois, and is on the editorial staff of *Advance for Nurses.*

Authors

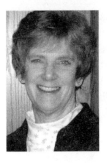

Catherine A. Andrews, MS, PhD, RN

Cathy was awarded a BS in nursing from the University of San Francisco and an MS in nursing and a PhD in Continuing and Vocational Education from the University of Wisconsin-Madison.

Dr. Andrews is an associate professor at Edgewood College, a small liberal arts college in Madison, Wisconsin, where she teaches baccalaureate nursing students, RNs studying for baccalaureate degrees, and nurses studying in the master's program. Cathy is a clinical examiner for Excelsior College, Albany, New York. She has been an educator in both hospital and academic settings for the past 20 years. Dr. Andrews is very dedicated to modifying coursework to include interpretive pedagogies and has a special interest in clinical education.

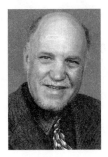

Joseph Barillari, BA, MA

Joseph Barillari is director of the Information Technology Office of Special Services at College of DuPage, Glen Ellyn, Illinois, where he manages the College of DuPage Press and the Library Learning Network, a satellite-broadcast training series for librarians in the United States, Canada, and the Caribbean. For 25 years, he has developed and managed nontraditional programs for Northern Illinois University and College of DuPage. He has taught history and humanities at Dundalk Community College, Essex Community College, Old Dominion University, and University of Maryland. Mr. Barillari received a bachelor's degree from College of Wooster, Wooster, Ohio, and a master's degree in history from Washington University in St. Louis, where he also completed additional advanced studies. A longtime photographer and film fan, Mr. Barillari writes a weekly movie review for a Chicago radio program.

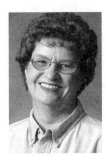

Carol Boswell, MSN, EdD, RN

Carol received a diploma degree from Methodist Hospital School of Nursing in Lubbock, Texas. After practicing for several years, she returned to school and was awarded a BSN from Texas Tech University Health Sciences Center in Odessa, an MSN from Texas Tech University Health Sciences Center in Lubbock, and an EdD in curriculum development from Texas Tech University in Lubbock.

Dr. Boswell frequently speaks at local, state, national, and international conferences. She has authored multiple publications related to health literacy, online teaching, research, and diabetes. She has been an educator for more than 10 years, working at multiple levels, including ADN, RN-BSN, graduate, and continuing education. She is currently on the faculty at the school of nursing at Texas Tech University Health Sciences Center.

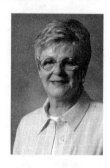

Sharon Cannon, MSN, EdD, RN

Sharon received her BSN from St. Louis University, and an MSN and EdD from Southern Illinois University, Edwardsville.

Dr. Cannon is a professor and regional dean for Texas Tech University Health Sciences Center in Odessa. She has been an educator for more than 20 years in various settings, including ADN, BSN, graduate and continuing education. She has presented at local, state, national and international conferences with an emphasis on healthcare literacy, leadership, curriculum, instruction, and online education. She has authored multiple publications on topics ranging from healthcare literacy to politics in nursing.

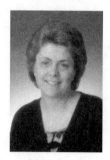

Linda Caputi, MSN, EdD, RN

Linda was awarded a BSN from Northern Illinois University, an MSN from Loyola University, and an EdD in instructional technology from Northern Illinois University.

Dr. Caputi has authored and co-authored more than 25 educational software programs, three books for nursing educators, and several journal articles. She won a 2004 Pinnacle award from Sigma Theta Tau for the software program *PhysWhiz II: Labor and Delivery*, and has won six awards from Sigma Theta Tau, two from American Journal of Nursing Company, and one from the Association for Educational Communications and Technology. Dr. Caputi was acknowledged for teaching excellence in the 1998 and 2002 editions of *Who's Who Among America's Teachers*. Dr. Caputi is a professor of nursing at College of DuPage, Glen Ellyn, Illinois, and is on the editorial staff of *Advance for Nurses*.

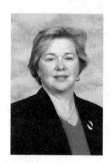

Glennys Compton, BSN, MSN, RN, ANP

Glennys received a diploma in nursing from Lutheran Hospital School for Nursing in Moline, Illinois, a BSN and adult nurse practitioner certification from Metropolitan State College, Denver, Colorado, and an MSN from the University of Wisconsin - Milwaukee. She is an associate professor of nursing at Alverno College in Milwaukee, Wisconsin, where she has taught pharmacology, foundational nursing, and intermediate courses in psychiatric and medical-surgical nursing. Her teaching expertise centers around care of acutely ill adults, critical care, care of chronically ill adults, and the use of technology in teaching.

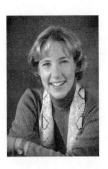

Susan Diehl, BSN, MSN, RN, FNP, APRN

Susan received her BSN from Cedar Crest College in Allentown, Pennsylvania, and an MSN from Saint Joseph College in West Hartford, Connecticut. She is completing her dissertation for an EdD in educational leadership at the University of Hartford in Connecticut.

Susan is a family nurse practitioner and assistant professor at the University of Hartford. She is a research consultant and grant reviewer for the State of Connecticut Children's Trust Fund, and is active in the development of community programs for children and families in Hartford and surrounding communities.

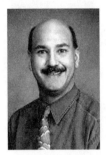

Ken W. Edmisson, ND, EdD, RNC, FNP

Ken received an ASN from Tennessee State University and an MSN and doctorate in nursing from the Frances Payne Bolton School of Nursing at Case Western Reserve University, with majors in family nurse practitioner, nursing administration, and clinical practice and inquiry. He received an EdD in curriculum and instruction from Tennessee State University.

Dr. Edmisson has worked at all levels, from staff nurse to director of nursing, in a variety of settings. He teaches medical-surgical and acute care nursing, research and theory, health assessment, pathophysiology, and management courses. He is a certified family nurse practitioner and medical-surgical nurse. Dr. Edmisson is an associate professor in the School of Nursing, Middle Tennessee State University.

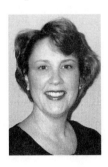

Lynn Engelmann, MSN, EdD, RN

Lynn was awarded a BSN from Marycrest College in Davenport, Iowa, an MSN from the Frances Payne Bolton School of Nursing at Case Western Reserve University, and an EdD in adult and continuing education from Northern Illinois University.

Dr. Engelmann is co-author of the book *Coaching Your Students to NCLEX Success* and co-editor of volumes 1 and 2 of *Teaching Nursing: The Art and Science*. She is a professor of medical-surgical nursing at College of DuPage, Glen Ellyn, Illinois. Lynn has presented nationally at conferences on program and NCLEX success. Curriculum and evaluation are her areas of special interest. She has been a faculty member in nursing education for more than 20 years.

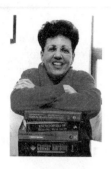

Marilyn Frank-Stromborg, MS, EdD, JD, RN, ANP, FAAN
Marilyn was awarded a BS from Northern Illinois University, an MS from the School of Nursing at New York Medical College, and a doctorate in educational psychology and a JD from Northern Illinois University. Marilyn is Presidential Research Professor and Chair of the School of Nursing at Northern Illinois University. Dr. Frank-Stromborg has presented 176 papers at national and international conferences, published 77 journal articles, 34 book chapters, and seven books, and has received more than $3 million in grant funding.

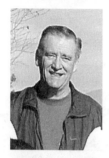

Doug Heaslip
Doug has worked 40 years in industry and business, focusing on the technical aspects of efficient production schedules and critical operation improvements. He operates two businesses, TechIssues and TechPro, which provide consulting services and technical solutions related to computers, applications, networks, and servers.

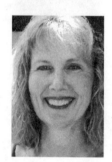

Donna Carol Maheady, MS, EdD, RN, CPNP
Donna graduated from the University of Bridgeport School of Nursing in Bridgeport, Connecticut. She received a certificate as a pediatric nurse practitioner from the University of Texas Medical Branch at Galveston, an MS in Nursing from the State University of New York at Buffalo, and an EdD in educational leadership from Florida Atlantic University. Dr. Maheady, author of *Nursing Students with Disabilities: Change the Course*, is an adjunct assistant professor in the Christine E. Lynn College of Nursing at Florida Atlantic University.
Donna is the founder of the nonprofit web site ExceptionalNurse.com, a resource for nurses and nursing students with disabilities. She has published numerous articles on disability-related topics. Pediatrics and developmental disabilities are her areas of special interest. She has been a faculty member in nursing education for more than 20 years.

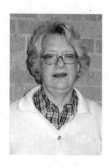

Julie L. Millenbruch, MS(N), RN, CRRN
Julie was awarded a BSN and MS(N) from the University of Missouri-Columbia School of Nursing. She is a nursing doctoral student at the University of Wisconsin-Madison. Julie is an associate professor of nursing at Alverno College, a private liberal arts college in Milwaukee. Ms. Millenbruch has presented at national conferences on topics related to rehabilitation nursing and has conducted several seminars and workshops on the design and implementation of nursing student assessment. She has also served as an on-site evaluator for the

Commission on Collegiate Nursing Education. Ms. Millenbruch has been a faculty member in nursing education for more than 15 years.

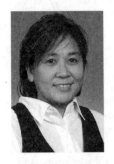

Janice A. Miller, BSN, MSN, RN
Janice received her BSN and MSN in community health nursing from Saint Xavier University, Chicago. She has more than 20 years of clinical experience in obstetric nursing, having served in various roles including clinician, preceptor, and instructor for neonatal resuscitation. Curriculum and continuing education are areas of special interest. Janice is an assistant professor at College of DuPage, Glen Ellyn, Illinois.

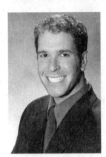

Bob Morgan, BA
Bob received his BA in political science from the University of Illinois in Champaign. He is working toward a JD at Northern Illinois University College of Law. Bob is a research assistant for Dr. Marilyn Frank-Stromborg, focusing on nursing education and the law.

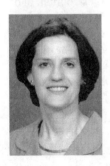

Arlene Morris BSN, MSN, RN
Arlene was awarded a BSN from Harding University, Searcy, Arkansas, and an MSN from Troy State University in Troy, Alabama, and is pursuing an EdD in adult education at Auburn University in Auburn, Alabama. Arlene is a faculty member for both the BSN and the RN-to-BSN nursing programs at Auburn University in Montgomery, Alabama, teaching professional development, advanced holistic assessment, and gerontology courses in both classroom and web-based formats. She has presented at regional, national, and international conferences on topics related to critical thinking, the affective domain of learning, and technology in nursing education.

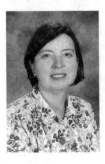

Ainslie Taylor Nibert, MSN, PhD, RN, CCRN
Ainslie earned a BSN from Texas Christian University in Fort Worth, an MSN from the University of Texas Health Science Center in Houston, and a PhD in nursing from Texas Woman's University, Denton. Dr. Nibert is the director of research at Health Education Systems, Inc., a nationally known producer of standardized nursing exams, and faculty associate, College of Nursing, Texas Woman's University. Her articles have appeared in *Computers in Nursing*, *Critical Care Nurse*, *Critical Care Nursing Clinics of North America*, and *Nurse Educator*, and she

has lectured nationally on critical care and nursing education topics. Her previous positions include critical care staff nurse, nurse manager, and nursing education coordinator, associate professor, and department chair of a baccalaureate nursing program.

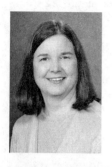

Lynn Norman, BSN, MSN, RN

Lynn was awarded a BSN and an MSN from the University of Alabama at Birmingham School of Nursing. Lynn is an assistant professor of nursing at Auburn University, Montgomery. Previously, Lynn was an education consultant at the Alabama Board of Nursing and served on the National Council of State Boards of Nursing Examination Committee. She has published and presented information on the National Council Licensure Examination process and test plan. Affective learning and nursing program evaluation are her interests.

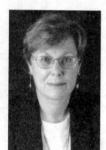

Marilyn H. Oermann, MSNEd, PhD, RN, FAAN

Dr. Oermann was awarded a BSN from Pennsylvania State University and an MSNEd and PhD from the University of Pittsburgh. Dr. Oermann is a professor of nursing at Wayne State University in Detroit. She has authored or coauthored nine nursing books and more than 100 articles in nursing and healthcare journals. *Evaluation and Testing in Nursing Education* received a 1999 American Journal of Nursing Book of the Year Award, Best Books of the Year Award from Doody's Journal, and Best Picks Award for Top-Rated Books for 1998-1999 from Sigma Theta Tau. Her newest book is *Writing for Publication in Nursing*. She is editor of the new series *Annual Review of Nursing Education*. Her current research focuses on teaching consumers about quality health care using the Internet. She is also the editor of *Outcomes Management* and is a member of the American Academy of Nursing.

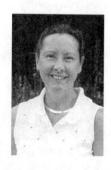

Kathleen Ohman, MS, EdD, RN, CCRN

Kathleen was awarded a BS in Nursing from the College of St. Benedict in St. Joseph, Minnesota, and an MS from St. Cloud State University with a focus in health care education. She earned an MS in nursing and an EdD in educational policy and administration from the University of Minnesota.

Dr. Ohman is professor of nursing at the College of St. Benedict. Her teaching focuses on the care of adults and critical care nursing. She has authored nine journal publications (two of which received writing awards), contributed to three software programs and a review book for the National Council Licensure Examination for Registered Nurses (NCLEX-RN), and twice served as item writer for NCLEX-RN. Dr. Ohman has presented nationally on topics such as teaching-learning strategies and transformational leadership.

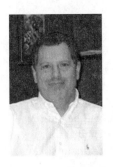

Jeffrey Papp, MS, PhD, RT (R) (QM)

Jeff was awarded a BS from DePaul University in Chicago, an MS in health science from Governors State University in University Park, Illinois, and a PhD in health science from Columbia University. Dr. Papp, author of *Quality Management in the Imaging Sciences*, is a professor of diagnostic imaging at College of DuPage in Glen Ellyn, Illinois. Jeff has presented nationally at conferences on quality management and is the author of three books and numerous journal articles. He has been a faculty member in diagnostic imaging for more than 25 years.

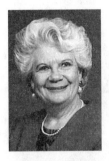

Gay Reeves, MSN, EdD, RN

Gay was awarded an ADN and BSN from Mississippi University for Women in Columbus, an MSN from the University of Alabama, School of Nursing at Birmingham, and an EdD in educational leadership from Mississippi State University. Dr. Reeves is director of the associate degree nursing program at College of the Mainland, Texas City, Texas. She has also served as coordinator of an RN-to-BSN transition program. She has been a faculty member in nursing education for more than 15 years.

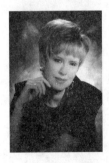

Jeanette Rossetti, MS, EdD, RN

Jeanette was awarded a BSN from Lewis University in Romeoville, Illinois, an MS from St. Xavier University in Chicago, and an EdD in adult education from Northern Illinois University in DeKalb. Dr. Rossetti is an assistant professor at Northern Illinois University School of Nursing. Her specialty area is mental health psychiatric nursing. In addition to her teaching experience, Dr. Rossetti worked at Riveredge Psychiatric Hospital for 12 years in a variety of nursing positions. Dr. Rossetti is a member of the Illinois Guardianship and Advocacy Commission, Human Rights Authority.

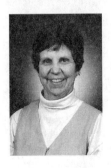

Enid A. Rossi, MSN, EdD, RN

Enid earned a BSN and MSN from California State University at Los Angeles and an EdD in curriculum and instruction from Northern Arizona University. Her dissertation evaluated an action research approach for nursing faculty teacher development. Dr. Rossi is an assistant professor at Northern Arizona University and has been teaching family and community health nursing for 18 years. Enid has presented nationally at conferences about action research. She also produced two cultural videotapes for Navajo Community College. Her poem, "Charge," was published in *The HeART of Nursing: Expressions of Creative Art in Nursing*.

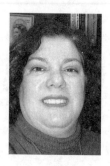

Donita T. Ruggiero, BSN, MN, RN
Donita earned an ADN from Nicholls State University in Thibodaux, Louisiana, a BSN from Loyola University, and a MN from Louisiana State University Health Sciences Center in New Orleans. She has been a member of the nursing faculty at Delgado Community College in New Orleans for more than 10 years. She has presented nationally at conferences on various topics including test anxiety and online tutoring and has contributed to medical-surgical and National Council Licensure Examination review books. The use of technology in teaching nursing is of special interest to her.

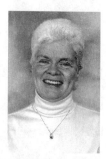

Kathleen Twohy, BSN, MPH, PhD, RN
Kathy received a bachelor's degree in nursing from the University of Maryland as part of the Walter Reed Army Institute of Nursing program, an MPH from the University of Minnesota School of Public Health, and a doctorate in family social science from the University of Minnesota. She has been a faculty member in nursing for almost 30 years and has thrived on curriculum development and design and assessment of learning. Her clinical areas of interest include maternal-child health, public health, and family nursing.

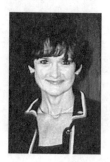

Anne Wendt, MSN, PhD, RN
Anne Wendt was awarded a BSN from the University of Minnesota in Minneapolis, an MSN from Loyola University of Chicago, and a PhD in psychometrics from University of Chicago. Dr. Wendt has been a staff nurse in clinical practice, held positions in education at all levels of undergraduate programs, developed continuing education and online programs, and led numerous research studies. She works for the National Council of State Boards of Nursing as the National Council Licensure Examination (NCLEX) Content Manager and is responsible for all aspects of examination development of the NCLEX for both registered nurses and licensed practical nurses. Dr. Wendt has authored multiple articles on NCLEX and testing-related publications and given national and international presentations.

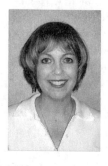

Luanne Wielichowski, MSN, RN, ARNP, BC, FNP
Luanne earned a BSN from the University of Wisconsin - Milwaukee, an MSN with a focus on nursing education and maternal-child nursing from Marquette University, and completed a post-master's family nurse practitioner certification program at the University of Wisconsin - Milwaukee. She has been an associate professor of nursing at Alverno College in Milwaukee for 14 years and continues to practice hematology and oncology nursing at a private clinic. She has recently presented on women's health issues, traveling with students, implementing an ability-based curriculum, and assessment as learning.

Reviewers

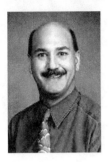

Ken W. Edmisson, ND, EdD, RNC, FNP

Ken received an ASN from Tennessee State University and an MSN and doctorate in nursing from the Frances Payne Bolton School of Nursing at Case Western Reserve University, with majors in family nurse practitioner, nursing administration, and clinical practice and inquiry. He received an EdD in curriculum and instruction from Tennessee State University.

Dr. Edmisson has worked at all levels, from staff nurse to director of nursing, in a variety of settings. He teaches medical-surgical and acute care nursing, research and theory, health assessment, pathophysiology, and management courses. He is a certified family nurse practitioner and medical-surgical nurse. Dr. Edmisson is an associate professor in the School of Nursing, Middle Tennessee State University.

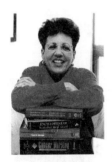

Marilyn Frank-Stromborg, MS, EdD, JD, RN, ANP, FAAN

Marilyn was awarded a BS from Northern Illinois University, an MS from the School of Nursing at New York Medical College, and a doctorate in educational psychology and a JD from Northern Illinois University. Marilyn is Presidential Research Professor and Chair of the School of Nursing at Northern Illinois University. Dr. Frank-Stromborg has presented 176 papers at national and international conferences, published 77 journal articles, 34 book chapters, and seven books, and has received more than $3 million in grant funding.

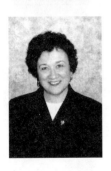

Nancy Kron, BSN, MS, RN

Nancy was awarded a BSN from Marycrest College in Davenport, Iowa, and an MS from the University of Minnesota. Nancy has worked as a staff nurse, assistant unit manager, and clinical nurse specialist in medical-surgical, intensive care, home care, and hospice settings. She has been teaching nursing since 1981. Nancy is a member of the nursing faculty at Milwaukee Area Technical College. She has been working with a statewide committee to develop a new curriculum for the technical college system in Wisconsin.

Key to Credentials

Abbreviation	Definition
Degree	
BA	Bachelor of Arts
BSN	Bachelor of Science in Nursing
EdD	Doctor of Education
JD	Juris Doctor
MA	Master of Arts
MN	Master of Nursing
MPH	Master of Public Health
MS	Master of Science
MSN	Master of Science in Nursing
MSNEd	Master of Science in Nursing Education
ND	Nursing Doctorate
PhD	Doctor of Philosophy
Certification	
ANP	Adult Nurse Practitioner
APRN	Advanced Practice Registered Nurse
ARNP	Advanced Registered Nurse Practitioner
BC	Board Certified
CCRN	Critical Care Registered Nurse
CPNP	Certified Pediatric Nurse Practitioner
CRRN	Certified Rehabilitation Registered Nurse
FAAN	Fellow of the American Academy of Nursing
FNP	Family Nurse Practitioner
RT(R)(QM)	Registered Technologist in Radiography and Quality Management

Table of Contents

Unit 1: Teaching Roles and Responsibilities

Chapter 1: The Nursing Faculty Shortage   2
    Linda Caputi, MSN, EdD, RN

Chapter 2: You've Already Got the Skills to be a Nurse Educator   24
    Joseph Barillari, BA, MA

Chapter 3: Writing for Publication in Nursing: What Every   32
    Nurse Educator Needs to Know
    Marilyn H. Oermann, MSNEd, PhD, RN, FAAN

Chapter 4: Getting Started with Grants   55
    Susan Diehl, BSN, MSN, RN, FNP, APRN

Chapter 5: Negotiating Faculty Politics   70
    Ken W. Edmisson, ND, EdD, RNC, FNP

Unit 2: The Educational Process in Action

Chapter 6: Inspiring Students   90
    Jeanette Rossetti, MS, EdD, RN

Chapter 7: Planning and Implementing Short-term Travel   101
    Courses and Cultural Immersion Experiences
    Luanne Wielichowski, MSN, RN, ARNP, BC, FNP,
    and Julie L. Millenbruch, MS(N), RN, CRRN

Chapter 8: Revitalizing for Success with Active   125
    Learning Approaches
    Kathleen Ohman, MS, EdD, RN, CCRN

Chapter 9: Online Clinical Discussions: An Opportunity   146
    for Reflective Thought
    Glennys K. Compton, BSN, MSN, RN, ANP

Chapter 10: Reflective Writing: A New Approach   163
    in Clinical Assessment
    Catherine A. Andrews, MS, PhD, RN

Unit 3: Focus on Students

Chapter 11: Online Tutoring to Foster Student Success   193
    Donita T. Ruggiero, BSN, MN, RN
Chapter 12: Teaching Nursing Students with Disabilities   209
    Donna Carol Maheady, MS, EdD, RN, CPNP
Chapter 13: The National Council Licensure Examinations   237
    Anne Wendt, MSN, PhD, RN

Unit 4: Focus on Curriculum

Chapter 14: Engaging Students for Affective Learning   282
    Throughout the Curriculum
    Arlene Morris, BSN, MSN, RN,
    and Lynn Norman, BSN, MSN, RN
Chapter 15: Using Educational Theory as a Basis for Leveling   296
    Nursing Laboratory Simulation Experiences
    Arlene Morris, BSN, MSN, RN
Chapter 16: Benchmarking for Progression: Implications for   314
    Students, Faculty, and Administrators
    Ainslie Taylor Nibert, MSN, PhD, RN, CCRN
Chapter 17: Academic Program Review   336
    Jeffrey Papp, MS, PhD, RT (R) (QM)

Unit 5: Focus on Critical Thinking

Chapter 18: Critical Thinking Online: Can It Be Conquered?   355
    Carol Boswell, MSN, EdD, RN,
    and Sharon Cannon, MSN, EdD, RN
Chapter 19: Ideas to Develop Critical Thinking   367
    in the Classroom and the Clinical Setting
    Lynn Engelmann, MSN, EdD, RN,
    and Linda Caputi, MSN, EdD, RN

Unit 6: Focus on Accreditation

Chapter 20: The Nuts and Bolts of CCNE Accreditation   391
     Kathleen Twohy, BSN, MPH, PhD, RN
Chapter 21: The Nuts and Bolts of NLNAC Accreditation   411
     Gay Reeves, MSN, EdD, RN

Unit 7: Faculty Support and Development

Chapter 22: Nursing College Evaluation Systems   423
     and Their Legal Implications
     Marilyn Frank-Stromborg, MS, EdD, JD, RN, ANP, FAAN,
     and Bob Morgan, BA
Chapter 23: Action Research to Develop   440
     Evidence-Based Teaching
     Enid A. Rossi, MSN, EdD, RN
Chapter 24: Starting an Email Discussion List   459
     Doug Heaslip
Chapter 25: Empowering One Another   477
     Lynn Engelmann, MSN, EdD, RN,
     and Janice A. Miller, BSN, MSN, RN

Index   493

Tables   499

Figures   500

Appendices   502

Teaching Roles and Responsibilities

Unit 1

Chapter 1: The Nursing Faculty Shortage
    Linda Caputi, MSN, EdD, RN

Chapter 2: You've Already Got the Skills to be a Nurse Educator
    Joseph Barillari, BA, MA

Chapter 3: Writing for Publication in Nursing:
        What Every Nurse Educator Needs to Know
    Marilyn H. Oermann, MSNEd, PhD, RN, FAAN

Chapter 4: Getting Started with Grants
    Susan Diehl, BSN, MSN, RN, FNP, APRN

Chapter 5: Negotiating Faculty Politics
    Ken W. Edmisson, ND, EdD, RNC, FNP

Chapter 1: The Nursing Faculty Shortage

Linda Caputi, MSN, EdD, RN

I might not want to admit it, but under that expensive hair coloring and youthful appearance lies the truth: I'm part of the graying professorate—the growing number of faculty whose impending retirement is contributing to a major faculty shortage in the United States. For those of us who have spent 20 years or more in the profession, one question resonates: Who will take our place? Most readers of this text are experiencing this phenomenon from one of two vantage points. They are members either of the graying professorate or of the faculty who are replacing us. – Linda Caputi

Introduction

"As nursing looks forward to providing care for an increasingly chronically ill, dependent population with demands for nursing care, will the educators be available to prepare future generations of nurses?"

"Rising nurse salaries in practice settings have attracted potentially new nurse educators into nursing service. A PhD heading a hospital's nurse education and research department is no longer an oddity."

"The term 'faculty shortage' however does not adequately capture the entire problem. The problem is not only that there are faculty shortages but rather shortages of faculty who are educated as teachers, let alone experienced teachers of nursing. The shortages nonetheless are as severe as they have ever been, due

Educational Philosophy

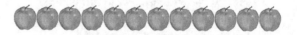

My educational philosophy is succinct: Give the best educational experience possible. I feel faculty should continuously challenge themselves to provide creative, interesting, and sound education—students soon learn that education doesn't have to be boring; they become self-motivated, enthusiastic, and interested…learning then follows. – Linda Caputi to the complicated interplay between the need to increase student enrollments (to increase the numbers of practicing nurses), and the need to turn qualified applicants away from many schools due to limited faculty and financial resources."

Reading these quotes, do you feel like you've just picked up the latest nursing education journal? Think again. The first two were published in the *Journal of Professional Nursing*, 1990, written by Mullinix (p. 133), and the last appeared in *Nurse Educator,* 1992, written by Princeton (p. 34).

The *American Journal of Nursing* reported in 1991 that the National League for Nursing (NLN) estimated that about 5 percent of the full-time teaching positions were vacant in all kinds of nursing programs (*News,* 1991). In 2002 the *American Nurse* reported that an October 2000 survey by the American Association of Colleges of Nursing (AACN) found that 7.4 percent of faculty positions were vacant (Trossman, 2002). These vacancies are for "heavy lifting" faculty positions; that is, positions that require both classroom and clinical teaching.

"The 'writing's been on the wall' for many years, so to speak, in terms of documenting the need for more well-prepared teachers of nursing and anticipation of future needs.... It is clear what measures need to be taken immediately to turn the teacher crisis in nursing around to prevent it from becoming more severe. What we must do is obvious; the challenge is to begin, now" (Princeton, 1992, p. 37). This quote, too, is from 1992—more than 10 years ago! Clearly, it is time for all stakeholders to get off the mark and do something!

A colleague who travels extensively to consult with nursing schools recently shared with me that most schools are reporting that 50 percent of their faculty will retire in the next five years. This comment is supported by AACN statistics indicating that in baccalaureate and graduate nursing programs in 2001, the mean age of full-time, doctorally prepared faculty was 53.2; it was 48.7 years for master's-prepared faculty (Berlin & Sechrist, 2002). With the average age at retirement for nursing faculty at 62.5 years, this indicates a tremendous need for educators over the next 10 years as further retirements occur. The shortage that existed a decade ago is still with us.

This chapter discusses the current nursing faculty shortage and ways to minimize its impact.

Causes of the Current Faculty Shortage

Interestingly, many of the basic causes of the current faulty shortage are the same as those indicated in the literature 10 years ago (Berlin & Sechrist, 2002; DeYoung & Bliss, 1995). The primary causes are:

- **Aging of the present faculty.** According to AACN (2003) the mean age of full-time doctorally prepared nursing faculty rose to 53.5 in 2002 from 49.7 in 1993; for master's prepared, the mean age rose to 48.8 in 2002 from 46 in 1993. At the same time, the percent of faculty aged 36 to 45 dropped to only 10 percent in 2002 from 30 percent in 1993. The faculty are aging with no younger faculty taking their place.
- **Fewer graduate students choosing teaching careers.**
  - In 1977, 24.7 percent of graduates from nursing master's programs were education majors.
  - In 1994, 11.3 percent of graduates from nursing master's programs were education majors.
  - In 2002, 3.5 percent were education majors (AACN, 2003).

It is apparent that the number of nurses who declared an education track in graduate school has diminished over the last two decades. Interestingly, the faculty who will be retiring over the next five-plus years were graduates of these programs. Therefore the faculty who were socialized into the role of the educator during graduate school will be eliminated, replaced by new faculty who are master's prepared as nurse clinicians, not as nurse educators. Even the most committed, clinically competent nurse is not able to teach and evaluate student learning by simply presenting and processing information (Zungolo, 2002). A substantial effort is required to socialize these excellent clinicians into the role of the educator; learning and applying the art and science of nursing education. Special programs for master's-prepared clinicians are in order (Berlin & Sechrist, 2002).

- **A limited number of programs preparing nurses as teachers.** This has contributed to the shortage, although the number of such programs is currently on the rise.
- **An exit of master's- and doctorally prepared nurses from academia to clinical and private sectors offering greater financial rewards.** Over the last decade, considerable budget cuts at academic institutions have placed constraints on faculty salaries. Academia cannot compete with private-sector

healthcare organizations competing for nurses educated at the graduate level (AACN, 2003).

- **Workload and workplace issues.** It is not unusual for nursing faculty to have the heaviest teaching load in terms of contact hours among college or university faculty. This is often because clinical hours are not assigned a one-to-one ratio; that is, one clock hour of clinical instruction is not considered one contact hour of teaching load. Some faculty must teach two or more hours to equal one hour of teaching load. Clinical teaching is extremely labor-intensive and should merit one hour of contact for one clock hour of teaching. New faculty will find this more attractive. Additionally, to retain older faculty, clinical teaching assignments may need to be adjusted relative to faculty's physical and energy limits (Brendtro & Hegge, 2000).
- **Unrealistic role expectations.** New faculty struggle to fill all the roles expected of them by administrators, colleagues, and students. Because most new faculty do not have a background in nursing education, it is impossible for them to meet expectations, which contributes to the stress of new faculty.
- **Advanced practice registered nurses (APRNs) are unable to maintain their clinical practice and certification while in full-time faculty positions.** Perhaps more APRNs would consider a teaching position if they had time to maintain their certification.

In addition, other contemporary factors are impacting the workload and role expectations of faculty teaching undergraduate nursing students. Health care has changed dramatically, requiring more education in the same amount of time. Faculty struggle to find ways to teach all that needs to taught. Additionally, the passing standard for the NCLEX® continues to rise. Although this is justified in terms of preparing safe practitioners, it nevertheless puts pressures on nursing faculty. When a student fails the NCLEX, faculty often feel responsible. This contributes to faculty not enjoying their positions.

Faculty must create teaching approaches that meet these rising educational expectations. These teaching approaches must be designed based on:

- Budget constraints;
- Time constraints;
- Evidence-based educational strategies; and
- The diversity of learners with myriad learning styles.

To create such teaching approaches is a challenge for the most experienced teacher and most likely overwhelming for the novice with no formal educational background in teaching nursing.

Consequences of the Faculty Shortage

Inability to Accommodate Burgeoning Student Applications

The consequences of the faculty shortage are both obvious and subtle. The most obvious consequence of the faculty shortage is the inability to accommodate all students applying for admission to undergraduate nursing programs. This, in turn, exacerbates the nursing shortage, threatening the health care of all our citizens.

In recent years the number of applicants to schools of nursing has increased dramatically. For example, College of DuPage in Glen Ellyn, Illinois, saw applications rise from 200 per year in the late 1990s to nearly 1,200 for 120 positions for the 2004-05 academic year. Neighboring colleges are experiencing the same influx of applicants, all at a time when the institutions that employ these graduates are begging for more nurses. College of DuPage and other schools around the country are working with healthcare institutions to devise means for accommodating more students.

Weekend programs or accelerated programs are possible solutions. These programs require creative scheduling to accommodate clinical experiences. However, more students require more faculty. Plans for new programs and increasing student positions are not viable if there are no faculty to teach these programs.

Nursing Research

A less noticeable result of a faculty shortage is its effect on nursing research. Research in all areas of nursing will be affected. Traditionally, doctorally prepared faculty produce the lion's share of nursing research. With senior faculty retiring and an insufficient number of junior faculty taking their places, who will conduct this research?

Another important consideration relative to nursing research is the degree required for tenure. Many institutions require a doctorate in nursing. These credentials are extremely helpful to generate research that will enhance the knowledge base of nursing. However, these programs generally do not develop effective teachers (Brendtro & Hegge, 2000). There is a real need for **educational** research. The NLN (2003), addressing this issue, has issued a position statement noting the need for the design of "evidence-based curricula." Among its recommendations for faculty were:

- Explore new pedagogies and new ways of thinking about nursing education.
- Conduct pedagogical research to document the effectiveness and meaningfulness of innovations being undertaken.
- Create an evidence base for nursing education that embraces innovation, identifies best practices, and serves to prepare a diverse nursing population that can transform nursing practice (p. 5).

Educational research is indeed important to the development of a science of nursing education. To this end, it is imperative that faculty hold doctorates in education. Institutions should not limit tenured faculty positions to those holding nursing doctorates. A mix of doctorates would be ideal. "There also continues to be a need in our academic communities for scholars and researchers in education.... As a discipline, nurse educators need research in nursing education" (Tanner, 1999, p. 51).

Opening tenure-track positions to nurses doctorally prepared in education would add to the pool of potential faculty and bring into the profession scholars in the art and science of education who can develop an evidence-based science of nursing education. Additionally, it may be a worthwhile experiment for universities to grant doctorates in nursing education.

Solutions for the Nursing Faculty Shortage

The solution to this shortage will be as complex as the causes. One approach to conceptualizing solutions is to consider the causes of the shortage and the environment in which nursing faculty work.

The causes of the shortage are an obvious area of concern and will be addressed throughout this chapter. The problems with the environment in which nursing faculty work is equally important, but solutions are perhaps more elusive. However, it will be difficult to attract new faculty if the current faculty "....don't enjoy their day" (Berlin & Sechrist, 2002, p. 55). AACN (2003) reports that 54.7 percent of faculty at the assistant professor, instructor, or lecturer levels reported dissatisfaction with their workloads. Many of these faculty leave teaching due to this dissatisfaction, and, more disconcerting, would not recommend teaching to nurses considering entering the teaching profession. Schools of nursing with a "good work climate" will have greater success recruiting and retaining faculty (Hinshaw, 2001).

Several changes that have occurred over the last 10 years may contribute to this dissatisfaction (AACN, 2003). They include:

- **Changes in the way higher education is conducted.** The triad of teaching, service, and research remains. However, the service and research requirements are becoming more intense as faculty are required to obtain extramural funding and publish extensively. These requirements put additional pressure on the shrinking faculty workforce.

- **Changes in the characteristics of today's students.** Today's college students are increasingly diverse and represent many different cultures. For many students, English is a second, third, or foreign language (Sutherland, 2004). This diversity enriches the classroom, but requires additional skills for the teacher. In addition, students now are more likely to be at different stages of life as they enter undergraduate nursing programs; 73 percent of undergraduate nursing students are considered nontraditional. With an average age of 30.9 years, more students are delaying their entry into higher education, and have jobs and families competing for their time and attention. Although adult learners bring a multitude of talents and skills, they challenge the faculty to develop creative, relevant critical-thinking and problem-solving experiences. Faculty must relate to students with varying learning styles and needs (Forrest, 2004).

These changes create challenges for faculty. Junior faculty who were prepared as nurse practitioners, rather than as nurse educators, may find they are not prepared to fill all these roles and ultimately leave teaching.

The Current Pool of Potential Faculty

The current pool of potential faculty consists largely of nurses educated at the master's level with an emphasis on clinical practice. In 1969 the American Nurses Association (ANA) identified a shortage of practitioners prepared at the graduate level. The ANA called for graduate education to emphasize clinical practice rather than teaching and administration. Schools listened and the number of nurses educated at the graduate level for advanced practice increased while those schooled in teaching and administration

8

decreased (Krisman-Scott, Kershbaumer & Thompson, 1998). This trend resulted in more practitioners but fewer educators.

It became apparent that a skilled clinician is not necessarily a skilled educator. Nearly a decade and a half after its 1969 recommendation, the ANA voiced concern that there would not be an adequate supply of nurses prepared to teach. That trend continues today. Only 64 of the 375 master's in nursing programs in the United States have an education track or postmaster's program (Bonnel, 2003).

So, the bottom line is that there is a pool of potential faculty with excellent clinical skills. What can be done to help these practitioners become educators? What do they need to know and how will they learn it?

Faculty Mentors

How does a person without teaching experience learn to teach? How would a new teacher know **how** to teach without any formal coursework? For many, teaching is like parenting: One parents as one was parented and one teaches as one was taught. In this case, the new teacher may emulate a teacher from the distant past; the teaching approach may be decades old and not reflective of current educational theory. Then how should a new teacher learn? One of the best resources for practitioners entering teaching is a faculty mentor.

The faculty mentor facilitates the orientation and enculturation of the new teacher into the specific academic setting. This person provides guidance, assistance, and positive feedback, and is a friend who is willing to listen and offer support. (For more information see Chapter 25, "Empowering One Another," by Engelmann and Miller.) However, the mentor does **not** provide a graduate degree in nursing education. Unfortunately, many faculty who are asked to be mentors are expected to teach the new faculty everything the mentor knows about teaching. This approach tends to cause resentment and disdain among the experienced faculty, and could eventually diminish the pool of willing mentors.

One way to avoid overloading senior faculty with additional mentoring duties is to hire new faculty a year before the date another faculty member retires. The junior faculty can work side by side with the retiring teacher. This allows time for both people to achieve a successful mentoring experience.

The New Faculty Team

The idea of a faculty team is one that has been employed in clinical nursing for many years. Some institutions provide newly employed nurses with educational time, a preceptor, and extended orientation. Schools of nursing might benefit from such a plan tailored to the needs of new faculty. A new-faculty team would comprise the following members:

- The new faculty;
- The mentor, a senior faculty; and
- The department administrator.

Together, this three-person team develops an action plan that outlines the specific needs of the new teacher and the means to meet those needs. This plan may cover a period of several years, and should be **individualized** to each new teacher. The plan should focus first on the teaching aspect of the triad of faculty responsibilities " teaching, research, and service" and should be designed so the new faculty first becomes a competent, able teacher. Research and service can then be addressed after a few years of teaching experience. To expect the new teacher to perform all aspects of the position while learning to be a teacher may very well drive the new person out of education completely. New teachers' committee responsibilities should also be minimized for their first three years.

The tenure clock should be paused for those finishing doctoral degrees to allow time to complete their coursework and dissertation. It is nearly impossible for a master's-prepared teacher to fill the triad of service, teaching, and research while also completing a doctoral degree. The tenure clock can be reset when the teacher has completed the doctoral work.

Developing the Individualized Plan of Action

When deciding what areas of content to include in the action plan for the new faculty, the team should start by considering core competencies. The NLN (2003) has developed a list of core competencies for nurse educators. The complete list can be found at www.nln.org/profdev/competency.htm. The major categories of competencies include:

- Facilitate learning;
- Facilitate learner development and socialization;
- Use assessment and evaluation strategies;

- Participate in curriculum design and evaluation of program outcomes;
- Function as change agents and leaders;
- Develop educator role;
- Engage in scholarship; and
- Function within the educational environment.

Although it is important for all educators to acquire each of the competencies listed within each of the above categories, the list may appear somewhat daunting to the novice educator. Among the many new faculty with whom I have worked and consulted over the last decade, several common areas emerge as priorities:

- Curriculum development;
- Conducting classroom sessions;
- Grading research papers; and
- Test item writing.

Following are some suggestions to help the novice educator in each of these areas.

Curriculum Development

An important first endeavor for the new faculty is to gain an understanding of the nursing program curriculum. This helps the teacher appreciate the bigger picture, and understand how all the pieces fit together to make the whole. It is important for the new faculty to understand basic concept such as:

- Program philosophy;
- Conceptual framework;
- Conceptual threads;
- Course structure and sequencing; and
- Content flow.

A sound understanding of these points will provide a framework within which the new teacher can develop educational experiences (Toms, 2004).

Conducting Classroom Sessions

A common learning need of new faculty is how to conduct classroom sessions, whether in lecture, case study discussion, or small group settings. Students may complain the new teacher only talks about the topic without providing visuals, examples, or application to client care. These deficiencies may stem from a lack of knowledge about instructional design. Therefore, it can be extremely helpful to focus the action plan on instructional design, steps of the design process, and application to the classroom.

Grading Research Papers

A common complaint of students is the inconsistency among teachers when grading research papers and other subjective assignments; inexperienced teachers often struggle with this task. The teacher can use a grading grid to determine topics the students must cover in an assigned paper. See Figure 1.1 for an example of such a grid for grading a term paper. When such a grid is used, the teacher can be confident with the grades awarded and is empowered when discussing the grade with the student.

Test Item Writing

One of the most difficult tasks for a new teacher is constructing valid and reliable multiple-choice tests. Currently in undergraduate nursing education, there is a need not only for valid and reliable multiple-choice test items, but also for tests to be written at the analysis and application levels.

Writing valid and reliable questions is also important because poorly written questions can lead students to fail, even if they understand the subject matter. Teachers must take the responsibility of ensuring that items are well-written, fair, valid, and reliable so they can be confident that students who fail do so because of deficient knowledge and not because of poorly constructed tests.

Helping New Faculty Navigate Conferences

Although new faculty can learn much from their colleagues at their home institutions, it is important for them to tap the wealth of information and learn the value of networking that comes from attending conferences. The mentor should encourage the new teacher to take advantage of such opportunities. At a recent nurse educators conference, I spoke with a senior faculty from another college whom I had met at a previous conference. As I approached her, I noticed a

Figure 1.1 - Grid for Grading a Term Paper

Total Points: 25	Points Allowed	Points Deducted	Points Given
I. Introduction	1		
II. Assessment: Effects of Illness on Growth & Development	6		
III. Nursing Diagnoses	1		
IV. Planning and Intervention			
A. Goals and outcome criteria	1		
B. Nursing management			
1. Care during admission	5		
2. Child/family teaching and discharge planning; evaluation for long-term management	3		
3. Activity therapy appropriate to child's age	3		
V. Conclusion	1		
VI. Format			
A. Composition	2		
B. APA Format	2		
C. One point off for each page over 12 pages			X
D. One point off for each of four professional nursing journals not used.			X
E. Two points off if submitted after due date and time.			X
F. Any paper received more than one week late will receive zero points. Failure to submit a paper will result in a failing grade for the course.			X
G. Plagiarism – See syllabus.			X
Additional Comments:			
TOTAL POINTS:	25		

young woman with her. I remarked, "How nice to bring your daughter with you!" She replied, "Oh, this isn't my daughter! This is one of our new faculty."

After the blushing subsided, I commented that it was wonderful to see a seasoned faculty attending a conference with a novice faculty. What a great way for the new person to learn how to get the most out of a conference. Fitzpatrick (2003) offers these suggestions for deriving the greatest benefit when attending a conference:

• Attend the keynote. This sets the stage for the conference.

- Attend informal activities and network with other attendees.
- Attend the poster sessions and discuss the work of these presenters; collect the abstracts.
- Make connections and network during educational offerings.

When I attend a conference, I make a point to get to know at least one new person. Over the years, the people I have met at conferences have become colleagues and have provided an invaluable network. Staying in touch with them has provided me with a continual source of new thoughts and innovative ideas, none of which I would have gained without first having met them at conferences.

Resources for Implementing the Faculty Development Plan for New Educators

If a mentor is not available to teach the new faculty the content listed on the action plan, then who is? Fortunately, there are many resources for the novice educator. In addition to formal coursework at local universities, the following are excellent resources.

NLN's Teaching in Nursing Certificate Program

The NLN offers several courses toward a certificate in teaching nursing. Courses are web-based so they are readily accessible. Some of the courses are:
- Teaching in nursing;
- Evaluation in nursing; and
- Computer technology for nurse educators.

In addition to the formal coursework, NLN offers two certification examinations for nursing educators. One examines teaching, learning, and evaluation, and the other covers the full scope of the faculty role. For more information, visit their website at: www.nln.org.

American Association of Colleges of Nursing

The AACN offers a faculty development resource called the Education Scholar www.educationscholar.org. The Education Scholar is a web-based program that covers the following topics:

Teaching Nursing: The Art and Science

- Personal working philosophy;
- Facilitating learning in a traditional classroom setting;
- Active learning strategies;
- Distance learning;
- Problem-based learning;
- Outcomes assessment; and
- Promoting change in the educational institution.

National Council of State Boards of Nursing

The National Council of State Boards of Nursing offers two web-based courses 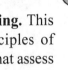 for nursing faculty on test item writing at www.ncsbn.org. They are:

- **Basic assessment strategies: test development and item writing.** This course offers information about measurement statistics, principles of multiple-choice item writing, basic techniques for writing items that assess higher-order cognitive processes, guidelines regarding potential item bias, and a critique of sample NCLEX examination questions.
- **Advanced assessment strategies: assessing higher-level thinking.** This course teaches nursing educators how to write items that assess critical thinking. It also offers suggestions for converting items to a higher cognitive level.

It may be best to take a basic course on test construction and measurement before beginning these courses.

Other Web-Based and Distance Education Courses for New Faculty

Some universities are offering complete web-based nurse educator programs. A sampling of these programs is listed below.

The University of Kansas School of Nursing

The University of Kansas School of Nursing offers an online nurse educator certification program at classes.kumc.edu/son/nursedu. Courses in this program include:

- Teaching strategies: designing a student learning environment;
- Curriculum/program planning and evaluation;
- Teaching with technology; and

- Nurse educator preceptorship. (In this course the student works with a mentor in the student's home community.)

University of Pennsylvania Teacher Education Program

The Teacher Education Program at University of Pennsylvania is a post-master's certificate program. This program is designed for advanced nurse practitioners who are interested in teaching. The major goals of the program are to prepare "master clinicians as master teachers" and applying educational theory to the adult learner. Visit www.nursing.upenn.edu/teachered/program.

Duquesne University School of Nursing

Duquesne University School of Nursing in Pittsburgh also offers an online program for nurse educators at www.nursing.duq.edu/gradmsneducurr.html. The program requirements include a core curriculum of 23 semester hours in both theory and clinical. An additional 14 semester hours covers courses on the following topics:
- Curriculum and instruction;
- Advanced clinical nursing;
- Evaluation in nursing education; and
- Nursing education role practice.

Retirees: A Resource to Deal with the Faculty Shortage

Once the experienced faculty has successfully mentored the new teacher, it may be time for the senior faculty to retire. As is the case in private industry, many faculty are being offered attractive retirement packages—this is good for them, but not good for the system. In some cases, administrators, fueled by the bottom line, actually encourage their faculty to retire. After all, a doctorally prepared professor with 25 years of tenure earns twice as much as an assistant faculty with a master's degree (Acord, 2000). But this practice is very short-sighted on the part of the administration.

The traditional all-or-nothing retirement approach needs an overhaul. Senior faculty have much to offer. Administrators and faculty must develop strategies for retaining the senior faculty's expertise. The aging professorate may not have the physical energy of their more youthful junior faculty, but their intellect and wisdom are qualities that should not be retired.

As an eager student of nursing education in the early 1980s, I studied at Loyola University, Chicago. I witnessed the value of our aging experts in nursing. Ann Zimmerman, a retired professor and former president of the ANA, was invited to teach a class in the graduate school. It was most exciting to learn about her early years in nursing and listen to her wisdom on nursing education. She was inspiring and an outstanding role model. Retired faculty serving in this capacity should be the norm throughout nursing education.

By phasing a person's retirement, the exiting faculty enjoys all the benefits of their retirement with an opportunity for part-time employment as an expert member in nursing academia (AACN, 2003). This idea already is used in the practice setting. I recently was talking with a nurse manager of an intensive care unit, who was describing all the new graduates she had recently hired for the night shift. This very insightful manager realized the new nurses outnumbered the experienced nurses on that shift. She contacted a recently retired, 30-year veteran of the night shift and asked her to return on a part-time basis.

When this graying professional said she no longer felt able to deal with the physicals demands of the job, the manager explained her plan: "You will be the expert, the night shift resource person. You will read charts, talk with the nurses about their assessments and plan of care for the shift. You will not be providing any direct client care."

Not only did the "retired" nurse accept the position, but she felt honored and valued for her expertise.

It should be noted that this clinical manager developed this idea along with all the managers in that hospital as the institution was considering strategies that would move them forward in their quest for ANA magnet status (www.nursingworld.org/ancc/magnet.html). Sometimes innovative programs like the magnet program encourage innovative ideas. The NLN's Center for Excellence in Nursing Education (www.nln.org/profdev/excellence.htm) may be analogous to the magnet program for healthcare organizations. Perhaps as schools of nursing seek to attain excellence status through the NLN, innovative and creative ideas will emerge.

It would be wonderful for schools of nursing to bring back retired faculty in an expert advisory role. The professor emeritus might do the following:

- Attend lectures and critique the teacher's delivery;
- Facilitate case study discussions and concept mapping;

- Guide new faculty in grading subjective assignments such as research papers;
- Help new faculty complete clinical evaluations; and
- Tutor at-risk students.

This list is only a beginning. What a valuable resource—those entering the ranks of professor emeritus. These faculty would not only assist novice faculty in developing quality instruction and learning experiences, but they also can play a valuable role in helping students succeed. The end results—novice faculty who are truly mentored and at-risk students assisted to complete the nursing degree —would be outcomes no one could fault.

Additional roles for retired faculty that would help lessen the workload of full-time faculty include:
- Supervise in the nursing skills laboratory;
- Assist with research projects;
- Teach selected classes; and
- Attend conferences and share information and proceedings with faculty.

An interesting way to utilize the knowledge of senior faculty is a faculty development center for nursing. This center can be staffed by a cadre of retired faculty who may have retired from other institutions within a community or region. Such a consortium can provide the benefit of varied faculty interests and expertise and a pooling of resources for new faculty. Workshops, seminars, and web-based courses can be developed by these faculty and offered as a means of financial support for the center.

Teaching Web-Based or Hybrid Courses

Another exciting area for retired faculty is helping teach web-based courses. Many schools have completely shifted the theory portions of their courses to the web or are developing hybrid courses that employ a mix of face-to-face and online instruction. Retired faculty may be interested in teaching the online portion of the course. This also can decrease the full-time faculty's workload.

Part-Time Faculty

The shortage of faculty often is met with an increase in part-time faculty. Budget cuts in higher education are also fueling the trend toward hiring part-time teachers. Currently, there is one part-time nursing faculty for every 1.7 full-time faculty (Zungolo, 2003). Employing part-time faculty is a short-sighted solution because part-time faculty typically have a very limited role. It is helpful to employ part-time faculty to avoid cancellation of a class; however, the increased use of part-time faculty puts an increased burden on the smaller core of full-time faculty (DeYoung, Bliss & Tracy, 2002). As more part-time faculty are used as replacements, the work of the decreasing number of full-time faculty increases proportionately. The work of academia continues with fewer people to carry the increased workload. The work this entails includes:

- Reviewing prospective student files. In one nursing program, the number of applicants has increased from 200 per year in the late 1990s to nearly 1,200 in Fall 2004. However, the school employs no additional assistance to sort through all these student files. Implementing an office of selective admissions is a strategy used by some nursing programs to provide needed assistance.
- Reviewing program policies and procedures.
- Updating curriculum to meet the changing practice arena.
- Developing weekend and fast-track programs to accommodate more students.
- Integrating technology, such as developing Web-based courses, to meet the needs of changing student populations.

And the list goes on. This can lead to an overworked full-time faculty, and might prompt early retirement for some who might otherwise work beyond the usual retirement age. Unfortunately, disgruntled full-time faculty often paint an unpleasant picture of the workload, which can further discourage nurses from entering the teaching profession.

Attracting Younger Faculty

A problem commonly cited in the literature is that nurses enter faculty positions at a much older age than faculty in other disciplines. On average, a person entering nursing academia is 10 years older than teachers of other disciplines (DeYoung, Bliss, & Tracy, 2002). This typically leaves only time for the faculty to teach for 15 to 20 years before reaching retirement age (Hinshaw, 2001). "Thus, a new professional tradition needs to be considered in order to lengthen the number of years nursing faculty have to be productive in academia" (Hinshaw, 2001, p. 11). We must entice nurses to enter teaching at a much younger age so they can provide more years of teaching throughout their careers.

One suggestion is to entice younger nurses into graduate education with a focus on nursing education. We must guide and mentor these students into academia or risk losing them to the practice arena. Additionally, the idea that a nurse must practice for several years before entering a master's program further discourages students from earning graduate degrees during the early years of their careers. Institutions should create fast-track programs that allow students to move from bachelor's to doctorate degrees in a reduced time. These programs are necessary to ensure master's graduates advance into doctorate programs. Accessibility is also important. Web-based master's and doctoral programs may create more opportunities for nurses to join the teaching profession, regardless of their proximity to colleges and universities.

Young, promising nurses should be encouraged to consider careers in education, but this may be difficult given today's nursing shortage. Many nurses are enjoying attractive salaries and benefits. They may be deterred from entering graduate programs to eventually teach, when they might earn less than they are earning in a staff nurse position. In fact, Trossman (2002) reports that some new graduates accept clinical positions at which they earn more than the faculty who taught them. Interestingly, this creates a self-destructive cycle for the teaching profession. If nurses do not continue their education to become nurse educators, the number of students denied admission to nursing schools will continue to increase. According to an AACN (2001) survey of baccalaureate and graduate programs, 4,967 students were denied admission due to insufficient faculty, insufficient clinical sites, and budget constraints.

Faculty would do well to share with potential nurse educators the satisfying aspects of a career in academia which include opportunities to (Hinshaw, 2001, p. 7):

- Develop and shape new professionals;
- Engage in creative, intellectual discussions with faculty colleagues and students;
- Pursue a research and/or scholarly program of professional and personal interest;
- Contribute to improving health care through student education and the generation of new knowledge;
- Provide professional, disciplinary, and interdisciplinary leadership; and
- Shape health policy based on professional and scholarly expertise.

Summary

The causes of the nursing faculty shortage are multifaceted and complex. Both short-term and long-term strategies must be considered if the shortage is to be reversed. Reversing the faculty shortage is imperative to increasing the number of practicing nurses providing direct client care. Unfortunately, the faculty shortage has been present for more than a decade and continues to grow. To date, attempts to change the situation either have not worked or have not been seriously considered.

Learning Activities

1. AACN provides more suggestions for relieving the faculty shortage in its 2003 white paper, *Faculty Shortages in Baccalaureate and Graduate Nursing Programs: Scope of the Problem and Strategies for Expanding the Supply* (www.aacn.nche.edu/publications/whitepapers/facultyshortages.htm). Analyze its suggestion to use non-nursing faculty and courses to satisfy nursing course requirements. Discuss this option with a colleague.
2. Visit the websites listed in this chapter in the section ***Resources for Implementing the Faculty Development Plan for New Educators***. Compare and contrast the components of each program.
3. Survey the nursing schools in your state. How many full-time faculty do they employ? How have the schools handled faculty retirements? How many faculty will be retiring in the next five years? Are these schools experiencing difficulty hiring new faculty? If so, are they implementing any policy changes to address this problem?

References

Acord, L. G. (2000). Education. Help wanted—faculty. *Journal of Professional Nursing, 16*(1), 3.

American Association of Colleges of Nursing (2003). *Faculty shortages in baccalaureate and graduate nursing programs*. Washington, DC: Author.

Anderson, C. A. (2002). From the editor. Nursing faculty—going, going, gone. *Nursing Outlook, 50*(2), 43-44.

As enrollments rebound, schools face a growing faculty shortage. (1991). *American Journal of Nursing, 91*(4), 108,112-113.

Berlin, L. E., & Sechrist, K. R. (2002). The shortage of doctorally prepared nursing faculty: A dire situation. *Nursing Outlook, 50*(2), 50-56.

Bonnel, W. (2003). Nurse educator shortage: New program approach. *Kansas Nurse, 78*(3), 1-2.

Brendtro, M. J., & Hegge, M. (2000). Nursing faculty: One generation away from extinction? *Journal of Professional Nursing, 16*(2), 97-103.

DeYoung, S. (1995). Nursing faculty—an engendered species? *Journal of Professional Nursing, 11*(2), 84-88.

DeYoung, S., Bliss, J., & Tracy, J. P. (2002). The nursing faculty shortage: Is there hope? *Journal of Professional Nursing, 18*(6), 313-319.

Fitzpatrick, J. (2003). Professional development: Getting the most from the summit. *Nursing Education Perspectives, 24*(3), 221.

Forrest, S. (2004). Learning styles. In L. Caputi & L. Engelmann (Eds.), *Teaching nursing: The art and science* (pp. 389-405).Glen Ellyn, IL: College of DuPage Press.

Hinshaw, A. (2001). A continuing challenge: The shortage of educationally prepared nursing faculty. *Online Journal of Issues in Nursing 6*(1). Retrieved March, 2004, from http://www.nursingworld.org/ojin/topic14/tpc14_3.htm.

Krisman-Scott, M. A., Kershbaumer, R. M., & Thompson, J. E. (1998). Faculty preparation: A new solution to an old problem. *Journal of Nursing Education, 37*(7), 318-320.

Mullinix, C. F. (1990). The next shortage—the nurse educator. *Journal of Professional Nursing, 6*(3), 133.

National League for Nursing (2003). *Position statement: Innovation in nursing education: A call to reform*. New York: Author.

Princeton, J. C. (1992). The teacher crisis in nursing education—revisited. *Nurse Educator, 17*(5), 34-37.

Sutherland, L. (2004). Teaching students from culturally-diverse backgrounds. In L. Caputi & L. Engelmann (Eds.), *Teaching nursing: The art and science* (pp. 446-468). Glen Ellyn, IL: College of DuPage Press.

Tanner, C. A. (1999). Developing the new professorate. *Journal of Nursing Education, 38*(2), 51-52.

Toms, R. (2004). Curriculum development: Pulling the threads together. In L. Caputi & L. Engelmann (Eds.), *Teaching nursing: The art and science* (pp. 469-486). Glen Ellyn, IL: College of DuPage Press.

Trossman, S. (2002). Who will be there to teach? Shortage of nursing faculty a growing problem. *American Nurse, 34*(1), 22-23.

Zungolo, E. (2003). President's message. The predicament of nursing education: The faculty censes. *Nurse Education Perspectives, 24*(2), 62.

Zungolo, E. (2002). President's message. The preparation of nurse educators: Developing the knowledge base to transmit the discipline of nursing. *Nurse Education Perspectives, 23*(5), 210.

Bibliography

Lang, M. (2002). Online faculty help address shortage of nurse educators. *Patient Care Staffing Report 2002, 2*(9), 10.

Lowe, N.K. (2002). How shall they learn without a teacher? *JOGNN, 31*(4), 391.

Mundiner, M. (1994, Fall-Winter). Endangered nursing school. *Advanced Practice Nurse, 46-47,* 59.

Wieck, K. L. (2003). Faculty forum. Faculty for the millennium: Changes needed to attract the emerging workforce into nursing. *Journal of Nursing Education, 42*(4), 131-158.

Zungolo, E. (2002). President's message. Cultivation of a scarce resource: nursing faculty. *Nursing Education Perspectives, 23*(1), 2.

Zungolo, E. (2002). President's message. Paradox, incongruity, and a new vision for our profession: remarks from the opening session of the NLN Education summit 2002. *Nursing Education Perspectives, 23*(6), pp. 274, 307.

Chapter 2: You've Already Got the Skills to be a Nurse Educator

Joseph Barillari, BA, MA

A new venture, such as entering nursing education, often produces mild anxiety and self-doubt—doubt about one's ability to perform in a new position. However, new nurse educators arrive at the doors of academia with skills derived from many nursing experiences. Mr. Barillari very graciously explains how the new nurse educator can apply those skills to jump-start a teaching career.
– Linda Caputi

Educational Philosophy

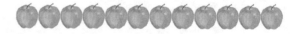

My philosophy of teaching begins with the premise that phrases like *philosophy of teaching* are conceits that get in the way of effective teaching. I am more comfortable putting it more simply: that there are values, goals, and attitudes that buttress my teaching.

I feel strongly that a good general education that samples the wide range of human knowledge is essential for all. Such an education gives students a confidence in learning that is the foundation for real growth, both as individuals and citizens. I insist that communication (oral, written, and artistic) be clear and to the point, that it be free of jargon and cant. Imprecise communication is the enemy of sound learning. I believe teaching must always be fair to the students, but should be vigorous and challenging to both students and teacher. As a person whose job is the encouragement and support of the creativity of others, I know that smugness, provincialism, and familiarity are all enemies of true knowledge and barriers to personal growth. When I teach, I challenge students to jettison the commonplace and avoid the familiar or easy—risk taking is as essential for teaching and learning as it is for all life's endeavors.
– Joseph Barillari

Introduction

I have a theory—it's not something that's going to be a compelling ice breaker at a cocktail party, but it could be a useful one to new teachers of nursing. The theory is simple and maybe a little audacious. Most nurses, by dint of education or experience, have learned skills that predispose them to be good teachers, at any level and with any groups of nursing students. It's not mystical and it's not a gimmick, nor is it cheerleading. It's a theory based on facts, simple ones to be sure. But a little context will make the theory clear and meaningful.

If you are about to teach your first class in nursing and your experience is all in clinical nursing and not teaching, I am sure you are feeling a little trepidation. For many, the feeling may border on terror. That's hardly unusual. I have known many fearless practitioners: soldiers, artists, movie producers, and the like who were just plain scared when asked to teach a college class for the first time. Generally, if there is any comfort in the fact, their fear is directly proportional to their competence in their own field. Achievers like to achieve—a classroom is a new environment and no competent person likes to appear less than competent, particularly in front of an audience.

Wise, well-trained people tend to seek counsel. My job in this little essay is to provide that counsel. Yet the last person many of you would come to for advice would be someone like me. I am not a nurse. I have never worked in any of the health professions. All my formal postsecondary education and teaching experience is in fields as far from nursing as any can be—nursing is practical, straightforward, goal-oriented, and demanding of consistency. I was trained in the liberal arts—a field that seems to many in practical fields to be ill-defined, vague, and inconsistent.

Yet, I know I can be of help to the first-time college teacher. First of all, although I may know very little about the formal field of nursing education, I know a lot about teaching. I have nearly 40 years' experience teaching a wide variety of postsecondary students in history, humanities, film, and writing. I have taught in prestigious (and some not-so-prestigious) places. I have taught in secure military intelligence facilities where burn bags were passed around after class to collect scrap paper. I taught in a mess area passageway aboard a Navy ship at sea while firemen-sailors in full regalia streamed through the middle of my class. I have taught in maximum security prisons where classes were cancelled because the institution was in lockdown. I have taught in two-year, four-year, and graduate institutions. I have taught developmental students and gifted students. I know teaching; or rather, I know students. And all teaching comes down to a series of transactions with students. These transactions are varied—information exchange, motivation, problem-solving, leadership, and even playing Cupid, teaching reluctant suitors to love learning. So, from this vantage point I offer my thoughts.

The Teaching-Learning Environment

Teaching is a field that offers many roads to competence and success. Think of your best teachers—not necessarily the ones you found the most likeable, but the ones that taught you the most—and what you learned from them stuck. Probably, they are a small group and in many cases, as different from each other as you are from them.

Teaching is a field where the old truism, **Be yourself**, works and works well. Perhaps the better way to put it is: **In teaching, don't try to be someone you're not.** The lectern of a college classroom is best likened to a glass microscope slide. The only difference is that 20 or 30 pairs of eyes are looking through the microscope's eyepiece. It can be an unforgiving environment that can magnify a person's flaws. Incompetence is hard to hide. Inconsistency has no shelter. Even the least astute student can spot a phony. If you like yourself and your judgment is pretty good, just be yourself. Students will sort the rest out for themselves. They will cut you the slack you'll need to get started and make the class a success.

Teaching is an environment that allows, even prizes, honesty and directness. "I don't know but will find out" is a perfectly reasonable and acceptable answer to students—in fact, it is sometimes the only responsible answer. If a teacher can communicate it with some sensitivity, candor about a student's shortcomings is infinitely preferred to mealy-mouthed silence or gratuitous indulgence of a student's ego.

Skills You Already Have

What's most important to me is that nurses already have a pretty sophisticated skill set that predisposes them to succeed in the classroom. Let's look at these skills. Depending on your background, some of your skills from this list will be stronger than others, but it is safe to say that all of these are skills almost every nurse learns either in formal education or on the job.

- **Triage.** Competent nurses and competent teachers both need this skill. For nurses, it means examining a newly arrived patient and not doing anything until an assessment is made and patient needs are identified. Good teachers must triage their students. It can be formal, with some form of pre-testing. Teachers can assess students individually or as a group in a class. Whatever the process, most nurse educators do some form of triage more consistently than most other teachers. Knowing a student's deficiencies or strengths empowers teachers and can result in the difference between a student's success and failure in a class.

- **Charting.** Many teachers could gain a lot from a course on patient charting. Charting skills are essential to good caregiving. The same skill set makes for better teachers and, more importantly, better learning outcomes. In a modern setting, particularly one that teaches clinical skills, the old-fashioned grade book is not enough. Students are an increasingly diverse group, not only in terms of background and demographics, but also in terms of abilities and talents. Like you, they are motivated; and, like you, they know enough to ask questions. It is useful to keep good notes on your meetings with them. It is a good assurance of consistency and a way of assessing your advice. It is a way to make sure you don't forget a commitment to a student. Finally, like all good charting, it is a way to be accountable.

- **Problem solving.** Good nurses are problem solvers. So too are good teachers. Teachers and nurses, for all that is routine in their jobs, can not—when it comes to solving student-related problems—assume that one size fits all. The best teachers and the best nurses are those who know when to look beyond the pat procedure or the time-honored habits. As a teacher, I truly earn my pay solving problems with learners who do not neatly fit the bell-shaped curve or conform to the latest taxonomies of personality types determined by standardized tests.

  As a nurse, you know that there are asymptomatic patients who can be very ill. Experienced nurses know to read subtle or secondary signs for illness, to probe a little more deeply, and to develop an inner alarm system to help you treat patients in your care. Student needs can be equally elusive. Experienced teachers know how to make intelligent guesses about why a particular student isn't learning. More often than not, these problems have little to do with the traditional reasons for poor performance—lower ability or poor motivation. Adult learners and traditional-age learners alike live in complex worlds filled with many stressors—money, family, and difficult schedules—that often affect academic performance. You should be ready and able to learn the roots of students' problems and, even if you are unable to help solve them, you should give students a context in which to understand their problems.

- **Monitoring.** One of the primary skills teachers use to help them diagnose students' problems is ongoing monitoring. Like nursing, teaching relies on regular monitoring. It requires care and ongoing attentiveness, but it pays good results. Some teachers rely on only two tests per term (a midterm and a final exam) to monitor and assess students' progress and performance. Better teachers use more inputs—quizzes, short practice tests, class discussion, and attendance—to create more complete pictures. Relying on a couple of exams each term is akin to monitoring patients using only a thermometer. Good nurses and good teachers both may find monitoring can be tedious, but both know it is effective.

- **An ethical base.** In a way, the discussion so far can be put into ethical terms. Teachers, no less than nurses, have ethical standards that govern their work. They may not be as formalized, but it is important for teachers to do right by their students and do things for the right reasons. Going the extra mile for students to help them do their best is a part of the teacher's ethical framework. Clearly, college students are on their own and must take responsibility for their own learning; but teachers have a similar responsibility to enable student learning. Like nurses, the foundation for teachers could easily be that of nurses: "First, do no harm." Teachers at all levels, even postsecondary teachers, have enormous power either to help students better themselves or to send them in the wrong direction. Teaching may not present the same clear-cut alternatives between life and death, good health and poor, that exist in nursing. But we all know from our own experiences how important good teachers have been and, how harmful poor ones can be. One thing that all competent teachers should know is a sense of caution and forbearance. Judgments about students should always be carefully weighed—a teacher's personal ethos should preclude precipitous or whimsical behaviors. The forbearance nurses learn, that sense of caution makes "First, do no harm" as important for those at the front of the classroom as it is for those at the patient's bedside.

- **Currency.** An old saw is that teachers should write their lectures or class notes on yellow legal paper, so as the years go on, students won't be able to judge the lessons' age by the color of the paper. There might have been a time a generation ago when teachers felt they could get away with using notes or material they themselves learned in college. Today's nurses know better. The health profession swims in a stormy sea of change: Medications, procedures, policies, and even ethical concerns are all changing, and are all in need of continuing, professional updates. In many ways, nurses have a big advantage over the teaching profession—they are accustomed to the need to keep current. Large bodies of nursing knowledge—basic physiology, basic clinical practices, and good work habits—have not changed dramatically. But those who teach most effectively are those whose knowledge is most current, not only in their clinical specialty, but also in teaching methodologies and tools. For example, even though personal computers have been around for 20 years, there are many teachers who only use one for word processing or presentations. The Internet has been part of our lives for a decade, yet most teachers have not worked regularly in an intensive, web-based learning environment. In all enterprises, change is the handmaiden of progress. In clinical nursing, embracing change is not a choice, but an imperative. At some colleges and universities, change comes at glacial speeds. Nurses can help be a force for change and improvement in teaching. Staying current can make a dramatic difference in your patient's quality of care; it will have enormous impact on your students' learning achievements. It might even be a force for change at the institution where you teach.

A Change in Environment

The previous section demonstrated that nurses have an impressive array of tools and attitudes that can make them highly effective teachers. In fairness, some things about teaching are different, and could be surprising. Supervising a student nurse's clinical practicum will hold no surprises for the experienced nurse. Teaching in a classroom will. The nature of the setting and the generally respected philosophy of academic freedom translate to a work environment that is largely unsupervised. Student evaluations each term and administrative evaluations every year, even at their most rigorous, do not come close to the close supervision and accountability nurses are used to in the healthcare industry.

At first blush, academia might seem an enviable place to be; but, for the new teacher, this great freedom means there may not be enough feedback on your performance. There is a solution for this. Get to know the respected, experienced teachers. Ask to be invited to their classrooms. Ask them to come to yours. Attend seminars on teaching—the quality will vary enormously, but attending many will give you a quick look at those skills all good teachers have.

Your most important resource may be the most easily accessible. This takes us back to the beginning of this chapter. Think back on your own education and on those teachers who made a difference in what and how you learned. They won't necessarily be the most popular, the most entertaining, or the most caring; but they will be the ones who put across the subject matter that encouraged your learning and enabled your mastery. What did they do? Could you do it?

Finally, the best thing you can do is know who you are. You needn't be an accomplished lecturer or performer. You may not be a comfortable counselor. And, if you are shy or diffident to public speaking, you may never feel fully comfortable in front of a class. But, knowing yourself and your limitations will enable you to develop a teaching style that works for you and your students. Don't forget in your self-analysis to remember your strengths. Think about how well you work with patients. Think about how you performed when you precepted new nurses for your unit. Think about how well you communicated complex patient information to the other members of your health team—to the other nurses, the pharmacist, the lab, other specialized technicians, the physicians, and even the occasional administrator. What are the qualities that made those communications effective? Odds are that what made them effective will also make you effective as a teacher.

Summary

The intent of this chapter is not to trivialize the task of teaching, to make it seem easy, or to rob it of its greatest attraction, its challenge. But in many respects, the best teachers grow best in the rich topsoil of good content knowledge. And it's my opinion that experienced nurses know their stuff and know it well. You may be shy in front of a class, you may be apprehensive about your teaching abilities, and you may even fear your unwillingness to suffer fools; but when you are a nurse and everyday people trust their lives to your knowledge and your skill in applying it, you bring a lot more to teaching than do people from many other fields.

I still teach a course each term because I enjoy the challenge. I have many colleagues who still enjoy the task even though they are well into their 70s. All I can say before your first teaching experience is that I hope you quickly get over your apprehension and enjoy one of the richest challenges available in any profession—to pass on its knowledge and skills. It may be modest, but it is still a sure ticket to a form of immortality. Good luck on your first class. Future generations of nurses are counting on you.

Learning Activities

1. Reflect on your strengths as a nurse in clinical practice. What strengths can you use in your role as an educator?
2. Visit a class conducted by a fellow nurse educator. What instructional strategies used by that teacher are strategies you could use?

Chapter 3: Writing for Publication in Nursing: What Every Nurse Educator Needs to Know

Marilyn H. Oermann, MSNEd, PhD, RN, FAAN

The work of nursing faculty is always creative and often truly amazing. This work needs to be shared for all to use and enjoy. One way to disseminate one's work is to publish. Publishing is an absolute necessity if the profession is to grow and evolve. It is truly a pleasure to have Dr. Oermann, a prolific writer and leader in nursing education, contribute this chapter on what nurse educators need to know about writing for publication. – Linda Caputi

Educational Philosophy

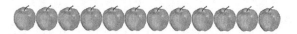

Teaching in nursing involves the assessment of student learning needs, development of experiences to meet those needs, and evaluation of student achievement. As such, it is a diagnostic process beginning with knowledge of the students—their capabilities, interests, and motivations. Teaching requires the involvement of the learner and a supportive learning environment. Developing the learning environment involves not only the setting in which learning occurs, but also the interpersonal relationships between teacher and students. Teaching is an interactional process; the ability to work effectively with students in varied settings is critical in promoting their learning and developing a climate in which they can try out new ideas and approaches to care.

Teaching strategies in nursing foster development of not only knowledge and skills for practice but also problem-solving and critical-thinking abilities. For this reason varied teaching methods are essential. In the clinical setting, the teacher guides student development of competencies within an environment in which the student is comfortable asking faculty for guidance. While students help select learning experiences for clinical practice, the course and clinical objectives should guide student experiences in this area. – Marilyn H. Oermann

Introduction

As faculty prepare themselves for teaching in schools of nursing, they develop their abilities to lecture, design instructional methods for classroom and clinical teaching, evaluate students in the clinical setting, and construct tests, among other skills. Another competency faculty need to develop is the ability to write for publication. It is essential for faculty to disseminate their educational innovations and new initiatives to other teachers and to build our knowledge base about nursing education. By writing for publication, teachers share their knowledge and expertise with other faculty.

This chapter describes the process of writing for publication, from deciding what to write through completion of the final draft. It also addresses what happens once the manuscript reaches the editorial office and how to revise the manuscript to improve chances of acceptance.

Benefits of Writing for Publication as a Nurse Educator

Through writing for publication, nursing faculty share their educational innovations and new ideas about curriculum, distance education, clinical teaching, evaluation, and other topics about which other faculty also are concerned. When projects and initiatives related to nursing education are published, other faculty can use that work in their own schools of nursing. Writing for publication allows educators to share best practices rather than recreating the same initiatives for their students and programs.

The most effective way to communicate nursing education research—not only formal studies conducted by faculty but also projects that faculty planned, implemented, and evaluated—is publishing the findings. The benefit of writing for publication is that by sharing problems they addressed through research and what they learned, faculty can guide other teachers facing similar problems. By disseminating nursing education studies in journals, books, and online resources, faculty build evidence for practice as a teacher in nursing. Without this evidence there is no basis for the decisions we make as nurse educators, and studies' findings can only be used widely if they are published.

Another reason to learn about writing for publication is that in many nursing schools, publishing is essential for promotion and tenure. While each school has its own criteria for promotion and tenure, including the number and types of publications required for different faculty ranks, there are some general principles for publishing that faculty should know. Research articles published in refereed (peer-reviewed) journals carry more weight in promotion and tenure decisions than do descriptive articles about teaching, curriculum development, and other educational topics. In refereed journals, such as *Nurse Educator*, *Journal of Nursing Education*, and *International Journal of Nursing Education Scholarship*, experts critically review each submitted manuscript, identify needed revisions, and recommend to the editor whether the paper should be accepted. Because of peer review, publication in refereed journals—no matter what type of article—carries more weight than it does in non-refereed journals and book chapters.

Because of the research required to write for publication, faculty gain new knowledge that they can use to develop their lectures and course materials. Conversely, faculty can use their own lectures and teaching materials as the basis for new articles.

Why Faculty Do Not Write for Publication

Many innovations in nursing education are known only by the faculty and students in a particular school of nursing. What are the barriers to writing for publication as a nurse educator?

First, writing is a skill that takes practice and time to develop. The added time it takes novice writers to develop a paper may diminish their motivation to write. It may be helpful for a novice faculty to partner with a teacher who has experience publishing. The experienced writer can help the novice improve as a writer and help expedite the publishing process.

Second, not understanding the process of writing—how to move from ideas to a finished manuscript—may also be a barrier. Faculty may be unsure how to develop a manuscript, what to expect during the review process, and what steps to take when a manuscript is returned for revision. Having one's paper and ideas rejected is sometimes difficult but it is a part of the process. If faculty understand how to handle editors' rejections, they may be more encouraged to continue writing (Oermann, 1999b).

A third problem facing educators, with their busy work and personal schedules, is finding the time to prepare a manuscript. With all the steps involved, beginning with reviewing the literature, writing the draft, editing the paper, and revising it based on reviewers' feedback, time is often an issue.

Strategies to Resolve Barriers to Writing

The more faculty write for publication, the easier and faster it becomes. The problem of finding time to write is especially difficult to manage, but there are some strategies faculty can use to build time for writing into their teaching schedules.

For example, it is important to set due dates for completing the manuscript and each of its sections (Oermann, 1999a, 2002). With this strategy the author can view each section of content as an individual writing project. The due dates should be recorded on the manuscript outline and they should be realistic, taking into consideration the faculty's teaching schedule and other responsibilities. The key to this strategy is to not waver from the deadlines; once a due date is moved back, the easier it becomes to delay the entire process.

Faculty need to find the time when they are most productive, and use that time for writing (Oermann, 1999a, 2002). The best time for writing varies for each person—some authors write best early in the morning while others are most productive late at night. Some faculty may need large blocks of time for writing; others may find an hour a day works best. Teachers must make a concerted effort not to use the time for preparing classes, meeting with students and other faculty, or completing personal responsibilities. In addition to reserving this time for writing, the author should create an environment without distractions; avoid answering telephone calls or checking email.

Phase One: Planning

Understanding the process of publication makes it easier to work through writing a paper and responding to peer review. The unpublished document that is submitted to the journal or publisher is called the manuscript or paper (American Medical Association [AMA], 1998). When published, the manuscript is referred to as an article.

Identifying the Purpose of the Manuscript and Importance of the Topic

The most important early step in writing for publication is to identify the purpose of the manuscript. The purpose may be to describe an innovation for teaching developed by faculty, a new program in the nursing school, a research study, or other topics of interest to nurse educators. Knowing the purpose of the manuscript guides two major processes:

- Reviewing existing literature to determine if the topic already has been addressed; and
- Keeping the paper focused on the selected topic.

Faculty should be clear about the intended outcome of the manuscript for readers: What will they gain from it?

In addition to clarifying the purpose of the paper, the author must confirm the importance of the topic for nurse educators and determine whether it is appropriate for publication in any existing journal. Faculty should ask themselves if proposed papers will present new ideas not yet in the literature (Oermann, 2002). If others have written about the topic, what is new and different about the proposed manuscript? The paper should make a difference in teaching, evaluation, curriculum development, working with students, and other areas of nursing education; otherwise it is not worth writing. It is best to assess the importance of the topic before beginning rather than preparing a paper that has a limited chance of publication.

Review the Literature

Journal editors are interested in publishing new ideas about nursing education and innovations that have not been reported in the literature. Although faculty may think their ideas and innovations are new, a review of the literature may prove otherwise. For this reason, the next step is to review the literature on the topic. A literature review has two objectives:

- To determine if the proposed topic or slant of the manuscript has been described already in the literature; and
- To gather information that can be used in writing the paper.

There are many bibliographic databases for the author to use in reviewing the literature, but typically the two most useful databases are MEDLINE, available through PubMed, and the Cumulative Index to Nursing and Allied Health Literature (CINAHL). Both of these databases index nursing journal articles and are easy to search. If the topic is broader than nursing education, the literature review should be extended into databases that publish papers on that subject.

Usually, reviewing the literature from the previous three to five years is sufficient. However, if there are a limited number of publications on the topic within that timeframe, the author can search earlier literature. Authors should record all of the information needed for preparing references, no matter what reference style is used by the journal, to avoid having to recheck the information later. By keeping a list of articles, books, and other materials that were not relevant to the paper, the author can avoid having to review the same sources in a different database or at a later time.

Because of the extensive number of references discovered in most literature searches, authors need ways to keep track of source materials so they can be retrieved when needed for future use. Faculty can use the results of literature searches for several other purposes, such as:

- Lectures;
- Development of course materials and strategies for teaching;
- Research projects; and
- Other writing projects for publication.

However, to do this, authors need a way to store and keep track of the references. One way is to record bibliographic information in a computer file. Authors can develop their own files to store reference information or can use commercial bibliographic management software such as EndNote, Reference Manager, and ProCite (Thomson ISI ResearchSoft, 2004). These programs allow authors to search online bibliographic databases, store reference information in a database, create reference lists, and automatically format bibliographies for manuscripts.

Select a Journal

Too often, faculty first write their manuscript, then search for a journal that might be interested in publishing it. However, those steps should be reversed. After deciding on a topic, an author should have a clear idea of the paper's likely publisher and target reader. If the topic is how to develop a portfolio, is the audience any nurse educator in a school of nursing, novice teachers with limited knowledge of portfolios, or staff nurses who can develop a portfolio for career advancement? The intended audience is important because it helps the author select possible journals for submission. Keeping the audience in mind also should guide the author's decisions about depth of content, types of examples to use, how the information is presented, and writing style.

Once the target audience is clear, the manuscript can be submitted to a journal that publishes papers on that topic for those readers (Oermann, 2002). Thus, rather than writing a paper and then trying to find a journal interested in publishing it, the author should select journals that cover that content area and reach the intended audience, then write for that journal. Some journals publish only original research or only clinical practice articles; other journals publish articles on clinical practice and research in that clinical specialty. *Nurse Educator* publishes more non-research articles than does the *Journal of Nursing Education*. Some journals carry short articles focusing on application of new ideas in practice without the background information and supporting rationale for those ideas, while others publish more detailed and comprehensive reviews. It is up to the faculty to choose the best fit for the manuscript.

As the educator reviews journals, it is helpful to maintain a file of each publication's author guidelines. For each manuscript, the author might have a file with information about three to five journals for possible submission. If an editor has no interest in reviewing the paper, or if the paper is rejected by the first journal to which submitted, the author can send the manuscript to another journal in the file.

Information for Authors

Author guidelines provide information about the content areas the journal covers and the types of articles it publishes. No manuscript should be written without these guidelines because they indicate the maximum page count, reference style, submission format, and other details about how to prepare the paper. Most journals have author information pages on their websites. For example, all of the information needed to prepare a manuscript for submission to *Nurse Educator* can be found at www.nursingcenter.com/upload/static/230542/educauthor.html#prep.

This URL can easily be launched from the CD accompanying this book. Simply launch your Internet browser, put the CD-ROM in the drive, go to Chapter 3 on the CD, and click on the website address.

Strategies for Identifying Possible Journals

There are hundreds of journals in which faculty can publish. One useful technique for identifying which journals are likely targets is to use an online directory of nursing and healthcare journals (Table 3.1). The journals are listed alphabetically and, in some directories, also are categorized by specialty. The ONLINE Nursing Editors website has email links to more than 200 nursing journal and book editors and provides links to author guidelines for many of the journals (Johnson, 2003). Faculty can search through this list for potential publishers, query the editors about their interest in the topic, and gather author guidelines, all at one website.

(Each of these URLs can be easily launched from the CD accompanying this book. Simply launch your Internet browser, put the CD-ROM in the drive, go to Chapter 3 on the CD, and then click on the website address.)

Another way to identify appropriate journals is to search bibliographic databases of nursing and healthcare articles such as CINAHL and PubMed. Faculty can search for the topic they want to write about and identify journals that publish in that content area for the intended audience. A quick literature search to explore possible journals also will reveal whether articles on that topic already have been published.

Writing the Query Letter to the Editor

The next step is to write query letters to the editors of the journals that are possible outlets for the manuscript. The intent of the query letter is to determine whether the editor is interested in reviewing the paper. While faculty can prepare and submit a manuscript without first querying the editor, the author can waste time preparing the paper to fit that journal and waiting for a response from the editor if the journal is not interested in the paper.

Manuscripts can be sent to only one journal at a time. If the paper is rejected, it can be sent to another journal, but only after the author is notified that it is no longer under consideration by the original journal. Query letters, in contrast, can be sent to several editors at a time. One advantage of online directories like ONLINE Nursing Editors is that most have email links to the editors, which make it easy for the author to send multiple query letters at once. Oermann (2002) recommends that after deciding to submit the article to a particular journal, the author should notify the other editors that the paper will not be submitted to

Table 3.1 - Online Directories of Nursing and Healthcare Journals

Journal Directories	URL
ONLINE Nursing Editors website provides email links to more than 200 nursing journals and book editors. Also has links to author guidelines for many journals.	members.aol.com/suzannehj/naed.htm
Academic Journal Directory of University of Texas Medical Branch School of Nursing (Galveston, Texas) lists more than 400 nursing and healthcare journals. User can navigate site via alphabetical lists of journals, journals grouped by subject (with nursing education as category), and keyword search. Site also provides links to journal's home page.	www.son.utmb.edu/catalog/catalog.htm
Medical College of Ohio website has links to author guidelines for more than 3,500 health and life sciences journals. Journals are listed alphabetically. Menu provides links to other resources for authors, eg, Uniform Requirements for Manuscripts Submitted to Biomedical Journals and Journal Impact Factors.	www.mco.edu/lib/instr/libinsta.html

them. Query letters should be brief and should indicate the purpose of the manuscript, whether the paper is a research report, and the author's contact information and professional position. Figure 3.1 is a sample query letter.

Figure 3.1 - Sample Query Letter

John Doe, MSN, RN, C
245 Hill Street
Pittsburgh, Pennsylvania 15228

January 1, 2004

Marilyn Oermann, MSNEd, PhD, RN, FAAN
Editor, *Journal of Nursing Care Quality*
5557 Cass Avenue
Detroit, Michigan 48202

Dear Dr. Oermann:

I am interested in submitting a manuscript to the *Journal of Nursing Care Quality*. The purpose of the manuscript is to describe a teaching intervention for asthma patients that we developed and evaluated systemwide. I was the coordinator of the team that developed the intervention, and I have extensive experience in caring for patients with asthma.

We anticipate completing the manuscript by March 2004. Thank you for your consideration.

Sincerely,

John Doe
John Doe, MSN, RN, C
Advanced Practice Nurse
Asthma Clinic

Deciding Authorship Credit

The standard for determining the authors of a manuscript is specified in the Uniform Requirements for Manuscripts Submitted to Biomedical Journals by the International Committee of Medical Journal Editors (ICMJE) (2003). Individuals can only be listed as authors if they participated in writing or substantially revising the paper. If the manuscript describes a research study, each author must have been involved in the study. It is inappropriate to include any other names on the manuscript.

It is not appropriate to include honorary authors on a manuscript. Honorary authors are colleagues—eg, the dean, program director, or faculty advisor—who are listed as authors without having participated in the paper's research, writing, or editing. Authorship is never assigned as a courtesy (Davidhizar, 2004). Ghost authorship, when the paper is actually written by an editor or a medical writer rather than the author, also is inappropriate. Individuals can only be listed as authors if they meet all three of the following criteria:

- Contributed substantially to the conception and design of the study, acquisition of data, or analysis and interpretation of the data;
- Participated in writing the manuscript or substantially revising it for important intellectual content (not editorial revisions); and
- Approved the final version (ICMJE, 2003).

There are many stories about faculty who ask or demand that their names be added to a paper written by one of their students. For this to occur, the faculty, like any other author, must meet all three conditions for authorship. A teacher can not ask a student to write a paper and list the faculty as sole author, or—even worse—submit as one's own work a paper written by a student for a course. Most colleges and universities have policies to cover these situations.

In a situation in which the faculty and student together planned a project or study, and both participated in writing the manuscript, both are listed as co-authors. It is advisable to agree on which author will be listed first on the manuscript **before** writing begins.

There are times, however, when authors want to acknowledge the help they received with a study or project, or with writing the manuscript. In these instances, acknowledgments are used. In a manuscript, the acknowledgement appears on the page preceding the references. Every person mentioned in the acknowledgment needs to give written permission for his or her name to be cited in the paper. Similarly, agencies, health systems, and institutions can not be named in the text without their written permission.

An example of an acknowledgment is: "The author acknowledges the assistance of Mary Jones, EdD, RN, in developing the tool and pilot testing it with students in her program." In this example, Mary Jones needs to provide written permission to cite her name in the acknowledgement.

Phase Two: Writing

By this point in the process, the author has decided on the purpose of the manuscript, identified the potential readers, polled editors who might be interested in reviewing the manuscript, prioritized these journals, gathered author guidelines, and completed the literature review.

Before beginning a first draft, the author should carefully review the journal's author guidelines and decide how to present the content considering the journal's readership and writing style. Some journals in nursing use more formal, academic writing styles, often with passive voice. For example:

Despite extensive research on patient education, there are few studies on patients' perceptions of the role of the nurse in their education. Most research has examined the effectiveness of different teaching interventions and approaches, but few have explored the importance of nurses delivering that teaching from the point of view of the patient.

Other journals use a more informal writing style with active voice. For example, "We developed a research study in which we asked patients to rate the importance of having nurses provide their education during their hospitalization." Journals with an informal writing style often use sentences in the second person, which refer to the reader as "you." For example, "You can best teach the patient by dividing the material into smaller content areas and using visuals to supplement your teaching."

Now, the author moves into the second phase: writing the paper. Gene Fowler, the journalist and screenwriter, wrote: "Writing is easy: All you do is stare at a blank sheet of paper until drops of blood form on your forehead" (BrainyMedia.com, 2004). Before beginning work on the manuscript, the author should write a detailed outline. This will serve as a guide for the paper and should help the author avoid those drops of blood.

Develop an Outline

The outline is a general plan of the content to be included in the manuscript and its order (Oermann, 1999b, 2000, 2002). Outlines may be formal (developed using Roman numerals) or informal (a list of topics and their order). The outline is critical because it guides the author in deciding what content to include in the paper and how to organize it. The outline is a working document, able to be revised as the writing proceeds, which is far easier than rewriting the entire manuscript.

Oermann (2000) identified advantages of outlining before beginning to write. An outline:

- Identifies the content areas to include in a manuscript;
- Organizes the content in a logical order;
- Facilitates the identification of missing content before beginning to write;
- Suggests headings and subheadings to use with the manuscript;
- Keeps the author on the topic; and
- Helps the author complete the paper on time by assigning due dates.

The goal of the outline is to group content together and encourage the author to decide on the best order to present it. If the organization of the content is not apparent, the author can record key content areas on index cards, then rearrange them until he or she is satisfied with the order (Oermann, 2000). Or, the author can develop a concept map—similar to what students prepare as a clinical learning activity—that links content areas together. This sometimes helps the author decide how to present the content.

Writing the First Draft

Once the outline is complete, the author can start writing the draft. The approach to writing the first draft should be to write quickly and get the content down rather than worry about grammar and writing style (Fondiller, 1999; Oermann, 2002). By revising for grammar while writing, authors shift their thinking away from the content and how to present it, which can disrupt the train of thought.

How many drafts to write depends on how clearly the author can express his or her own ideas. With practice, writing becomes easier and fewer drafts are needed.

Although the title and abstract are the beginning pages of a manuscript, some authors write the draft of the text first, then the title and abstract. Others write the title and abstract first (Huth, 1999). Either way, the title and abstract are works in progress that may need to be revised later.

It is important to include the citations while typing the initial draft. Otherwise, in later revisions, the author may not recall the source of the information. In the draft, the authors' names and publication dates can be listed in parentheses, which then can be formatted easily for journals using the American Psychological Association (APA) reference style (APA, 2001). When writing for journals that use a numbered system for the citations, the author's last name and publication date still should be recorded in the draft. The references can be numbered later. Otherwise, the citations would need to be renumbered every time a new reference is added somewhere in the paper. However, initially include **all** information on references; this saves having to retrieve the information at a later time.

Revising the Draft

Once satisfied with the content, the author edits the draft for grammar, punctuation, spelling, and writing style. It is best to start by revising the paragraphs before checking each sentence and choice of words (Oermann, 2002). Proceeding in this manner moves the author from broad aspects of the paper to more specific ones.

Each paragraph should begin with an introductory sentence that captures the content in the paragraph. Authors also should check the organization of the paragraphs to ensure that the content is sequenced clearly. This is a good time to check for smooth transitions between paragraphs. After revising the paragraphs, the author edits the sentences and transitions between them, ensures that they are grammatically correct, reviews the length and structure of the sentences within each paragraph, and checks the choice of words. At some point the author needs to be satisfied enough with the writing to submit the manuscript and avoid editing the paper beyond what is necessary to improve the writing. It may be helpful to have another faculty read the paper at this point to validate that it is ready for submission.

Preparing References

Not all journals to which faculty submit manuscripts use APA style. Many journals use a numbered citation format such as the *Uniform Requirements* (ICMJE, 2003) or *American Medical Association (AMA) Manual of Style* (AMA, 1998). The journal's author guidelines should indicate the style to use when preparing references.

The name-year system, such as the APA style used in this text, records the name of the author and year of publication within the text. Another common reference style is the citation-sequence format in which Arabic numerals are used for the citations in the text, which are numbered consecutively. In some styles, the numerals are placed in parentheses; in others they are set in superscript. For example:

...developed and tested the clinical evaluation form.(1-2)
...developed and tested the clinical evaluation form.[1-2]

By numbering the citations rather than including author names and publication dates, the text is not interrupted by a list of references within a sentence. These formats may be adapted by the journal, and for this reason the author needs to follow the author guidelines for each journal.

Authors must verify the accuracy of their references against the original publication. Studies have found errors in nursing publications in the spelling of authors' names, order of names, title of the article, and journal in which published (Oermann, Cummings, & Wilmes, 2001; Oermann, Mason, & Wilmes, 2002; Oermann & Ziolkowski, 2002). Authors also should check that the citations are placed with the correct content in the text and that they correspond to the correct reference on the reference list.

Preparing Tables and Figures

When the author has detailed information to present, it is sometimes best to develop a table for those data. Tables should not be used if the information can be reported clearly in the text. The principle is to develop tables for complex and detailed information that can be displayed and understood more clearly in table form rather than narrative. Tables are used to:
• Report exact values;

- Present detailed information;
- Display quantitative values; and
- Show relationships among data (Oermann, 2002).

There are different types of tables. A tabulation table is a short, informal table that is included as part of the text. It sets the information off from the text (AMA, 1998). Another type is the traditional, formal table with columns and rows. This type of table typically is used for presenting quantitative values, statistical data, and detailed information. A third type of table, often used in non-research articles, is a word table or text table. A text table could be used to illustrate different program evaluation models; their characteristics, advantages and disadvantages; and nursing programs that have used each one. Information such as this is too detailed for the text and is better presented in a table. Table 3.1 is a text table. Text tables, like statistical tables, should be used only if the information can not be clearly presented as part of the text.

In the text, the author highlights major findings from the tables and includes summary statements about them but does not repeat information from the tables in the text (Oermann, 2002). The text should refer readers to the tables by using a phrase such as "shown in Table 3.1" or "…program evaluation models (Table 3.1)."

Figures include graphs, diagrams, photographs, and other illustrations. They are valuable in showing trends in data, changes over time, and comparisons (Oermann, 2002). Because editors often must reduce the size of figures for publication, the information on the figures should be large enough that it can be seen at a reduced size.

Preparing and Submitting Final Copy

Before submitting the paper to the journal, the author should complete one final check to confirm that the format is consistent with the journal requirements. For many journals, the manuscript can be sent via email. If submitting the paper as a hard copy, the author should be sure that the correct number of copies are sent along with any additional materials required, such as the copyright release and a disk containing the manuscript.

Manuscripts—including the title page, references, tables, and figure captions—generally should be double-spaced. The author information page will indicate the margins to use, but if this information is not provided, 1 inch to 1½ inch margins should be used on all sides. No spaces should be left between paragraphs, hard returns should not be used, and pages should be numbered as indicated in the guidelines. Some journals use running heads and others do not; once again it is the author's responsibility to follow these guidelines when preparing the final copy for submission.

When the manuscript is ready to send to the journal, the author prepares a cover letter (Figure 3.2) that indicates:

- The title of the paper;
- That the paper is original and has not been published previously;
- The materials enclosed in the envelope or attached to the email message; and
- The corresponding author's full name and contact information.

If the journal has different departments, the cover letter should specify the department for which the paper was prepared. Some journals have authors sign the transfer of copyright form when submitting the manuscript. For journals that do not follow this procedure, the author should include in the cover letter a statement that the paper is original, is not under review by another journal, and has not been published elsewhere. The following statement can be used: "Neither the entire paper nor any part of it has been published or has been accepted for publication by another journal. The manuscript is not under review by another journal and is submitted only to [name of journal]."

In most instances journals will confirm receipt of the manuscript with an email to the author. If unsure of the procedure, the author should include a self-addressed, stamped envelope for this purpose. Manuscripts are not returned when rejected.

Phase Three: Publishing

After it is submitted to the journal, the manuscript is reviewed by experts in the content area. If the manuscript is a research report, it will be reviewed by someone with expertise in research methods or statistics. This process is called peer review. Manuscripts are critiqued by reviewers who are experts and by the editor who decides whether to publish the paper. The peer review process ensures that quality papers with accurate content and up-to-date information are accepted for publication.

Figure 3.2 - Sample Cover Letter

March 1, 2004

Marilyn Oermann, MSNEd, PhD, RN, FAAN
Editor, *Journal of Nursing Care Quality*
5557 Cass Avenue
Detroit, Michigan 48202

Dear Dr. Oermann:

Attached please find the manuscript, "Evaluation of an Educational Intervention for Patients with Asthma," for your review for possible publication in the *Journal of Nursing Care Quality*. Neither the entire paper nor any part of it has been published or has been accepted for publication by another journal. The manuscript is not under review by another journal and is submitted only to the *Journal of Nursing Care Quality*.

Thank you for your consideration.

Sincerely,

John Doe

John Doe, MSN, RN, C
245 Hill Street
Pittsburgh, Pennsylvania 15228
412-111-2222
jdoe@aol.com

Peer review is usually a blind review process. Identifying information about the author is removed from the manuscript, creating less chance of bias, and authors are unaware of who reviewed their manuscript (Oermann, 2002). With anonymity, reviewers can more honestly critique a paper than if they know who

Figure 3.3 - Sample Manuscript Review Form

Journal of Nursing Care Quality
Manuscript Review Form

Return review to: Marilyn Oermann moermann@msn.com or moermann@comcast.net
Title:
Due   Reviewer #

As you read the manuscript, write positive, negative, and developmental comments on the manuscript pages. Return manuscript pages with comments; destroy remaining pages. Please send the completed review to the person indicated above.

YES NO   COMMENTS

____ ____   Does the paper present new findings or ideas?
____ ____   If no, does it present old material better?
____ ____   Is the content timely/relevant?
____ ____   logically and clearly developed?
____ ____   sophisticated enough for our readers?
____ ____   innovative?
____ ____   Introduction: Is the purpose of the paper clear?
            Methods (*research paper*)
____ ____   Are the sample and sampling method adequate?
____ ____   Are the instruments reliable and valid?
____ ____   Are statistical tests appropriate?
            Methods (*other types of papers*)
____ ____   Were the objectives of the project clearly identified?
____ ____   Were the outcomes evaluated adequately?
____ ____   Do conclusions and implications go beyond what findings support?
____ ____   Are the references current?
____ ____   Is the content's application/utility made explicit to the reader's
                 practice setting?
____ ____   Was the paper interesting to read?

Recommendation:
    ( ) Accept for publication without revision
    ( ) Accept for publication after satisfactory revision
    ( ) Review again after major revision
    ( ) Reject

Please circle the number that best indicates the overall quality of this manuscript:

1	2	3	4	5	6
Outstanding	Excellent	Good	Acceptable	Uncertain of acceptability	Unacceptable

Comments/Suggestions: Print or type on reverse side or separate page.

wrote it. Reviewers complete a form to summarize their critique, which is returned to the author with the editor's comments. Figure 3.3 is a sample review form.

A manuscript can be accepted without or with revision, the author can be asked to revise the manuscript and resubmit it for another review, or the paper can be rejected. Huth (1999) identified five criteria typically used to decide whether a paper is accepted for publication:

- Relevance of the manuscript considering the journal's mission and readers;
- Importance of the content;
- Originality of the content;
- Strength of the evidence to support the conclusions of the paper; and
- Usefulness to the journal in relation to the other topics it covers (p. 258).

Novice writers must not become discouraged if the editor asks for revisions or rejects the article. Publishing requires perseverance and faith that the article eventually will be accepted.

If the article requires revisions, the author should make the suggested changes or provide a rationale for not making them. A summary of the revisions proposed and made in the paper should accompany the manuscript. An example is provided in Table 3.2. By developing a summary such as this, the author improves the paper's chances of publication because the summary lists the proposed revisions and where they were made in the manuscript or explains why they were not done. If the manuscript is rejected, the author should revise it, using feedback from the peer review process, and submit it to another journal. Once the manuscript is accepted for publication, the author answers the editor's queries, carefully reads the page proofs to find any errors, and returns all materials to the publisher before the journal's deadline.

Summary

Writing for publication is an important skill for faculty to develop. Not only is it essential in many schools of nursing for promotion and tenure decisions, but publication allows faculty to share their initiatives and innovations with others. Publishing one's work is the best way to advance nursing education.

Table 3.2 - Sample Summary to Accompany Revised Manuscript

Oermann MH; MS # 111 Accuracy of References in Three Critical Care Nursing Journals

Revisions Proposed	Revisions Made
Reviewer #1: Where are references #5 and #11 cited in mss?	Reference #5 on p. 4, line 19; reference #11 on p. 6, line 16
Omit last line of mss.	Omitted; last paragraph revised (p. 11, lines 4-7)
Reviewer #2: On p. 5, define criteria	Sentence rewritten with criteria for major and minor errors defined (p. 6, lines 15-23)
On pp. 8 and 9, only issue errors mentioned	Statement added on volume errors (p. 7, line 21)
Reviewer #3: References 1, 2, 10-12, 15 not found in PubMed	Abstracts of 1, 2, 11 enclosed; 10 - article enclosed and reference list updated; 12 is AMA Style Manual book; 15 - reference updated with publication date (book)
Reviewer #4: p. 5, under design, specify criteria	Rewritten for clarity (see p. 6, section beginning on line 14)
Why were these particular journals selected?	Because widely read nursing journals; discussion added on p. 5 (line 21)
Why so few references from *JOPAN* checked compared to *AJCC*?	*Journal of PeriAnesthesia Nursing* had 481 citations in 31 articles. *American Journal of Critical Care* had 1181 references in 48 articles. 10 percent of the references from **each** journal were analyzed consistent with earlier studies. With this method the same **proportion** of references reviewed in each journal. Described on p. 6, lines 3-9
Omit last sentence of text	Omitted; paragraph rewritten
Reviewer #5: General Comments 1. & 2a. Expand on why correct citation is important	Introduction (pp. 3-4) expanded and rewritten
2b. Conclude in article with how to do an effective search	Discussion expanded; strategies to avoid reference errors included on p. 9 (lines 22-23) to p. 10 (lines 1-19)
3. Avoid redundancy in portions of text	Introduction and discussion rewritten. Sentence with phrase "accounted for the majority" deleted in revision
4. Bias	Discussion revised so it does not focus on reference errors "wasting time" (see introduction p. 3 [lines 15-21] through p. 4 [lines 1-3]; discussion p. 9, lines 12-16). Strategies for searches added on p. 9 line 22 - p. 10 lines 1-19

Learning Activities

1. Go to each of the online nursing journal directories (Table 3.1), review the type of information available, and bookmark the websites for later use.
2. Develop an idea for a manuscript. Go to the online nursing journal directories (ie, websites reviewed in Activity 1). Select three journals to which you might submit this manuscript. Obtain the author guidelines for these journals, using at least one of these directories.
3. Write a query letter to one of these journals and check that it is complete.
4. Who deserves authorship of a paper? What three criteria must be met? Think about a group with whom you have recently worked. If you decided to write a manuscript about this work, which group members would meet the criteria for authorship and who would be acknowledged instead for their contributions? Why?
5. Select an article from a nursing or healthcare journal that you read recently. Read the first paragraph of the article. Can you determine from the first paragraph what the article is about? Why or why not? Did the paragraph get your attention? Did it make you interested in reading further? Now skim the article. Was it easy to read? What did you learn about the writing style?

References

American Medical Association. (1998). *Manual of style: A guide for authors and editors* (9th ed.). Baltimore: Williams & Wilkins.

American Psychological Association. (2001). *Publication manual of the American Psychological Association* (5th ed.). Washington DC: Author.

BrainyMedia.com. (2004). *Gene Fowler quotes*. Retrieved Jan. 21, 2004, from http://www.brainyquote.com/quotes/authors/g/gene_fowler.html.

Davidhizar, R. (2004). Guidelines for citing multiple authors. *Nurse Author & Editor, 14*(1), 1-4.

Fondiller, S. H. (1999). *The writer's workbook* (2nd ed.). Sudbury, MA: Jones and Bartlett.

Huth, E. J. (1999). *Writing and publishing in medicine* (3rd ed.). Baltimore: Williams & Wilkins.

International Committee of Medical Journal Editors. (2003). Uniform requirements for manuscripts submitted to biomedical journals: Writing and editing for biomedical publication. Retrieved Jan. 23, 2004, from http://www.icmje.org/index.html#author.

Johnson, S. H. (2003). ONLINE Nursing Editors. Retrieved Jan. 21, 2004, from http://members.aol.com/suzannehj/naed.htm.

Oermann, M. H. (1999a). Extensive writing projects: Tips for completing them on time. *Nurse Author & Editor, 9*(1), 8-10.

Oermann, M. H. (1999b). Writing for publication as an advanced practice nurse. *Nursing Connections, 12*(3), 5-13.

Oermann, M. H. (2000). Refining outlining skills: Part 1: The topic or sentence method. *Nurse Author & Editor, 10*(2), 4, 7-8.

Oermann, M. H. (2002). *Writing for publication in nursing.* Philadelphia: Lippincott, Williams & Wilkins.

Oermann, M. H., Cummings, S. L., & Wilmes, N. A. (2001). Accuracy of references in four pediatric nursing journals. *Journal of Pediatric Nursing, 16*, 263-268.

Oermann, M. H., Mason, N. M., & Wilmes, N. A. (2002). Accuracy of references in general readership nursing journals. *Nurse Educator, 27*, 260-264.

Oermann, M. H., & Ziolkowski, L. D. (2002). Accuracy of references in three critical care nursing journals. *Journal of PeriAnesthesia Nursing, 17*(2), 78-83.

Thomson ISI ResearchSoft. (2004). Home page. Retrieved Jan. 25, 2004, from http://www.risinc.com.

Chapter 4: Getting Started With Grants

Susan Diehl, BSN, MSN, RN, FNP, APRN

Research, the scholarship of discovery, advances our knowledge and provides evidence-based best practices for the development of a science of nursing education. Grants can assist in this noble endeavor by providing the resources necessary for conducting research. This chapter provides an interesting, easy-to-read explanation of what procuring a grant is all about. – Linda Caputi

Introduction

Grant writing. The mere sound of the words is likely to raise fear and doubt in the mind of the nurse educator. This is a common and completely normal reaction to the topic of grant writing in higher education. It is, however, unfortunate on two counts. First, external or alternative funding is becoming increasingly important because of market pressures and resource constraints in higher education. While academics are familiar with obtaining individual research and training grants, there will be increased demand to attach funding to service and teaching activities that support both the institution's mission and individual scholarly pursuits. In fact, in some institutions revenue generation is an expected part of the faculty role (Hensen, 2003; Lindeman, 2000). Second, by focusing on the complaints of grantsmanship (too confusing, frustrating, time-consuming), educators often fail to see the true value of incorporating grantsmanship in their work. The obvious benefit to receiving grants is the reward of being paid for special talents and ideas. The less obvious—but equally wonderful—benefit is that the discipline of grant seeking itself can actually help shape the career of the nurse educator. Thinking like a grantseeker forces the academic to plan in organized ways that bring ideas to fruition. Many have begrudgingly admitted

Educational Philosophy

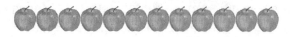

If a teacher sets the table with energy, experience, sound knowledge, and a welcoming spirit, learners will pull up a chair. – Susan Diehl

that being an active grantseeker has been invaluable in framing their daily activities of teaching, research, and service. It is not just a way to obtain dollars; it is a way to think.

The purpose of this chapter is to introduce nurse educators to the idea of grantsmanship so they feel confident enough to incorporate grant seeking into their professional lives. Most nurses do not realize how well positioned they are to be successful players in the grant world, so it is the intent of this chapter to provide the background that will encourage nurses to start to participate. The grant world is large. In the United States, there are more 60,000 funding institutions from the private sector alone that gave away $30 billion in 2002 (The Foundation Center, 2003). It is reasonable to believe that nurse educators can be highly successful in obtaining funding to support their ideas and dreams.

The Four Elements of the Grant Process

Although the grant process is admittedly confounding at times, there are really only four elements that need to be understood to begin participating in the grant world. They are:
1. **The Great Idea.** A way to solve a problem or address a need.
2. **The Grantseeker.** The person who seeks out funding to support the great idea.
3. **The Grantmaker.** The organization whose purpose is to fund great ideas.
4. **The Proposal.** The document that brings the first three elements together.

The Great Idea

The purpose of grants is to award money to support worthy causes. Although what is considered a worthy cause varies among grantmaking institutions, they all are interested in projects or programs that address some sort of human need. Every funded project started out with an idea.

Ideas are simply the plans and schemes that live in our heads. Whether through teaching, research, or service, nurse educators are constantly using ideas to solve problems to make things better for students, patients, and communities. It is easy to get careless with ideas, using them to serve a purpose and then letting them go. More times than one can imagine, those ideas were potential grant proposals. So, keeping track of ideas that one is interested in pursuing further is a first step to thinking like a grantseeker. Just as one keeps track of accomplishments and activities as a nurse educator, one must record potential proposal ideas as a grantseeker.

A good suggestion for storing ideas is to keep an **idea drawer**, where ideas of interest can be filed. To highlight the benefit of keeping an idea drawer, a colleague's story follows:

As a pediatric nurse, I used to have a file drawer where I would keep things that interested me. Articles from journals and magazines, notes about things that happened at work, famous quotes, pictures, interesting programs or projects. They were in no particular order, in fact, the drawer became the place where I put things that I wasn't sure what to do with. Well, one day, I couldn't get the drawer closed, so I was forced to clean it out. A newspaper clipping about the rise in child abuse and neglect got put in a pile next to a random newsletter from a child welfare organization. Somehow, I knew that nurses needed to be involved in this issue, and I knew I might be able to do something to help. It took a lot of focusing and reframing but I kept those two pieces of paper in front of me, wrote successful grants, and began a career in developing programs to prevent child abuse and neglect. I love it. My advice? Keep an idea drawer. Just clean it out more often than I did.

This story illustrates an important principle of grantsmanship. Finding money to support ideas is a little more complex than having an idea and then finding someone to fund it. Grant cycles, current events, and changes in the nurse educator's professional life prevent the process from being this simple. This is why it is important to take care of ideas. While it is impossible to predict when an idea may become useful, there are ways to play with these ideas so they **do something**.

A way to add to the idea drawer is to keep a journal. A journal is a novice grantseeker's best friend. This is the place where brainstorming and dreaming can occur, as well as a place to practice writing skills needed to become more proficient in writing grants. How one keeps a journal is a highly personal affair, but there are many resources from the field of creative writing that can help the nurse educator become an effective dreamer on paper. Dwelling in the possibilities of passions and ideas should be an ongoing process in the life of a nurse educator. For those unfamiliar with journal writing, the book *Writing Alone and With Others* by Pat Schneider (2003) is recommended.

Keeping a journal also helps clarify the nurse educator's passions and true interests. Grant writing experts agree that the most successful projects are the ones that have a clear passion behind them. While nurse educators may claim to not have any ideas, it is unlikely they do not have passion for their work. Having a good sense of what delights and excites the educator is critically important to the development of a professional career and finding the support for it.

The acts of defining a passion, collecting ideas, and seeing possibilities translate well when adding funding into the mix. It is just a matter of seeing the connections. When the nurse educator sees an idea that repeatedly captures his or her attention, it is time to see if the idea is a **great idea**. This is usually intuitive, but there are some qualities that separate great ideas from good ones. Ideas that are worth pursuing have some originality. This does not mean that an idea has to be wildly innovative, but it means that there should be a spark to the idea that makes it different. A great idea also solves a problem. Most ideas start because of a need to change something, and a great idea shows a way to meet that need. If one has gotten this far, it is worth trying to envision the idea in practice.

Funding organizations look for opportunities to support ideas that attempt to solve worthy problems. The nurse educator should try to define the idea as a problem and then consider ways that one might solve the problem. The solutions are what funders are interested in learning more about. The time when an idea is percolating is exactly the right time to take this step. This means that when an idea is put in the idea drawer, one should immediately start to think about how this idea looks in a problem-solving context.

Several fundamental questions should be explored when thinking about putting an idea into action. There are many resources that can help the nurse educator turn ideas into fundable projects. One such book is *The Complete Guide to Getting a Grant* by Laurie Blum (1996). Another fun read is *Storytelling for Grantseekers: The Guide to Creative Nonprofit Fundraising* by C. C. Clarke (2001). Consider this adapted list of fundamental questions as a beginning:

- What is the problem or need that your idea addresses? How involved or expert are you in the problem?
- Where else have you seen this problem addressed?
- How do you plan to solve the problem or meet the need?
- How would things be different or better if your idea was implemented? Locally? Globally?
- How would you know if things were better?
- What do you need to implement your idea? Money? People?

By attempting to answer these questions, ideas become more realistic and more useful in planning for grant seeking. If the answers come fairly easily, one is well on the way to a successful—and fundable—adventure. It is important to remember this is an ongoing process. One should never throw away the ideas that do not quite fit, nor should one stop adding new ones. The grantseeking process does not have an even ebb and flow. One needs to rely on being ready when opportunities present themselves, whether the ideas eventually are funded or not.

When the nurse educator believes he or she has an idea worth pursing, it is time to let colleagues review the idea or project. Before one invests the time to pursue funding, it is wise to explain the project to a selected group of three different people, and ask for their feedback. The first person should be a colleague who knows you and understands why you are interested in this idea. This person can help evaluate and shape the nurse educator's commitment to the proposed idea. The second person should be an experienced grantmaker or someone who has had experience with grantseeking. This person will be able to provide feedback from a funder's perspective. The third person who should be consulted is someone who would likely oppose the idea. For example, if the idea is to design an online course, choose a person who is Internet-phobic. Although this seems odd, it is very important not to skip the third person. Nothing shapes the significance of your project more than the feedback of a dubious audience.

Explaining an idea to different people gives the nurse educator a chance to clarify and reshape the idea. One common mistake that grant writers make is assuming that everyone knows what they mean. Discussing the idea with different people is also an excellent way to perfect the organization and tone of the idea, which will be important when it is time to apply for funding. Probably the most important benefit of this exercise is that the nurse educator has begun to create a network of people who are interested in the idea. Networking is an efficient use of time, especially as the process moves to finding grants.

The Grantseeker

The term "grantseeker" may be unfamiliar to the reader. This term is used in the grant business to describe the person who looks for funding opportunities and finds ways to obtain the funding, ie, one who actually writes grants. In short, a grantseeker is a matchmaker.

The purpose of this chapter is to blur the line between the idea person and the grantseeker, as this is the reality of the grant world today. The explosion of information technology has changed relationships and roles in the grant world.

Grants have become less the domain of the professionals and more open to the people with the ideas. As recently as five years ago, professional grantseekers earned their money as matchmakers between idea people and funders. It was hard-earned money because the task was grueling. This is changing. Information about funding opportunities is available on the Internet for the person willing to invest the time to research them. While professional grantseekers continue to serve a valuable service in gatekeeping and provide assistance in writing grants, their role has become more consultative.

Above all else, funders want to support worthy causes that are likely to produce successful outcomes. To ensure success, most funders want to get as close as possible to the original source of the project or program. That means they want to deal directly with the actual person behind the idea. This means nurse educators must be accountable for their ideas, so it behooves them to become actively involved in the process of seeking out grants. This is the process nurses are least familiar with, so it should be made clear that the procedure has a bit of a learning curve. It is wise to be patient. The ability to find out about grant opportunities grows with time. As a beginner, one will need to know a little bit about the language of the grant world, adopt some behaviors of professional grantseekers, and, most importantly, decide on the type of grantseeker one wants to be.

There is no deficit of advice and guidance available on the subjects of grantseeking and grant writing. The fact that Amazon.com carries more than 60,000 titles on the subject is proof enough. Before one becomes overwhelmed with the good advice of others, it is critical for the nurse educator to know himself or herself when starting to propose projects for funding. To do this, the educator must think ahead and plan carefully what he or she truly wants to do and be. Try this short exercise:

Envision yourself five years from now. What do you see yourself doing with your passions and interests? Do you see yourself deeply involved in clinical nursing research? Will you be operating a health clinic at a homeless shelter? Will you be inventing curricula for long-distance learning in nursing?

Now do some careful soul searching about your work personality. Do you like to have a lot of things going on at once or do you prefer to focus on one project at a time? Do you prefer working alone or with others?

Whatever you see yourself doing in the future will help narrow the search for funders who will be interested in your proposals. Likewise, your work personality should define the types of grants that will be manageable for you. If you like to engage in short activities or have more than one interest, you should seek out grants that are time limited and intended for very specific purposes. If you enjoy the planning and commitment of long-term programs, your search could include larger grants that extend over longer periods of time. The real art of grantseeking lies in knowing what you want and to what you are willing to commit. It pays to be self aware from the start. Frustration with the grant process generally comes from people not taking this important step.

Although Internet searches make it easier to locate potential grantors, the sheer number of funding organizations makes it impossible to stay abreast of all of them. The beginning grantseeker should understand that time and networking will help to stay aware of opportunities down the road. One should not miss opportunities. Following is a good example:

Maureen has always loved technology. She was an intensive care nurse for years, and was always the first to learn the latest technology. When she became a nurse educator, she immediately became involved with instituting technology in the classroom. She designed websites and interactive electronic games for her students. Her classes were very popular with students and she continued designing teaching interventions with technology. She was enjoying her work, but it started to take a toll on her time. Someone suggested she write a grant for some release time so she could focus on a particular web project. Maureen was surprised at this suggestion. It had never occurred to her to seek help with her work.

Maureen applied for a small grant from a technology corporation. She used the money to get release time from teaching and developed a health assessment tool that is being used by many universities on the East Coast. Maureen continued to pursue larger grants, and her work is now almost completely funded by grant awards. She admits she initially avoided grantseeking because of the investment of time it would require. "The time I gained to pursue good things clearly outweighed the time it took to apply for the grants," she says. Maureen was successful because she incorporated a grantseeking attitude into her real work. She stayed focused on matching her exact needs to grant opportunities.

New nurse educators often are surprised at the large number of grant initiatives in which they are invited to participate. Grant talk is daily discussion in higher education, and it is sometimes easy to get caught up in participating even when it is not exactly the educator's cup of tea. Being flexible about opportunities but firm about passions is a way to avoid becoming overwhelmed or frustrated with the grant process.

The Grantmaker

Grantmakers, also known as funders or donors, are the organizations that give money to worthy causes. In general, worthy causes are defined as activities that result in making things better for society. These organizations are set up to review, evaluate, and give money to projects or programs that fit the mission of the institution. This section provides an overview of the categories of grant institutions, types of grants, and the characteristics of grantmakers, that make the work of the grantseeker quite interesting.

There are three basic types of grantmakers. Private foundations are organizations that are created with the money of wealthy philanthropists. Large foundations like the Hearst Foundation are familiar to the public, but there are many smaller private foundations. In 2002, private foundations gave away $30 billion (The Foundation Center, 2003). Government agencies are the second major type of grantmaker. Government grants can be obtained at the federal, state, and local levels. Nurses probably are somewhat familiar with some of the grant activity that takes place at government agencies such as the National Institutes of Health. Private businesses and corporations are the third type of grantmaker. Their money is usually given to support needs of their local community. The term "foundation" is also used to describe legal entities set up to meet philanthropic needs. Corporate foundations and community or public foundations are also types of funders. Nurses and their work have been funded from all of these types of institutions.

Grantmakers give away different kinds of grants, in amounts that can vary from a few thousand dollars to a few hundred thousand and more. It is important to understand the categories of grants that are available so the grantseeker can find the best fit (Brown & Brown, 2001):

- **Program grants.** These grants support the establishment of specific, targeted programs like support groups for teen mothers.
- **Start-up grants.** Also known as program development grants, these grants supply seed money for programs that are expected to become long-term and eventually be supported by other means.
- **Research grants.** These grants support the study of an issue. They are most often given to universities or nonprofit research facilities.
- **Endowment grants.** Endowment funds are invested to provide an annual flow of income to support a cause.
- **Consulting grants.** It is increasingly common for grantmakers to offer grants to hire consultants on valuable projects.
- **Training grants.** These grants support professional development and conference activities.
- **Scholarship and fellowship grants.** These grants support educational costs for individuals.

Having a sense of the type of grants an organization provides is a good start in the grantseeker's quest. However, while all funding institutions have the same goal of giving money to nonprofit organizations and their worthy causes, this is where the similarity ends.

Each institution has its own unique mission and interests. Depending on the founder's wishes, money is donated to support specific interests, such as health, education, community building, or the arts. They may also limit their funding to certain geographical locations or populations.

Each grantmaking institution has its own requirements and processes for organizations applying for grants. One institution might require query letters before the proposal is submitted; another might prefer to simply receive the proposals. Some institutions prefer individual narrative proposals; others have standard application forms. In addition, grantmaking institutions have their own timelines for distributing grants, called grant cycles.

Keeping up with each potential grantor's requirements mandates some research and accurate record keeping. The grantseeker should collect information about potential donors including a description of the institution's interest, types and amounts of grants offered in the past, and funding cycles. Annual reports and histories of funded grants can help the grantseeker determine whether to pursue a foundation for funding. Information about foundations is available in directories like *The Foundation Directory, The National Directory of Corporate Giving,* or regional directories, which are available at most libraries. The most updated information is best obtained from foundation directories on the Internet.

The Internet has made it much easier to collect information about prospective donors, especially in the last few years. The Foundation Center (www.fdncenter.org) has a sophisticated website that lists foundations and provides links to many foundation sites. (The Foundation Center website can be easily launched from the CD accompanying this book. Simply launch your Internet browser, put the CD-ROM in the drive, go to Chapter 4 on the CD, and click on the website address.) A subscription is required for access to detailed information about specific grants, but there is enough free information to send the grantseeker in the right direction. During online research, searches by keyword will help the grantseeker narrow the list of potential donors. Since the project should have a clear focus, and the grantseeker should know what kind of grant he or she is looking for, keywords are easily used to manage the search.

Trying to locate funders who will be excited about the project and researching their characteristics and requirements may seem like an imposing task. Instead of thinking of foundations as donors, it is helpful to think of them as partners. Brown and Brown (2001) describe the appropriate paradigm for the grantseeker.

Grants are not free money. Foundations and other grantmakers are organizations that have missions and goals just as you do. Funders award grants because what the recipients want to do with the money fits in with the funder's own goals, initiatives and dreams, and with their founder's stated wishes. It makes sense to see a grant as a fair deal between colleagues whose interests are similar but whose resources are different. (p. 5)

Partners are not givers and receivers. Partners invite each other to participate in a common venture, and partners try to understand each other. Using this concept helps the grantseeker to see the project from the grantmaker's point of view and be more attentive to matching the partners' goals and tone. This special attention will be rewarded when it is time to write the grant proposal.

The Proposal

Writing grant proposals is not a difficult task in itself, especially if one already has thought out the idea, and knows that the funder is likely to support the project's mission. The best approach for writing grant proposals is to be clear, consistent, concise, and compelling. Most grantmakers have very specific guidelines for how grant proposals should be presented. It is the grantseeker's job to carefully review the donor's expectations and answer the questions, complete the required forms, and create a cover letter. The details of a grant proposal can be overwhelming to the nurse educator, but there are two solutions to this perceived problem. One is to remember the purpose of the proposal. The nurse educator has a great idea and has found a funder who might help make it happen. The proposal is simply a way to give the funder a logical reason to choose to support this project.

The second way is to practice with a boilerplate proposal. The boilerplate proposal is a generic outline of the project—a template—written without any particular funder in mind. The boilerplate proposal allows the writer to practice translating the great idea into the language of grantmakers.

There are many resources on writing a good grant proposal using a boilerplate. Hensen's (2003) *Grant Writing in Higher Education* has a very detailed guide to writing proposals. This author presents seven basic components of a boilerplate proposal and a short description of what each component entails.

Another useful template is the Common Grant Application supplied by the National Network of Grantmakers. This document can be downloaded from www.nng.org. (This URL can easily be launched from the CD accompanying this book. Simply launch your Internet browser, put the CD-ROM in the drive, go to Chapter 4 on the CD, and click on the website address.)

Whatever boilerplate template the grantseeker uses, the point is to get the basic information on paper. Grantmakers may ask for more information or request the information in a different format, but the basics remain the same. The following components should be included:

- Introduction or summary of the project;
- Statement of need and goal of the project;
- Project objectives, project activities, and method of evaluation;
- Budget;
- Description of the grantseeker's organization and funding history;
- Supporting materials; and
- Cover letter.

The Introduction

The introduction is a summary of the project, which grant officers will read to get a sense of what the project is about. Expert grant writers limit this section to one page. After reading the introduction, grant officers should clearly understand the need and goal of the project, the people involved, the total budget, and how much money is being requested from their institution. The introduction is where quick decisions may be made, so this section must be written in language that is clear, concise, and confident. The best advice for writing this section of the boilerplate is to write it last.

Statement of Need

The statement of need describes why the proposed project is necessary. Grantmakers look for how the specific need that is being addressed fits the larger social issue with which their institution is concerned. The funnel approach is helpful here: Start with the general problem, and then describe how it affects a specific community. Hard data that show the existence of a problem should be incorporated here, and the writer should refer to the literature thoroughly and thoughtfully. Using too many statistics is confusing, but a synthesized body of evidence provides a clear rationale for the project. Follow the statement of need with the project's overall goal and a description of the community or population it will serve.

Work of the Project

The work of the project is described in this next section and tells exactly what the project will do. It should be written with:
- Clear objectives;
- A description of the activities that will meet those objectives; and
- An explanation of how success will be measured.

Writers often make two mistakes in this section. One is confusing **goals** with **objectives**. It is helpful to think of the goal as the endpoint, and the objectives as the intended ways to get there. Goals can be written as general statements whereas objectives are more concrete and measurable. The other mistake writers tend to make is including too many goals and objectives. One overall goal is sufficient for any grant proposal. The number of objectives may vary with the size of the project, but there rarely should be more than five.

Grantmakers prize innovation but look carefully for feasibility in grant proposals. This section is the writer's chance to demonstrate how the project can be completed successfully. Clearly defining how the activities support the objectives, how the objectives support the goal, and how the goal supports the needs statement is crucial in grant proposals.

The Budget

Since grantmakers are financial agents, the budget is vitally important to the success of a grant proposal. Most beginning nurse grantseekers struggle with this part of the boilerplate proposal, finding it difficult to attach dollar figures to the activities and people needed for the grant. There are many resources to assist in preparing a budget. The National Network of Grantmakers' *Common Grant Application* (www.nng.org) offers a good template to follow. (This URL can easily be launched from the CD accompanying this book. Simply launch your Internet browser, put the CD-ROM in the drive, go to Chapter 4 on the CD, and click on the website address.) *Storytelling for Grant Seekers: The Guide to Creative Nonprofit Fundraising* by C. C. Clarke (2001) offers straightforward and practical advice on creating budgets.

The key to grant budgets is to work through the basic budget components of revenue and expenses. By showing the difference in revenue and expenses, one is letting the funder know the amount of money that is requested. Grantmakers want to see that the project is supported, so it is wise to include any in-kind donations in the revenue column.

Grant budgets are generally one or two pages long. A budget narrative, describing the use of the money, may also be requested. The narrative should include plans for future funding and a report of any other funding options that the grantseeker has pursued for the project. Annual reports and a copy of the Internal Revenue Service 501(c) letter confirming nonprofit status should be attached to the budget narrative.

The Organization's History and Funding History

The next component is a short description of the organization's history and funding history. Grantmakers must be sure that the recipients of their donations are nonprofit organizations and must ensure that the person in charge of the grant is supported by an institutional structure, usually the academic institution where the nurse educator works. Universities are familiar with faculty grants and the administrative office normally has a boilerplate description of the institution's history and annual report suitable for grant submissions.

Supporting Documents

The section for supporting documents usually includes letters of support, relevant newspaper articles or research articles, and the resumes of people involved in the project. Letters of support and endorsements are important to the grant proposal. One should not underestimate the value of personal and professional testimonials of the person who will direct the project. Funders know that great ideas are only as good as the people who carry them out.

Cover Letter

The cover letter is perhaps the most important part of the proposal. Grant writers will spend 90 percent of their time writing the proposal, but the cover letter will make or break the grant request. The cover letter is the best opportunity for the grantseeker to connect with the funder and highlight the uniqueness of the proposal. A good cover letter should show that it was expressly written to the funder. This can be done by clearly responding to the needs and interests of the funder. When describing the project, one should present the most compelling ideas first. The letter should be visually appealing, concise, and professional, just as the rest of the proposal should be.

Final Thoughts on the Proposal

The proposal is what brings a great idea, grantseekers, and grantmakers together. A good proposal conveys that they belong together. There is no way to predict a funder's reaction to a grant proposal. If a proposal is rejected, it is important to try to get feedback from the grantmaker. Evaluating both the successes and failures in seeking grants is important learning for the nurse educator—learning that can help bring success with the next proposal.

Summary

Nurse educators are encouraged to actively incorporate grantseeking into their professional lives. Their roles in higher education will demand it, and their work will be better because of it. The nurse educator who takes good care of ideas and develops a grantseeking attitude is well prepared to enter the world of grants. The rest comes from experience. Getting started with grants is like everything else. Getting started is the hard part. As Blum (1996), an expert in the field of fund raising and grant writing, stated, "Anyone can learn to find grants, and I am the best example. I didn't go to school to learn to be a grantseeker, I learned by doing it. The point is that anyone can get a grant for an idea they really believe in" (p. 12).

Learning Activities

1. Identify some of your ideas about nursing or nursing education. Describe how you might turn those ideas into grant proposals.
2. Visit the website of a professional organization such as the National League for Nursing or Sigma Theta Tau International. Find the organization's guidelines for submitting a grant proposal. Print the submission guidelines and use them to write a grant proposal. Have a colleague critique your proposal.
3. Prepare a budget proposal for a specific project or program.

References

Blum, L. (1996). *The complete guide to getting a grant.* New York: John Wiley & Sons.

Brown, L. G., & Brown, M. J. (2001). *Demystifying grant seeking: What you really need to do to get grants.* San Francisco: Jossey-Bass.

The Foundation Center (2003). *Foundation growth and giving estimates: 2002 preview.* Retrieved Oct. 24, 2003, from www.fdncenter.org.

Hensen, K. T. (2003). *Grant writing in higher education: A step by step guide.* Upper Saddle River, NJ: Pearson, Allyn & Bacon.

Lindeman, C. A. (2000). The future of nursing education. *Journal of Nursing Education, 39*(1), 5-12.

Bibliography

Clarke, C. C. (2001). *Storytelling for grantseekers: The guide to creative nonprofit fundraising.* San Francisco: Jossey-Bass.

The National Network of Grantmakers. (n.d.). Retrieved from www.nng.org.

Schneider, P. (2003). *Writing alone and with others.* New York: Oxford University Press.

Chapter 5: Negotiating Faculty Politics

Ken W. Edmisson, ND, EdD, RNC, FNP

This chapter provides some personal insights into the workings of academia within a nursing school. Dr. Edmisson draws upon his years of experience to offer a candid look at what new faculty should consider when applying for and accepting that first position. This chapter provides a "heads up" for new faculty, one I could have used more than 20 years ago! – Linda Caputi

Introduction

Congratulations! You have decided to dedicate yourself to teaching the next generation of nurses. You are now a nursing professor. You have earned a master's degree in nursing, and perhaps even a doctorate. You are a highly skilled and knowledgeable clinical expert. You probably have held a variety of positions ranging from staff nurse to chief nursing officer of a medical facility. You have experienced and endured situations that have stretched you and helped you to grow. However, you are about to embark on a new, very rewarding, and incredibly challenging career as a nursing professor.

This chapter provides a guide for considering some components of the faculty role. This chapter does not attempt to address all aspects of the faculty role, but instead focuses on two of the most essential ones: contractual and social/political issues.

Educational Philosophy

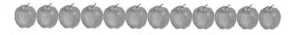

Teaching and learning go hand in hand; you can't have one without the other. My role as an educator is to facilitate the student's learning. Many times, that is merely rephrasing or presenting the material in yet one more way for the student to experience. At other times, I am the presenter of new material. No matter what, teaching and learning are lifelong processes. Socrates' methods are my favored means. – Ken W. Edmisson

Contractual Aspects for Faculty

The key contractual issues of academia include:
- The hiring process;
- Workload;
- Clinical practice;
- Level and amount of classroom responsibility;
- Clinical supervision;
- Tenure-track versus clinical-track appointments;
- Scholarly activity;
- Service; and
- Salary.

Hiring

The first consideration in the hiring process should be how you found the position. Was it advertised? Were you contacted by the school of nursing? Or, did you inquire about a position? In any case, contact was made, either with the chief academic nursing officer or a search committee for the school. You will no doubt be asked to submit references and a curriculum vitae and to forward transcripts to the school. Do not be offended by these requests. Accrediting bodies require that schools retain evidence that faculty members have qualifying academic degrees in nursing.

A search committee within the school of nursing may be established to coordinate the interview process. The search committee is typically composed of faculty representing a wide range of interests. This facilitates evaluation of all aspects of the candidate for a proper fit within the school. The search committee typically sets the schedule for the interview and establishes with whom the candidate will meet and interview. Typically, the search committee will be the candidate's primary point of contact for communicating with the school about the position. If a search committee is not used, then the chief academic nursing officer is usually the contact person.

The type of interview depends on the school's administrative structure and the position you are seeking. Most schools require an interview with the chief academic nursing officer. For some schools, this may be the only interview, particularly if the upcoming semester is approaching and there is an immediate need to fill the faculty position. Usually, however, other interviews ensue.

You may have communicated via telephone and email with the chief academic nursing officer. The chief academic nursing officer and senior members of the college administration determine if the new teacher will be compatible with the existing faculty and will want the candidate to meet, and even interview with, the nursing faculty.

The faculty interview may take several modalities. It may involve one interview with the search committee. The committee may require the candidate to perform a presentation, in front of the committee or the entire faculty, on a topic dictated by the search committee or chosen by the candidate. Presentations may cover one's teaching style, philosophy of teaching, philosophy of nursing, a current research program, or a clinical practice topic. Interviews also may involve visiting various faculty members within the school.

The interview may be brief—one meeting or one day—or it may extend two or more days and include a campus tour, additional meetings with other school representatives, and a tour of the community. Be prepared for an exhaustive interview process; it does get trying at times.

Once the formalities of the interview are over, the process of negotiating the contractual items begins.

Workload

Workload is somewhat difficult to define in academia. Faculty, as most are aware, do not typically go to school and sit in their offices from 8 AM to 5 PM Monday through Friday. College and university faculty typically are required to carry a predefined workload each semester. Typical workloads vary anywhere from nine to 15-plus hours per semester. Now, what exactly does that mean?

Workload Hours

A three-semester-hour theory course is a course that meets for three hours per week for the entire 15-week semester, or 45 hours. The faculty teaching this course receives three credits for their workload.

Nursing—like other science laboratory and practicum disciplines—differs from traditional liberal arts courses, because of its laboratory and clinical course requirements. For the sake of simplicity, let's consider laboratory and clinical courses the same for discussion pertaining to workload credit.

The intent is to enable the student ample time to acquire necessary skills needed without awarding equivalent credit for each hour spent during the laboratory work. This would increase the number of credit hours spent for the course and degree considerably. Nursing typically uses a ratio of credit hours to clock hours. Most schools use a credit hours-to-clock hours ratio of one-to-two or one-to-three for clinical and laboratory courses. In other words, for every two or three hours spent during the activity per week, the student is awarded one semester hour credit. Thus, a three–semester-hour **clinical** course with a one credit hour to two clock hour ratio would require the student to perform a total of 90 clock hours (3 semester hours credit x 2 clock hours x 15 weeks in the semester = 90 clock hours).

It is important to note that the time faculty spend in a clinical or laboratory course may be calculated in a variety of ways with respect to workload credit. Two eight-hour clinical days per week may be counted anywhere between eight and 16 hours of teaching workload, depending on the institution. Schools may or may not use the same formula to calculate faculty workload and student credit.

Most faculty workloads range from nine to 15 hours credit per semester. Some schools, however, calculate workloads on a yearly basis, meaning that faculty members are expected to teach a specific number of credit hours per year. These hours may be evenly distributed over both semesters or may be unevenly distributed depending on faculty, student, and curricular need. Some schools offer certain courses only during certain semesters and may have greater needs during those semesters.

Release time is another factor to consider when discussing workload credit. Situations that may warrant release time include administrative responsibilities, faculty advising, and faculty sponsorship of campus organizations, grant planning, and new course development. The chief academic nursing officer or a special committee with administrative approval may award the release time. Release time may be granted for a varied amount of credit. For example, you may be awarded three hours release time to work on a special project. A grant of three hours' release time means you will be expected to dedicate three to six clock hours per week for the entire semester to the project.

Scholarly Activities and Service

One other point to consider when discussing workload credit is time for scholarly activity and service activity. Ask what expectations are placed on you with respect to scholarly activity and service in your role as faculty. If the institution is research focused, you will be expected to perform some type of scholarly activity, whether it be independent research, collaborative clinical investigation, writing for publication, or another scholarly activity.

Some form of service is almost always expected from faculty, especially in the healthcare practice disciplines. Service may involve serving on school or college committees, advising a student organization, working with a community organization, participating at a local medical facility, or maintaining a clinical practice. Service also may include work with a regional, national, or international professional association. Sometimes there exists a fine line when having to distinguish between professional service in associations and boards and that associated with scholarly activity. That distinction should be determined by the practices of the institution where you are teaching.

The important consideration when contemplating scholarly activity and service is their impact on the time commitment and responsibilities of your faculty role. If you are expected to participate regularly and be productive in these activities, you must be given some workload credit for these activities. In return, you must demonstrate some product at the conclusion of the time granted for these activities.

One advantage of active participation in scholarly research and funded grant research is that the faculty member often is able to buy out some of the workload credit using grant dollars. This means the faculty may be able to receive release time to work on the grant because the teacher's participation was a calculated expense of the grant. For example, the faculty member may agree to dedicate 30 percent of a full workload to the grant. Based on a 12-hour workload, this means the teacher would receive 3.6 hours release time (30 percent of 12 hours) for workload credit, which the faculty member would be expected to dedicate each week to the grant activity.

Finally, consider what workload would be realistic. If the workload credit does not make sense to you or appears to be unrealistic, do not just ignore it. Ask other faculty or the chief academic nursing officer to explain. Understanding workload credit early in your teacher career may help clarify many questions and relieve some stress later on.

Clinical Practice

Questions to consider about clinical practice include the following:
- Will you be expected to maintain currency in clinical practice in addition to fulfilling your full-time faculty role?

- Will you be expected to participate in a clinical faculty practice already established within the school?
- Will you receive a joint appointment teaching in the school of nursing and practicing at a local medical facility?
- Will you be granted release time and workload credit to participate in an established faculty practice? Some schools of nursing allow release time so faculty may offer services in an established practice. This may also entail clinical supervision of students.

Some schools may grant release time for faculty to maintain clinical skills. This is especially important for advanced practice nurses, who are required to complete some clinical practice hours to maintain their certifications. If you receive release time for this, ask if you are allowed to keep the salary paid by the clinical facility during that time, or if you must pay it to the school.

Two additional responsibilities that typically are not calculated as workload hours are office hours and committee work. Most faculty at a college or university are required to hold six to 10 office hours each week. This allows face-to-face meetings with students and others who may need to interact with you. Typically, you can advise students, prepare for courses, perform committee work, and complete other projects during office hour time.

Another time-consuming activity is committee work. Nursing academia seems to be inundated with committee work. Typically there are standing committees for curriculum, scholarly activity, student services, and faculty development. There also are myriad other committees, such as a search committee, that might be formed during the course of the year. It is important to realize that committees accomplish much work and are essential for gathering the input needed to guide the nursing program. However, faculty should be mindful that no formal workload credit is assigned for this time. Often new faculty are not required to engage in committee work, especially during their early years of teaching.

Coursework Responsibility

Coursework responsibility is a major concern for both the faculty and the chief academic nursing officer. The chief academic nursing officer must ensure that all courses are covered and taught by qualified and credentialed faculty, while maintaining equitable workloads. The chief academic nursing officer also must maintain balance across the curricula and levels of instruction, and faculty must be mindful of their own strengths and weaknesses when considering their ability to teach across curricula and on different levels of nursing education.

Whether the faculty will teach at the graduate or undergraduate level is decided initially based on the candidate's academic preparation and expertise. Typically, a doctoral degree is required for graduate teaching, but some institutions may allow a limited number of master's-prepared individuals to teach at the graduate level, particularly if they have unique qualifications and expertise. A master's degree in nursing should be the minimal qualifying degree for teaching in a nursing program, even at the associate degree level.

Teaching Undergraduate Courses

Teaching and faculty expectations typically are different for associate degree programs than for bachelor's degree programs. Associate degree faculty are typically heavily involved in content, laboratory, and clinical instruction—teaching the basics of client care in preparation for the licensure examination. There is usually little to no expectation for faculty to be productive in scholarly activities.

Faculty at the bachelor's level work with a broader, more advanced curriculum and a wide array of duties to fulfill. Instruction is typically at a higher level. Bachelor's degree programs include courses not found in associate degree programs, such as those focusing on research methodology, community health, nursing theory, critical care, and nursing leadership and management. Elective courses also may be available, offering students opportunities for additional inquiry into the nursing profession.

Faculty at the bachelor's level tend to be more specialized than their peers teaching in associate degree programs. While associate degree faculty do teach courses in their specialty, those programs are more generic and often require faculty to collaborate and teach across the curriculum—leading a fundamentals course or helping with skills laboratories—during a semester when their specialty is not offered. This arrangement means faculty might teach course content with which they are not familiar. At the bachelor's degree level, however, faculty tend to teach only courses related to their specialty.

Teaching Graduate Courses

Teaching at the graduate level offers faculty a different venue to explore nursing. Graduate-level teaching requires more thorough examination of content than does undergraduate teaching. Faculty typically teach content in which they already have significant teaching experience, formal training, and clinical expertise. They also may teach some general courses such as nursing theory, research methodology, and trends and issues.

Some faculty have developed expertise in teaching certain advanced courses, such as pathophysiology, pharmacology, and health assessment. These are core courses in most graduate nursing programs, but they require an in-depth knowledge and expert delivery for students to excel.

At the graduate level, faculty also must determine in what concentration they will teach. Questions to consider include:

- What areas of concentration does the graduate program offer? Is there a nurse practitioner program? If so, what type? Is there a clinical nurse specialist track, a nurse anesthesia program, a nurse midwifery program?
- Does the program prepare nurse educators or nurse administrators?
- Where do you fit in?
- Are you so specialized that you can only teach in one type of program? Most nursing faculty are prepared as specialists in a single area.

It makes sense for courses such as advanced courses in pharmacology, health assessment, and pathophysiology be taught by an advanced practice nurse.

The rigors of teaching at the graduate level are different from those of the undergraduate level. While undergraduate students must learn a wide range of new tasks and psychomotor skills, many graduate courses require only a midterm and final examination and perhaps a research paper. Though the formal written assignments and tests might be fewer in number than at the undergraduate level, the courses require a greater depth of knowledge and, therefore, more acute research and study. The goal of internalizing content at the graduate level is not mere familiarity, it is mastery and expertise. Be prepared to be challenged during class discussions. This is the nature of the beast at the graduate level; this is a good thing.

Clinical Supervision Requirements

At most schools of nursing, some type of student clinical supervision is required of most faculty. The type of supervision, level of students supervised, and areas in which the students are supervised are important aspects of the teaching role. It is important to know how the clinical assignment figures into your workload.

One point to consider is the type of supervision required of the faculty member. Student supervision can take a multitude of forms. Commonly, faculty are required to be on the clinical unit directly supervising students. If this is the case, a few points should be addressed. You should be familiar with the clinical setting in which you will provide supervision; most accrediting agencies require that faculty are competent in the areas they teach.

Most nursing faculty should be able to supervise a fundamentals course. Beyond that, however, nursing care becomes more specialized. Pediatric rotations typically require a pediatric nurse specialist or practitioner for supervision in that area; likewise for clinicals in obstetrics, medical-surgical nursing, critical care, community health, and leadership.

What level of students will you be supervising? Are they undergraduate students requiring very organized, direct supervision, or are they graduate students? Even in graduate clinical courses, some students require direct supervision.

The clinical course you are teaching may allow for clinical supervision by preceptors. It will be your responsibility to ensure that all students are placed with an appropriate preceptor in the appropriate clinical area. This type of supervision can be viewed as less stressful to some faculty, and more stressful to others; it requires the faculty to be familiar with clinical agencies, resources, and qualified clinical preceptors. The teacher must become familiar with the requirements and policies for preceptors set by the school, accrediting and certifying agencies, and state nursing board.

Accrediting agencies typically require a master's degree in nursing as the minimum qualifying academic degree for a preceptor. Certifying agencies' requirements depend on what type of clinical course is being taught and what type of certification is being pursued. For advanced practice clinical preceptors, a master's degree in nursing along with the appropriate certification is required. Most state boards of nursing place restrictions on the number of students a practitioner may precept, just as they limit the number of students a teacher may directly supervise on a clinical unit.

Other specific questions to consider regarding clinical supervision include:

- How does clinical supervision contribute to your workload?
- Is the clinical supervision an independent course, or is it part of a course that combines didactic and clinical content?
- How are the students to be evaluated and graded?

Tenure-Track versus Clinical-Track Appointments

One important topic to understand—even before beginning your role as nursing faculty—is the difference between the tenure-track appointment and the clinical-track appointment.

The tenure track appointment is the role that typically comes to mind when university faculty positions are discussed. Tenure-track–appointed faculty have fulfilled academic and clinical requirements and achieved a certain level of experience at the institution. Many four-year colleges and universities have raised academic standards to require that faculty being considered for tenure-track positions have doctoral degrees. Some institutions may consider a teacher who is actively engaged in formal doctoral study with the real possibility of successful completion of the doctorate for a tenure-track position; in others, a doctorate may not be required for tenure.

Before earning tenure, faculty typically receive year-to-year contracts, with no guarantee of rehire for the following year. Tenure grants the faculty some security in the form of a permanent employment contract pending their continued performance of defined academic duties. Tenured positions are highly coveted in academia.

A teacher who receives a tenure-track appointment is in pursuit of tenure. There is typically a timeline of three to six years from the date of hire for the teacher to achieve tenure. During this time, the faculty member must be productive in the following arenas:

- Teaching;
- Scholarly activity; and
- Service.

Each institution defines these expectations differently.

A clinical-track appointment usually involves a heavy emphasis on clinical practice and student supervision. Most schools of nursing also incorporate didactic teaching in the clinical track role. Some clinical appointments require the teacher to continue to be productive in scholarly activity, focusing on more clinically oriented research; some also require service. The clinical-track appointment is widely used, but the responsibilities of these faculty vary greatly from institution to institution.

The type of appointment guides how faculty spend their time and energy. A clinical-track appointment usually affords a reprieve from course development, heavy didactic instruction, student advising, and other common faculty commitments. A tenure-track appointment typically requires all of those responsibilities, as well as service, scholarly activity, and classroom teaching.

Teaching, Service, and Research

Teaching, service, and research are the triad of the typical nursing faculty role. Most baccalaureate and higher degree nursing programs require faculty performance in all three areas. The academic institution sets the amount of productivity required in each of the three.

Teaching

Teaching is the cornerstone of the faculty role at all levels of nursing education. Most faculty are required to perform some amount of teaching. It may be formal didactic teaching, online course instruction, seminars, or clinical supervision; the specific teaching methodologies required are determined by the programs offered by the school.

Quality of teaching is an extremely important aspect of the faculty role. All academic institutions value quality teaching. However, the emphasis placed on quality teaching varies; some institutions make teaching performance a priority for faculty evaluation and some view it as equal to other components of the faculty role. Usually, the teaching abilities of each faculty member are evaluated at least once a year. This evaluation process may incorporate review by students, peers, or supervisors. It is important to question whether these evaluations influence promotion and tenure.

Questions to ask about teaching include:
- What amount of teaching will be required of you? At what level?
- How many courses will you be required to teach?

- Is the teaching load based on credit hours?
- What part of the workload is derived from teaching?
- What is the maximum number of students enrolled in each course?
- What is the student-to-teacher ratio in clinical courses?

Service

Service, the second area to consider, can also take on a wide range of activities. Service might be directed to the school of nursing, the college or university, the community, or another outlet. School-related service might entail student advising, committee membership, or administrative work. College or university service may entail those same functions as well as serving as faculty advisor to a student organization, or representing the university at official functions.

Community service can be time-consuming, but it can be fun and it is for the good of the community and provides great publicity for the school of nursing. As faculty providing community service, you might offer your expertise by serving on the board of a local community organization or medical facility. You might help coordinate a local walk for charity, CPR drive, or cancer screening. You might offer your services to a local clinic as a nurse or primary care provider. There are multitudes of ways to provide community service. It is important to make sure you follow the community service guidelines established by your school.

Professional service is available in many different fashions. Merely being a member of an organization does not qualify as professional service. If you are a member of the American Nurses Association and your state's association, are you a district, regional, or state officer? Do you perform a strategic role in the local, state, or national specialty association? Do you write questions for the National Council of State Boards of Nursing's NCLEX® examination?

Another form of professional service is serving on the editorial board, or as a reviewer, for a professional journals or text. Contributing to scholarly publications can help establish your expertise and improve your visibility among peers. These are just a few of the ways you can provide service.

Research

There are a wide variety of options for research and scholarly activity. Research may entail establishing a formal research agenda and program. This usually requires that the individual be doctorally prepared and capable of carrying out independent research and following through to publish that research. The faculty also must pursue external funding, usually from federal agencies. Writing grants and seeking federal funding is a very time-consuming ordeal. It is not unusual for the process to take two or three years. (See Chapter 4, "Getting Started with Grants," by Susan Diehl, for more information about procuring grants.)

Questions related to research and scholarly activity include:

- What types of research may be considered?
- Is locally focused research acceptable? Are small grants acceptable?
- Is each faculty member required to apply for or acquire a set amount of funding each year?
- Are promotion and/or tenure tied to the faculty's success procuring grants?
- What other types of scholarly activity are available and acceptable?
- Is authoring a chapter in a text acceptable in lieu of an article in a peer-reviewed journal?
- How many publications are faculty expected to achieve per year?
- How many publications are required for tenure and/or promotion?
- Does the institution accept poster presentations in lieu of podium oral presentations?
- How does research and scholarly activity count with regard to your workload? It seems unjust, and perhaps unethical, to require scholarly activity but not provide paid time to accomplish the task.

In considering faculty's responsibilities for teaching, service, and research, it is imperative to fully realize the impact this triad will have on your abilities and on the time and commitment you can offer. How do these activities factor into your workload? You will need to become acutely adept at time management and be able to allot specific amounts of time to each of these three areas weekly to accomplish your goals. Because you will be evaluated in each of these areas, you will need to demonstrate productivity in each of them.

Salary

Salary is typically not the reason one goes into teaching. This is especially true given the current economy and academic institutions' financial status. Generally speaking, faculty salaries are not competitive with clinical or administrative positions. Also, faculty salaries can vary within an institution across disciplines, with faculty in computer science, engineering, and business typically earning higher salaries than those in other departments. These salaries are usually market driven to attract faculty in these areas and compete with salaries in private industry.

Faculty salaries also vary depending on:

- Geographic location;
- Size of the institution;
- Focus of the school; and
- Type of degree granted.

A new registered nurse in the first year of clinical practice can earn a base salary of approximately $35,000 to $45,000 per year. With shift differentials, weekend differentials, specialty pay, and overtime, it is not inconceivable that a first-year registered nurse's take-home pay can reach $50,000 or $60,000. In that context, it is almost incomprehensible for colleges to expect to hire a doctorally prepared clinical specialist with years of nursing experience at a starting salary of $40,000.

Before long, nursing faculty salaries, too, will be market driven. Because of the national shortage of nurses and nursing faculty, faculty salaries may become more congruent with other disciplines. (See Chapter 1 "The Nursing Faculty Shortage," by Linda Caputi for more on the nursing faculty shortage.)

When discussing salary, the following questions should be asked:

- What factors influence starting salary?
- Is the salary for a full academic year?
- Is the salary for a nine- or 10-month contract? If so, can you elect to receive your salary in equal payments over 12 months?
- If you teach more than your required workload for a given semester, are you paid an additional amount? If so, how is the additional amount calculated?
- Are you required to teach during the summer? If so, how are you paid?
- Are you required to sign an additional contract for overload work or summer teaching?
- Does the institution provide full insurance coverage or do you have to pay a partial amount?
- Does the institution offer a 401(k) retirement plan?
- Are you eligible to receive tuition benefits? If so, are tuition dollars calculated as income?

When discussing and negotiating your salary, do not settle for an amount that is less than you feel is equitable.

Social and Political Aspects of the Faculty Role

The following section covers the social and political aspects of the faculty role, including the formal academic hierarchy, the power players on faculty, and the eternal tenured versus non-tenured faculty quandary.

Finding Your Way

You have been hired and are now walking into the school of nursing for the first time as a member of the faculty. You should become familiar with the clerical and administrative support staff within the university and specifically in the school of nursing. These individuals can save you time and can help you in many ways.

Campus support services are important as well. Does the school provide faculty with technology or library services support? Are student workers available in your department? Who does the photocopying? Who handles advising? Is it part of the faculty role or is there an advisor for the school of nursing? These are some of the questions to address as you begin your days as a faculty member. However, understanding the formal and informal leadership within the school of nursing and university also is important to your success.

Understanding the Leadership Hierarchy

Formality, structure, and chain of command are all familiar components of leadership; they also apply in academic settings. Faculty must be aware of which colleagues and administrators to approach—and when to approach them—to address departmental and intramural issues.

In some nursing programs, administrative protocols are less formal than in others. At smaller institutions, there may be only a department chair or coordinator who is responsible for the program. Course coordination is usually the responsibility of the primary teacher in each major course. Faculty in these programs typically meet to make joint decisions concerning the program. This simple structure eliminates layers of hierarchy found in larger programs.

Larger nursing programs typically have more than one person in administrative roles. These administrative positions may include a dean of the school of nursing and associate deans for graduate studies, undergraduate studies, academic affairs, research, student services, and other programs. In addition, below the associate dean for graduate studies there might be directors for the various programs, such as a family nurse practitioner program, nurse anesthesia program, master's degree program, and doctoral studies. Reporting to these directors, there may be coordinators responsible for particular courses, strands of courses, or certificate programs. Finally, the faculty are positioned under the coordinators.

It is important to know whom to consult when faced with a particular question or concern. You would not ask the dean about a particular course or major requirement for advising. Instead, you would consult with the course coordinator, program director, degree program director, or associate dean for academic affairs. Each administrator has specific responsibilities; it is wise to consult with each appropriately.

It is also important to understand that these positions bring with them a certain amount of prestige and power. People sometimes use this power and prestige inappropriately. Turf wars can occur when one person's area is encroached upon. These conflicts may stem from a variety of sources. Perhaps the individual in a certain position is insecure, unsure of his or her abilities, and feeling threatened. The individual may not want to be perceived as being unable to make smart decisions.

It is important to learn about the individuals in positions of authority within your program, to learn how they arrived in their positions, their styles of leadership, and how they make decisions. You have come across all types of individuals in positions of authority in your nursing practice; these individuals are no different in the academic setting. Go about establishing yourself sensibly and honorably.

Who Are the Power Players?

Knowing who the power players are is important for everyone involved. The power players may not be the people who are in charge. The chief academic nursing officer is undoubtedly a power player in any nursing school. However, others often cultivate positions of authority, either formally or informally.

Power players acquire their power in a variety of ways. A teacher may be a gifted researcher who continually brings in large grants. Other faculty may produce several published articles each year. These activities generally give faculty some additional prestige within the program.

Power players also may be those who have been at the school for a long time and are well known at the university and within the community. They may or may not be the best teachers or clinicians, but their longevity may give them added decision-making power in the school. Other power players are the tenured faculty.

Faculty members who hold endowed chairs also may be power players. These individuals are recruited to the school for various reasons. They might be well-established researchers or clinicians, deemed by the school to be the best of the best, and recruited to bolster the school's reputation. Funding for these chairs is usually from an outside source, and the professors' salaries typically are significantly higher than the average faculty's salary. These individuals may teach a small number of courses, and they usually concentrate their work around the endowed chair's focus, eg, research, clinical advancement, or community work.

There may be some faculty who are considered power players because of their command of content, aptitude for handling complex issues, speaking ability, clinical expertise, or involvement in professional organizations. These individuals may have connections with influential bodies such as the state nursing board, accreditation or certification agencies, or local legislatures. These individuals have the ability to greatly help the school.

The Tenured versus the Non-Tenured

Finally, it is important to understand the implications of the tenured versus the non-tenured faculty and the power tenured faculty often wield. Tenure is awarded faculty who have established themselves as:

- Accomplished teachers;
- Seasoned researchers and producers of scholarly work; and
- Professionals committed to service at various levels.

An implied responsibility of the tenured faculty is cultivating and helping those faculty who are on a tenure track, aspiring to tenured positions.

Faculty with tenure-track appointments are in a difficult situation. They are expected to be productive—very productive—and successful in all facets of their position. They are expected to teach courses expertly and earn outstanding evaluations. They are expected to generate research and provide service. These are all admirable goals, but many factors can create obstacles. What happens when students receive low grades and respond with poor evaluations of the faculty? What happens when a student does not like the counseling a teacher provides and damages the teacher's reputation by complaining to other faculty? These occurrences can have negative implications in decisions about tenure and promotion.

Tenure-track faculty, like all faculty, are evaluated yearly. However, tenure-track faculty evaluations are usually more involved. Performance is scrutinized in greater depth than for tenured faculty or those who are in clinical or temporary positions. The potential long-term **worth** of the teacher to the school and university is being evaluated. The many items considered during the evaluation of a tenure-track faculty include:

- The faculty member's own portfolio of published work, course syllabi, etc;
- Teaching and course evaluations;
- Peer evaluations;
- Administrative evaluations; and
- Evaluations by tenured faculty within the department, and even perhaps by tenured faculty from other schools or departments in the university.

It is this last type of input that needs to be dealt with cautiously. Tenured faculty often yield great power in decisions related to tenure-track faculty. Ideally, the relationship between tenured and tenure-track faculty should be supportive, guiding, and collegial; tenured faculty should work professionally with those in tenure-track positions in matters affecting the school of nursing, curriculum, and students. The tenured faculty should mentor their tenure-track colleagues, helping them to be successful when they are reviewed for tenure or promotion.

Generally, the whole faculty, or a smaller group of tenured professors, meets to evaluate tenure-track faculty. These seasoned faculty must maintain objectivity in their assessments and evaluations of the tenure track faculty under review.

Tenured faculty sometimes flaunt their positions to non-tenured faculty. These interactions create a sense of division among the faculty. Tenure-track faculty often are intimidated by tenured faculty and are afraid to disagree with them.

Most tenured faculty are older than their non-tenured counterparts and may have been away from clinical practice for some time. They may be entrenched in their views and rigid in their practices. The tenure-track faculty may be younger, have more current clinical experience, possess a wider range of educational training, or bring a fresh perspective to educational problems. This can be unsettling to the tenured faculty, but it does not mean you should be subservient; it merely means you should be aware that some faculty may be intimidated by you and that power plays may ensue.

Summary

This chapter provided a multitude of issues to consider when beginning your faculty role. Some of these are:
- Types of appointment and workload;
- Types and levels of courses to be taught and supervised;
- Institutional expectations for teaching, service and research;
- Salary; and
- Academic hierarchy.

This is not a complete list of items to contemplate. However, the chapter should provide some insight into the workings of academia within a school of nursing.

Learning Activities

1. Interview faculty who teach at the associate, baccalaureate, and graduate levels. Compare and contrast workload, role expectations, and salaries.
2. Interview faculty teaching in undergraduate nursing programs and faculty teaching in graduate programs. Compare and contrast expectations relative to publishing research and procuring grants.
3. Discuss the issue of service with several tenured faculty. What might you do to fulfill this expectation of the faculty role?

The Educational Process in Action

Unit 2

Chapter 6: Inspiring Students
     Jeanette Rossetti, MS, Ed D, RN

Chapter 7: Planning and Implementing Short Term Travel
     Courses and Cultural Immersion Experiences
     Luanne Wielichowski, MSN, RN, ARNP, BC, FNP,
     and Julie L. Millenbruch, MS(N), RN, CRRN

Chapter 8: Revitalizing for Success with Active Learning Approaches
     Kathleen Ohman, MS, Ed D, RN, CCRN

Chapter 9: Online Clinical Discussions: An Opportunity for Reflective Thought
     Glennys K. Compton, BSN, MSN, RN, ANP

Chapter 10: Reflective Writing: A New Approach in Clinical Assessment
     Catherine A. Andrews, MS, Ph D, RN

Chapter 6: Inspiring Students

Jeanette Rossetti, MS, EdD, RN

Inspiring students: Can it be done? Some faculty believe students must come motivated and inspired. Other faculty believe it is our responsibility to inspire those who are not. This author believes in the latter, and offers suggestions on how to inspire students. – Linda Caputi

Introduction

Motivating, enlightening, and inspiring students—and creating a passion for learning—are among the most important challenges for teachers. In the arena of adult higher education, much emphasis is placed on creative teaching strategies and the importance of engaging the learner. The use of instructional technology has received growing attention in the classroom, especially in the field of nursing, where it is important for the student to gain knowledge in a variety of complicated subjects. The nursing student must be competent and prepared to pass the NCLEX®. The stakes are high and nursing faculty have a heavy teaching responsibility.

However, good teaching is much more than a one-way pontification of ideas in an area of expertise. There is an important phenomenon that occurs between teacher and student that warrants serious consideration. This phenomenon has to do with inspiration. It is imperative to pass on to nursing students a love for learning, a love that will continue throughout their lifetime, a love of the profession that will enable them to be life-long learners.

Educational Philosophy

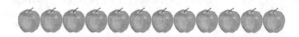

I believe in the importance of being able to motivate, enlighten, and inspire my students, thus creating a passion for learning. It is important to recognize that nursing students are adult, self-directed learners who excel in a nurturing, challenging, and supportive environment. – Jeanette Rossetti

Fostering this love for learning requires a special connection to the student. This chapter focuses on that connection—a connection with students through inspiration.

Inspiration: A Personal Reflection

"It is profoundly important that those who hope to be critical educators remain in touch with their lived worlds, their pre-understandings, their perceptual landscapes" (Greene, 1978, p. 102).

Being inspired by a teacher can have a positive and long-lasting effect on a student. It is important for nursing faculty to reflect on their experience as students and identify the effects of being inspired by their teachers. Personal reflection via autobiographical writing is an outlet for exploring one's connection to inspiration.

The following is the author's own reflection of being inspired, an event that took place some 20 years ago when she was an undergraduate nursing student.

As a junior student in a baccalaureate nursing program in 1983, I found myself questioning the profession for which I was preparing. I had just begun my first nursing clinical in medical-surgical and pediatric nursing, and I found the patient contact unfulfilling. I seemed to handle the tasks well, but I went from patient to patient, providing care without much time to make a connection with any individual person. I found certain nursing faculty stiff, rigid, and uncaring. I remember dreading clinical days and feeling relieved when they were over. I asked myself why I had gone into nursing in the first place! I wanted to connect and build rapport with patients and educate them about health and illness. I did not want to go from task to task, rushing through the day.

One day, after a particularly stressful clinical experience, I just wanted to quit, leave the hospital, and drop out of the nursing program, but as I explained my feelings to my teacher, she encouraged me to "pull it together" and "go back to work." Tears were "not necessary." Thank goodness for a supportive group of peers who encouraged me to continue with the program. I still felt uncertain and depressed. How could I quit now, three years into the program?

I decided to continue with the hope that something would change. I knew I soon would have different clinicals with new teachers and perhaps I would find an area of nursing that I enjoyed. The next semester I was scheduled to take the psychiatric nursing clinical, the clinical everyone feared, the One Flew over the Cuckoo's Nest clinical. I was very nervous and did not know what to expect. My teacher was an expert in her field who truly liked psychiatric nursing and teaching. I recall that all the other students were afraid of the first day of clinical just like I was, but our teacher immediately put us all at ease and acknowledged our feelings. She seemed to know what frightened us and gave us a chance to talk about it. I was very surprised. Always positive, she exuded energy. She had a way of engendering confidence, especially when it came to working with patients we were afraid of initially. Mental illness was new to many of us. The learning environment was challenging and rewarding, and I loved it. I felt alive. This was something I wanted to do. This was a moment of inspiration.

On the hospital units, my instructor was comfortable working with the patients. Watching her inspired me to feel that I could be a psychiatric nurse. She was available to listen and to discuss any thoughts or concerns I had about my experiences. I remember when I picked the patient I would work with one-on-one, an adolescent girl who was dealing with depression. I read as much as I could about her, the illness of depression, and the treatments scheduled. I learned a lot that semester, yet it was frightening to realize I soon would be a nurse, responsible for taking care of patients. My teacher and I had many discussions about patient care, the nursing process, and life in general. She was truly present for me and I felt I had found my place.

This teacher had a considerable effect on me personally and professionally: The effect she had on my self esteem and confidence would be difficult to overstate. I credit her with helping me get my first position in psychiatric nursing. It can be scary in nursing school when you are investing time and money and do not know what type of nursing you want to do, or for that matter, if you want to be a nurse at all. After I worked with this teacher, I knew for the first time what I wanted to be—a psychiatric nurse.

In the 1980s new nurses were told they needed medical-surgical nursing experience before entering the psychiatric nursing field. Psychiatric nursing was closed to new graduates because the managers of psychiatric units wanted to ensure that a new nurse would be competent in medical skills. My instructor gave me suggestions and advice about how to enter the field immediately after graduation. When we were finished talking, I always felt that I could do whatever I wanted, that nothing could stop me. She really helped me feel confident and motivated. She also helped me look **outside the box** to see things a little differently.

I felt good being around her and working and learning in my newly discovered clinical area. I felt motivated and enlightened. I was inspired, energized, and empowered.

She recommended, therefore, that I work very hard in my next critical care clinical. I was determined and earned an A. She told me not to give up, to be persistent. She gave me some concrete advice, including what to expect when I did get an interview. She asked me to let her know how my interviews went, and she told me that any hospital would be lucky to have me. Two semesters later, after many tries, I had a successful interview and got a job. I was one of the first graduates of my class to be hired.

I enjoyed my new position and stayed at the hospital for 12 years in a variety of nursing roles. Because of my teacher, I knew that someday I would want to teach nursing students. I wanted to have the same kind of connection and rapport, be present, and inspire students the way she had inspired me. The inspirational effect of past experiences has been far reaching in my life.

This is the author's story. What is your own personal story of inspiration? Have you had a powerful experience, one that has been long lasting? Is there someone in your history who has inspired you to be a nurse? A teacher? Explore the learning exercises at the end of the chapter to assist you in your personal reflection about inspiration.

Defining Inspiration

"If we can be a spirit-lifting presence among those with whom we work, we have begun to understand inspiration" (DePree, 2003, p. 170).

It is important to have an understanding about the phenomenon of inspiration. The word **inspiration** is used often and in many different arenas. There are inspirational works of music, inspirational quotations, and inspirational books, but what **is** inspiration? More importantly, what does it have to do with teaching and learning? The following definitions and descriptions are gleaned from literature in the areas of education, leadership, and psychology to help us understand what this phenomenon is all about.

The *Oxford English Dictionary* (1989) defines **inspiration** as:

1. The action of blowing on or into. 2. a. The action, or an act, of breathing

in or inhaling; the drawing in of the breath into the lungs in respiration. b. A drawing in of air; the absorption of air in the 'respiration of plants.' 3. The action of inspiring; the fact or condition of being inspired; a breathing or infusion into the mind or soul. a. A special immediate action or influence of the Spirit of God (or of some divinity or supernatural being) upon the human mind or soul; said esp. of that divine influence under which the books of Scripture are held to have been written. b. A breathing in or infusion of some idea, purpose, etc. into the mind; the suggestion, awakening, or creation of some feeling or impulse, esp. of an exalted kind.... 4a. Something inspired or infused into the mind; an inspired utterance or product. b. an inspiring principle. (p. 1036)

Relate the word **inspire** and the act of breathing. In a discussion of breathing techniques, Ornish (1996) illustrates how changes in one's breathing can affect the mind. Ornish demonstrates the power of language and the definition of **inspire**. "To some degree, our language reflects the importance of breathing and its influence on our mind. The term 'inspire' means both to inhale deeply and to become energized, creative, or motivated. 'Expire,' on the other hand, means to die" (p. 157). For the nurse, this connection has fascinating nuances. In client resuscitation procedures the airway receives the highest priority; all attempts are made to first ensure a client's airway and stimulate breathing. In education, is our first priority to ensure inspiration and stimulate energy, creativity, and motivation? This is a question that requires serious contemplation.

The word **inspiration** may mean catalyst, impetus, intuition, revelation, hope, purpose, and discovery. It is often synonymous with **motivation** (Hart, 1993), and is commonly used in artistic or problem-solving creativity. Inspiration is described as what gets one started on a project. Inspiration is related to creativity, which "swells far beyond its formal definition. It is a feeling, often of random occurrence, which produces a purely positive emotion within the inspired" (Council, 1988, p. 123). The moment of inspiration is brief but a truly inspiring event can be remembered long after the moment it occurs. From this brief point of inspiration one grows, builds, and expands. If the experience is used wisely the "inspired can become a more perceptive human" (Council, 1998, p. 123). Outcomes of inspiration are affective in nature and include a sense of joy and arousal. If one wants to preserve the reality of the experience, Council writes, one should communicate the resulting creative ideas. Of course drawing, painting, and poetry are some ways to communicate these ideas. Council powerfully writes,

"… if we as a species do not inspire, it would seem that we are destined to expire" (p. 130).

Inspiration and Leadership

Inspiration is not so much a quality in the leader (the inspirer), as it is a function of the needs of the inspired (Fairholm, 1994, p.161). Goleman, Boyatzis and McKee (2004) state that leaders who inspire offer a sense of common purpose beyond day-to-day tasks and they make work exciting. Leaders who inspire "create resonance and move people with a compelling vision or shared mission. Such leaders embody what they ask of others and are able to articulate a shared mission in a way that inspires others to follow" (p. 255-256).

Leadership literature is replete with examples of the ability of leaders to inspire. According to Fairholm (1994), inspiration means to "enlighten, exalt, and animate another person" (p. 161). Inspiration grows out of the interchange between leaders and followers. This interchange is similar to a relationship that offers new insight, new emotions, and/or new directions. The leader must truly appeal to the followers' emotions. A person is inspired when taken beyond routine ways of thinking and when the leader goes beyond facts by putting into words people's dreams and hopes and giving a sense of purpose and direction (Fairholm, 1991).

Charismatic or inspirational leadership has been identified as central to the transformational process (Bass, 1985). Inspirational leaders build confidence in their followers and use inspiration to increase the optimism and enthusiasm of the followers. The leader's inspirational influence on the followers is emotional and results in motivating followers to perform beyond what is expected of them. An ability to inspire is an essential characteristic of transformational leaders who are charismatic, intellectually stimulating, and individually considerate (Bass, 1998). Transformational leaders motivate others by tactics of influence (Yukl, 1994). These tactics include rational persuasion, inspirational appeals, personal appeals, and the use of symbolic behaviors.

It is essential that leaders motivate their followers and create a vision for them to follow. Giving guidance means little unless the organization's members also are inspired to reach for the new order described in the vision (Judge, 1999). To inspire others requires some knowledge and understanding of matters that are bigger and more lasting than day-to-day concerns.

It is important to note that what inspires some may not inspire others. We expect our leaders to be inspiring, enthusiastic, energetic, and positive about the future (Kouzes & Posner, 1987). "It is essential that leaders inspire our confidence in the validity of the goal" (p. 21). Leaders must have absolute and total personal belief in their dreams and be confident in their ability to make extraordinary things happen (Kouzes & Posner, 1995). Enthusiasm and passion are communicated by vivid language and expressive style: "Through their strong appeal and quiet persuasion, leaders enlist others in the dream. They breathe life into the shared vision and get people to see the exciting future possibilities" (Kouzes, et al., 1995, p. 318). Nursing faculty have the opportunity to inspire confidence in their students and help them meet their goals and dreams of becoming exceptional nurses.

Inspiration and the Teaching-Learning Transaction in Higher Education

"On the inspirational plane, I wanted to rekindle the sense of the importance and purpose of college teaching—the belief that college teachers can and do make a difference to their students and to society outside the classroom" (Brookfield, 1990, p. xiii).

Inspiration must be applied to higher education. It is essential for college and university teachers to reflect upon the purpose of college teaching, for "education at its best seems to both inform and to inspire" (Hart, 1993, p. 166). Education is so much more than just a presentation of facts and figures to be memorized for an examination.

The educational process that occurs between a teacher and student can be viewed as a connection, a synergy, an established rapport, or a transaction by which inspiration can occur. **Can occur** is the key. Inspiration does not occur in every teaching and learning situation. It may not be possible to **will** inspiration into being, but favorable conditions can encourage inspiration (Hart, 1993). An attitude of trust and faith, an ability to listen, and a willingness to allow events to unfold may lead to inspiration. If nurtured, inspiration can be a catalyst for learning. Inspiration will emerge naturally and regularly out of the process of learning (Hart, 1993). Inspiration should be invited into the classroom.

Inspiration is an event of such great pleasure and power as to provide a galvanizing and sought after experience around which to organize learning.

It not only provides new excitement and clarity for engaging in stimulating education but it decreases hopelessness and increases self-esteem at the same time (Hart, 1993, p. 166-167).

Inspirational teachers have a profound and long-lasting impact on their students. Students in educational programs were asked what they considered inspirational about former teachers (Burke & Nierenberg, 1998). Analysis of written narratives of more than 100 pre-service teachers revealed three dominant themes:

- Inspirational teachers were perceived to be caring toward the students.
- Teachers identified as inspirational generally had positive attitudes about life, teaching, and their students.
- These teachers inspired others because of their dedication to their jobs and their students.

Inspired teaching does not come from one particular theory, philosophy, or set of materials, but from teachers who can analyze their situation and create appropriate instruction to meet the needs of students (Duffy, 1992). Inspired teaching "originates in the creativity of teachers" (p. 444). Focusing on reading instruction, Duffy explains how direct instructional methods that are teacher-directed, sequenced, and repetitive, with the use of workbooks and frequent quizzes, can be "uninspiring, boring, dull, and essentially meaningless" (p. 442). Teachers need to be empowered and free to "create inspired instructional encounters" (p. 446) by using a variety of philosophical and theoretical approaches. Duffy describes inspired teaching as "at once conceptually coherent, responsive to students, and reflective of a broad range of professional knowledge" (p. 447).

Though it may be brief, a moment of inspiration can be remembered long afterward. For many, the moments of inspiration have long-lasting effects. "The imprint of good teachers remains long after the facts they gave us have faded" (Palmer, 1998, p. 21). Palmer also writes of the "mutual illumination that often occurs when we are willing to explore our inner dynamics with each other" (p. 23). This imprint and illumination describes the experience of inspiration.

Teaching is a complex and passionate experience comprising many different personal styles and approaches (Brookfield, 1990). Charismatic teachers are dynamic performers who "can hold audiences in the palms of their hands and in whose presence students are enthralled and inspired" (p. 8). However, charismatic teaching is but one of many teaching approaches. Teachers should be cautious about the myth of the perfect teacher (Brookfield, 1990). This point is significant because **inspiration** and **charisma** can be synonymous at times. Clarification is important because charisma is not necessary for inspiration to occur; however, the charismatic teacher is often inspirational.

"One is inspired to persevere by the presence of others" (Hooks, 1994, p. 56). Hooks shares how Paulo Freire inspired her after she witnessed him embody the practice he described in theory. "Freire's presence inspired me… it entered me in a way that writing can never touch one and it gave me courage" (p. 56). Hooks concludes by noting the need for courage as part of the formula:

> Throughout my years as student and professor, I have been most inspired by those teachers who have had the courage to transgress those boundaries that would confine each pupil to a rote, assembly-line approach to learning. Such teachers approach students with the will and desire to respond to our unique beings, even if the situation does not allow the full emergence of a relationship based on mutual recognition. Yet the possibility of such recognition is always present (p. 13).

Summary

This chapter explored the experience of inspiration via literature from the fields of education, leadership, and psychology. These definitions further the understanding of how inspiration is a factor in the educational process. Inspiration —a feeling, a spirit-lifting presence, a breathing in or infusion of some idea, a suggestion, an awakening—is an important factor when the teacher and learner interact. Results of inspiration can be increased clarity, energy, openness, and connection. In fact, inspiration **should** be nurtured and can be a catalyst for learning (Hart, 1993). In addition, the connection—viewed as a synergy and an established rapport between teacher and student—was shown to be an important component of the educational process, allowing for the opportunity for inspiration to occur.

It has been said that we teach who we are. This very well could be true. The experience of inspiration can be an important factor in a teacher's personal educational approach and can be part of the teacher's personality and approach to teaching. There is no doubt that every teacher can remember moments when they were inspired by former teachers and the illuminating effects they had. With inspiration a student can be truly energized by a teacher's presence and be motivated to seek out new knowledge. One has the opportunity to **breathe in** new ideas and feelings such as increased confidence, determination, and self-esteem.

In nursing students' education, faculty have the potential to go beyond imparting mere facts by giving their students the gifts of direction regarding career plans, increased motivation, and a sense of purpose. In the recent movie *Pay It Forward* (Reuther & Leder, 2000) a child's philosophy of life is that the world would be a better place if everyone tried to **pay it forward** by helping a stranger who would, in turn, help another. The results of this child's own generous gesture went far beyond his expectations. Ponder the possibilities if—instead of acts of kindness —the energy of inspiration were ignited in the classroom and passed on to students, then passed on again, and again. The effects of inspiration could become a vibrant and powerful force, reverberating to future nurses, igniting their dreams and energizing their healing touch.

Learning Activities

1. How has inspiration factored into your own transaction of learning? Reflect on

   your own education. Answer the following questions and make a personal connection to inspiration.
   - Think back through your own education. Were any of your teachers inspirational?
   - Can you remember the names of your inspirational teachers?
   - What were the effects of being inspired?
   - Do you feel you are inspirational?
   - If yes, what are the effects of inspiration on others?
   - If no, after reading this chapter, what ideas do you have to create an inspirational environment?
2. How can you apply the above information to your teaching?

References

Bass, B. M. (1985). *Leadership and performance beyond expectations*. New York: Free Press.

Bass, B. M. (1998). *Transformational leadership*. Mahwah, NJ: Lawrence Erlbaum Associates.

Brookfield, S. D. (1990). *The skillfull teacher*. San Francisco: Jossey-Bass.

Burke, R. W., & Nierenberg, I. (1998). In search of the inspirational in teachers and teaching. *Journal for a Just & Caring Education, 4*(3), 336-354.

Council, M. (1988). Creating inspiration. *Journal of Creative Behavior, 22*(2), 123-131.

DePree, M. (2003). *Leading without power: Finding hope in serving community*. San Francisco: Jossey-Bass.

Duffy, G. G. (1992). Let's free teachers to be inspired. *Phi Delta Kappan, 73*(6), 442-447.

Fairholm, G. W. (1991). *Values leadership: Toward a new philosophy of leadership*. Westport, CT: Prager.

Fairholm, G. W. (1994). *Leadership and the culture of trust*. Westport, CT: Prager.

Goleman, D., Boyatzis, R. McKee, A. (2004). Primal leadership. Learning to lead with emotional intelligence. Boston: Harvard Business School Publishing.

Greene, M. (1978). *Landscapes of Learning*. New York: Teachers College Press.

Hart, T. R. (1993). Inspiration: An exploration of the experience and its role in healthy functioning. (Diss, University of Massachusetts, 1993). *Dissertation Abstracts International, 54*(02), 1077.

Hooks, B. (1994). *Teaching to transgress*. New York: Routledge.

Judge, W. Q. (1999). *The leader's shadow: Exploring and developing executive character*. Thousand Oaks, CA: Sage Publications.

Kouzes, J. M., & Posner, B. Z. (1987). *The leadership challenge*. San Francisco: Jossey-Bass.

Kouzes, J. M., & Posner, B. Z. (1995). *The leadership challenge*. San Francisco: Jossey-Bass.

Ornish, D. (1996). *Dr. Dean Ornish's program for reversing heart disease*. New York: Ivy Books.

The Oxford English Dictionary. (2nd ed.). (1989). Oxford: Clarendon Press.

Palmer, P. J. (1998). *The courage to teach*. San Francisco: Jossey-Bass.

Reuther, S. (Producer), & Leder, M. (Director). (2000). *Pay it forward* [Motion Picture]. United States: Warner Brothers.

Yukl, G. A. (1994). *Leadership in organizations*. Englewood Cliffs, NJ: Prentice Hall.

Chapter 7: Planning and Implementing Short-term Travel Courses and Cultural Immersion Experiences

Luanne Wielichowski, MSN, RN, ARNP, BC, FNP,
and Julie L. Millenbruch, MS(N), RN, CRRN

What a challenging experience traveling with students must be! Especially as described in this chapter. Many nurses have known no other environment than a well-supplied medical center in a large city. This chapter reminds us that there is much nurses can do to bring health care to many who have none. And, because so many folks in this country are currently without health insurance, the nurse may not have to venture too far from home. – Linda Caputi

Educational Philosophy

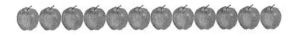

Good teaching is measured in your students' successes. Learning is a journey that I am fortunate to take along with my students. On this journey I support and guide students down the path to their ultimate goals. When teachers provide an environment that encourages engagement and motivation, students' success will follow. – Luanne Wielichowski

My teaching philosophy is centered on the fundamental belief that all individuals can learn if their learning environments are positive, supportive, and creative. I also believe that learning should be fun, and thus I strive to use humor—for example, cartoons—to illustrate core nursing concepts in classroom and clinical settings. – Julie L. Millenbruch

Introduction

The world is a book, and those who do
not travel read only one page.
– St. Augustine

Nursing literature is replete with articles and texts discussing the rationale and often the mandate for schools of nursing to prepare culturally knowledgeable and competent graduates to meet the health challenges of a multiethnic United States population (Leininger, 1994; Messias, 2001; Spector, 2004; Styles, 1993). Various methods have been used to meet this professional mandate. Faculty have analyzed and integrated content about diversity in health and illness throughout the lifespan within existing curricular offerings (Cotroneo, Grunzweig & Hollingsworth, 1986; Lindquist, 1990). They have assigned projects and designed assessments to provide students with an international and cross-cultural nursing focus (Kirkpatrick & Brown, 1999; Scherubel, 2001). Faculties have also offered study abroad programs that place nursing students in cultures different from their own while performing nursing functions (Beeman, 1991; Bond & Jones, 1994; Burnard, 1994; Colling & Wilson, 1998; Cummings, 1998; Frisch, 1990; Grant & McKenna, 2003; Haloburdo & Thompson, 1998; Lachat & Zerbe, 1992; Stevens, 1998; Story, Frederick, Hoornstra, Krob, Mayer, Meyers, & Smola, 1996; Walsh & DeJoseph, 2003).

This chapter describes how faculty can plan and implement a short-term study abroad nursing elective course. Practical suggestions address the process, from inception of the idea to the actual cultural encounter between students and individuals in the host culture. These suggestions are based on tried and true experiences of nursing faculty at a small, private, liberal arts, women's college who have led cultural immersion trips with nursing students to the Navajo Nation, England, Ireland, and Peru since 1998. The authors hope that other faculty can use these suggestions as they plan and embark on these exciting adventures with nursing students.

Plan Early

To ensure a successful student experience it is essential to plan thoroughly. Although planning times will vary depending on the experience, initial steps should begin as far in advance of the actual travel time as possible. This may be as much as two years or as little as six months, depending on the faculty's experience and available institutional and host-country resources. Faculty who teach travel courses commonly enjoy travel in their personal lives. They are often thinking about potential student experiences as they travel and network on their own, looking for future possibilities for students.

Both novice and experienced faculty can participate in a travel course. Novice faculty can bring experience from past cultural immersions, fluency in another language, or a passion for bridging cultures; all are critical attributes for fostering a positive student experience. Nursing faculty who have limited study-abroad travel experience with students will require more time to study the host culture's healthcare beliefs, practices, and lifeways and to initiate and establish international partnerships than faculty with experience in travel courses. Inexperienced faculty may benefit from a visit to the host country before traveling with nursing students. Face-to-face communication with host administrators and on-site assessment of learning opportunities enhances the planning process and provides both the host institution and the sponsoring college with reassurance that student learning and safety needs will be met.

When beginning to plan, consider connections already established between the home institution and the host country. Many colleges and universities have an international or study abroad office that can provide a wealth of knowledge as new programs are developed. Explore possible consortium relationships with other colleges or universities locally or overseas. Also, local church groups planning medical mission trips may be open to partnering with outside groups. Clear advantages to linking with another group are sharing resources, connections, travel planners, and group insurance. For the novice, this makes planning a first trip more manageable.

What, Where, When, Why, and Who

The next phase of the planning process is to consider each of the five Ws as they apply to the study abroad program.

What kind of course will be offered? It is important to link the travel course to the nursing and overall college curriculum. An elective course of one or two credits focusing on the health of the people in the area to be visited is invaluable and guides learning when the students arrive in the host country. This focus directs classroom and on-site activities to yield the biggest impact on individual, family, and community health.

Where will the destination be? Clearly, cultural immersion opportunities occur outside of the United States, but they also exist close to home. Within the United States, the American Indian nations and Mexican-American border communities provide rich cultural learning opportunities. Staying close to home keeps costs down and may allow greater student participation.

The destination's primary language also must be considered. In non–English-speaking communities or countries, bilingual students or interpreters are essential when providing direct client care.

Consider the type of experience the host country can offer. Will it be mostly observational or will students have hands-on experience? Developing countries generally allow more hands-on nursing experiences, especially when the course is connected with a medical mission. During the planning stage it is imperative for faculty to research the documentation of licensure and certification required in the host country to ensure the best experience and to meet the host government's expectations.

When will travel occur? When offering a short-term travel course, the most attractive scheduling is either between semesters or during spring break. This minimizes the disruption to students' schedules. Travel is usually for one to three weeks. If the faculty is on a nine-month contract and travel takes place outside that time, it is critical to have an extension contract in place to cover an accident or illness related to the trip.

Why invest the time and effort of developing and implementing an immersion experience? Because no amount of theory, videos, role playing, or reading about another culture is as rich a learning experience as a cultural immersion. The experiences nursing students have in the host culture last a lifetime and can encourage them to continue developing their skills in providing culturally competent nursing care.

Who should be allowed to participate? Any student with a desire to learn about another culture should participate. Ultimately, the goal should be to provide an opportunity for all students to experience a culture different from their own. Immersion experiences seem to naturally fit in upperclass courses because these students are further along in their nursing courses and therefore more ready for the experience. However, beginning students may have prior travel experience and may be bilingual. These students also can grow professionally and appreciate an immersion experience.

An often forgotten group of potential travel partners is the school's nursing alumni. Former students can offer both maturity and nursing experience. Inviting the alumni keeps them connected to the institution. Other faculty may also be interested in joining the group. Merging a variety of students and faculty also helps encourage mentoring.

When considering who will participate in the travel course, become familiar with the Patriot Act, anti-terrorism legislation enacted by the United States after the attacks of September 11, 2001. Information about the Patriot Act can be found at www.lifeandliberty.gov. This and all websites mentioned in this chapter can be accessed from the CD-ROM accompanying this book. Simply launch your Internet browser, put the CD-ROM in the drive, go to Chapter 7 on the CD, and click on the website address.

It is especially important to be familiar with the Patriot Act if non-American participants are traveling with the course. Non-U.S. citizens who leave the country may risk not being allowed to return. Also, check with your campus study abroad office to determine if there are institutional academic requirements that must be met for students to travel.

Setting Up the Course

Determine if the cultural immersion experience will be a separate course or treated as the culmination of another course. Other important steps when designing the course include:

- Decide which class year in the nursing curriculum the course will be held. If it is a junior-level course, decide whether freshman and sophomore students will be excluded from participating.
- Establish prerequisites for the course.
- Decide how many credits the course will carry. If this is an elective course, limit it to one or two credits, and definitely no more than three; an elective or enrichment course should not carry the same curricular weight as core courses.
- Determine how often the class will meet and for how long.
- Give the course a name, for example, *Cultural Perspectives in Health Care.*
- Determine a theoretical framework that supports the intended outcomes for students' cultural competence. For example, will the course teach and reinforce the concepts discussed in the Campinha-Bacote (1994) *Cultural*

Competence Model of Care? Or, will faculty achieve better student outcomes in developing cultural competence with Purnell's (1998) *Model for Cultural Competence*?

- Keep the course and outcomes broad so faculty can adapt the course to a variety of cultures in the future without having to rewrite it.
- Select readings to supplement course material. Professional journals and the Internet are great resources.
- For travel to non-English speaking countries, an optional language instruction text may be beneficial. For example, when on a medical mission in Peru, a text on Spanish for healthcare professionals may be required.

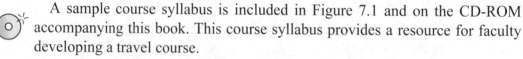

A sample course syllabus is included in Figure 7.1 and on the CD-ROM accompanying this book. This course syllabus provides a resource for faculty developing a travel course.

One of the most difficult tasks for faculty is establishing travel costs. These costs are in addition to course tuition. Inform students what is included and what is not included, eg, meals, lodging, on-site transportation, and entrance fees to attractions. Keep in mind the destination, cost of living, and exchange value of the dollar. Most importantly, estimate high. If the cost per student is set too high, the faculty can refund the students' money after the trip is over. Trying to collect additional money at the conclusion of the course is next to impossible.

Do not collect any money from students! Check the institution's policy regarding the handling of fees. If possible, establish an account through the campus business office for the travel expenses and have students make all payments directly to this account. Maintain accurate records of all money received and expenses paid. Keep all receipts. Set dates that money is due to the business office far in advance of actual travel. For example, if travel is scheduled for June, have all student money submitted by the middle of March. If airline travel is required, do not buy tickets until all money is received or there is at least enough to cover all student and faculty tickets. Air fare typically is not refundable; therefore, if a student decides to cancel, the ticket is the student's responsibility. Clearly communicate cancellation and refund policies and include this information in the orientation. Determine the minimum number of students that must be enrolled for the trip to be offered. Enrollment less than that number would necessitate cancellation of the trip. This information should be established at the onset so all parties are aware of the possibility of cancellation.

Figure 7.1 - Sample Travel Course Syllabus

Week One	Unit 1: Exploring the influence of culture and healthcare practices, shared belief systems and norms of a selected culture: *Cultural awareness*	Welcome and overview of the course.
Week Two	Unit 2: Developing a knowledge base of selected culture in relation to historical, political, social, economical, technological, and geographical factors: *Cultural knowledge*	Read assigned articles. MAP Due of: Campinha-Bacote, J. (1994). *The process of cultural competence in health care: A culturally competent mode of care.* (2nd ed.) Wyoming, Ohio: Transcultural C.A.R.E. Associates.
Week Three	Unit 3: Developing a knowledge base of selected culture in relation to healthcare beliefs, traditional healing methods, shared value systems, and religious practices: *Cultural knowledge*	Read assigned self-selected articles. Complete assigned projects.
Week Four	Unit 4: Comparing healthcare delivery systems of selected culture to local health service systems.	Read assigned self-selected articles. Complete assigned projects.
Week Five	Unit 5: Assessing health promotion programs that target high-risk health behavior within selected cultures: A primary healthcare strategy.	Read assigned self-selected articles. Complete assigned projects.
Week Six	Unit 6: Professional nursing practice within a cultural competence framework: Using cultural assessment tools in the provision of culturally competent nursing care: *Cultural skill*	Read assigned and self-selected articles.
Week Seven	Unit 7: Preparing for the cultural encounter/immersion experience: Language skills and other key activities	Read assigned and self-selected articles. Complete assigned projects.
Week Eight	Unit 8*: Bringing it all together	Final presentation.

*Travel Dates: To Be Announced.

Advertise, advertise, advertise! Create excitement about the course and travel. Hang posters, distribute pamphlets, send letters to alumni, and hold information sessions. Advertising must occur the semester prior to course registration to recruit students for the program.

Know Your Resources

Become best friends with departments on campus that can help plan the travel. Become familiar with the department for international studies and the business office. Talk with other faculty at the institution who have taken students abroad. These faculty can offer suggestions and insight. Investigate how the institution's travel agency can help. Invite guest speakers from the host country or healthcare professionals who have traveled to the country to share their experiences with the students. These discussions are especially important for novice faculty without previous travel experience to the destination. If the destination is a non—English-speaking country and the faculty and students are not bilingual, consider allotting part of the course time to basic language instruction by a qualified teacher. Most importantly, identify any connections in the host country that can facilitate student experiences. For example, it may be helpful to hire a guide who can act as a culture broker for the group throughout the stay.

Passports, Immunizations, and Insurance

The moment students decide to participate, they should apply for a passport, if they do not already have one. The passport application form is available at any U.S. post office or online at www.usps.com/passport. The cost is $85. It takes about three to four weeks to process the application; the application can be expedited for a $60 additional fee. A certified birth certificate, two passport-size pictures, and the fee must accompany the application.

Fortunately, nursing students receive a number of immunizations as a nursing program requirement. In addition to these standard immunizations, students enrolled in a travel course must update their tetanus immunization, complete the Hepatitis B series, and consider receiving Hepatitis A immunization. Two doses of the Hepatitis A vaccine are needed with the first dose given at least three months prior to travel and the second dose six months after the first. It is critical to check the websites of the Centers for Disease Control and Prevention, (www.cdc.gov), and the U.S. State Department Bureau of Consular Affairs, (www.travel.state.gov), for other immunization requirements or recommendations specific to the destination so all participants secure the required documentation.

Students should check with their individual health insurance companies to determine coverage outside of the United States. Some insurance policies do not cover a person traveling abroad. Insurance companies may offer a rider that can be purchased to cover expenses incurred while traveling outside of the United States. Hospitals and healthcare professionals in many countries require cash or credit card payment upfront prior to treatment and will not process insurance claims. In this case individuals with receipts can be reimbursed by their insurance companies upon their return. Insurance companies that require the insured to call within 24 to 48 hours of treatment for reimbursement often have a toll-free number printed on the insurance card; however, these numbers may not be accessible outside of the United States. Students should request a phone number to use abroad. For elderly participants, Medicare generally does cover people traveling abroad. Some institutions include short-term health insurance coverage as part of the overall cost of the trip. One advantage of including health insurance coverage in the course fee is that the faculty knows the extent of the students' coverage. This type of insurance often covers emergency travel home along with return of mortal remains.

Trip cancellation or interruption insurance can be included in the cost of the trip or faculty may allow individuals to decide whether they wish to purchase it. It is important to carefully read what events are reimbursable, as many situations do not qualify. A helpful tool is the website at www.insuremytrip.com, which compares 44 different travel insurance plans from 13 different companies. You can access this website from the CD-ROM accompanying this book. Simply launch your Internet browser, put the CD-ROM in the drive, go to Chapter 7 on the CD, and click on the website address.

Forms

Institutions that have established learning abroad programs most likely have a variety of forms for the student to complete prior to travel. These may include forms related to:

- General health and medical information;
- Permission for emergency medical treatment;
- Emergency contact notification; and
- Release and waiver forms.

Consult the school's attorney for assistance in developing forms if none are currently available.

Satellite Phones and a First Aid Kit

When traveling to remote areas or developing countries, a satellite phone is essential. These phones are big, bulky, heavy, expensive, and only work outdoors, but they are invaluable in emergencies and work in areas like mountains where regular cell phones cannot pick up a signal. Students can share in the responsibility of transporting the phone. A satellite phone can be rented or one can be purchased for approximately $1000. Some colleges are requiring the phones for every travel course. Become familiar with the phone prior to travel and have all important phone numbers and country codes with the phone at all times. The phones are rechargeable and come with a variety of outlet adapters.

A basic first aid kit is another must. It should include disinfectant or an antibacterial agent or ointment, hydrocortisone cream, bandages, gauze with tape, elastic bandage, small scissors (which cannot be packed in carry-on luggage), tweezers, soap, alcohol, and a flashlight. Individuals may want to pack aspirin, acetaminophen, or ibuprofen and vitamins, medications for constipation and diarrhea, antacids, antihistamines, decongestants, and normal saline eye drops.

What If…

Several "What if" situations are recurring themes in travel courses. Some of these situations are listed below. It is best to develop a plan in advance for dealing with each of these situations.

What if a student is late paying the fee? Drop the student from the class. Good intentions and empty promises do not pay the bills. If a student loan is delayed, and this can be confirmed with the financial aid department, an extension may be warranted.

What if a student misses the flight? Because of increased security at airports, passengers must arrive at the airport three hours before an international flight is scheduled to depart. Passengers must adhere to this rule. Once the flight has departed for overseas, it is difficult for faculty to follow up with a student who has missed the flight. Make plans ahead of time to have a contact at the college who can handle this situation locally. This person can locate the missing student and decide whether the student can join the group on a later flight. The student may lose the money invested or incur further costs depending on the action taken. The contact person at the college can speak with the faculty the next day to finalize arrangements.

What if a student becomes homesick? It is not uncommon for students to become homesick. For many students, this may be their first trip abroad or their first time away from family and familiar surroundings. The faculty may find themselves taking on additional roles such as confidant, friend, or parent figure. It is important to validate these students' feelings and either help them work through their feelings or make a decision about the student returning home early. One very homesick student can disrupt the experience for the whole group.

What if illness hits your group? Know where you are going and be familiar with the potential major illnesses there. In a developing country it is not unusual for students to experience several days of constipation followed by traveler's diarrhea. Depending on the severity of symptoms, the diarrhea may lead to dehydration. Treatment with anti-diarrheal agents can prolong the illness. In some countries prescription medications are cheap and easily obtained over the counter. Students traveling to other countries should come prepared with all medications they might have to take. Medical missions not only offer wonderful experiences, but also provide care by team physicians and nurses if students or faculty become ill.

What if you survive a dangerous situation? In the event the group or an individual experiences a dangerous situation it is important to validate the experience. It is natural that the student will want to call home to share the event with family members. Caution the student that full disclosure may be very upsetting to the family and they may request the student return home immediately. If the student is not prepared for immediate departure, it may be best to spare some of the details of the event until the group has returned home and the family can see the student is indeed safe. Of course, if a student has been physically harmed or hurt in any way, the student may require an immediate return home and family members will need to be notified to assist with the arrangements.

What if you experience an increase in terrorism in the country? Stay informed about political events and terrorist activity in the country you are planning to visit for at least six months before traveling by checking the State Department website, www.travel.state.gov. Is there dangerous activity near where you will be? If so, you may want to cancel the trip. If the situation appears stable and you choose to travel, you may need to decide whether to stay or to return home early if the situation changes. The school does not refund the money if travel is interrupted by acts of terrorism or war.

Course and Immersion Activities

Course activities can be divided into those that take place before traveling, while traveling and after traveling. The following section suggests learning activities for each of these timeframes.

Before Traveling

Group Discussions and Sharing

Students take responsibility for learning about a topic related to the country to be visited and share their findings with peers. Topics that focus on the host country's economy, government, geography, religion, history, healthcare system, and health and hygiene concerns help students develop their knowledge of the host culture.

Guest Speakers

Guests from the country to be visited are typically well received by students. Speakers can provide insights not easily found in published material. They can instruct students on monetary systems, commonly eaten foods, and political correctness.

Stages of Culture Shock

No matter how well the students have been prepared for the travel experience, they can never be totally prepared. Prior to travel review the feelings they may experience during the trip and emphasize that each stage is common (Johnson, 2004). Students move through these stages at different rates. Figure 7.2 lists these stages along with characteristics of each stage.

Staying Safe and Making Good Decisions

Take time to have a serious discussion about health and safety information

Figure 7.2 - Stages of Culture Shock

Honeymoon stage: Everything is Beautiful
- Planning to enter the culture
- Simultaneously excited and wary
- Anticipating new experiences
- Sense of excitement, pleasure, and satisfaction—"I'm here!"
- Everything appears wonderful
- Perhaps minor anxiety, sleeplessness
- Enthusiasm and curiosity abound

Crisis stage: Everything is Awful
- The honeymoon is over
- Anxious, restless, impatient
- Language difficulties become burdensome
- What was "charming" now seems "irritating"
- Differences are heightened
- Loneliness, decrease in cultural contacts

Recovery stage: Everything is Better
- Problem-solving skills get better
- A level of predictability helps the student adjust
- Language facility improves
- Anxiety and discomfort levels lessen

Adjustment stage: Everything is OK
- Seeing negatives and positives in a more balanced manner
- Becoming accustomed to differences
- Reaching out more to people from the new culture
- An acceptance of self and others

prior to departure. The following suggestions are from Alverno College (2002):

- To avoid problems going through customs, all prescription and over-the-counter medications should be stored in their original containers and kept in carry-on luggage.
- Establish safety of drinking water in the host country. If the water is not safe, neither is the ice. Use bottled water to brush teeth and avoid fruit and vegetables that cannot be peeled or are not fully cooked.
- In areas with poor sanitation, avoid street vendors, milk and milk products, raw fruit, raw vegetables, lettuce, raw fish, and raw meat. Bring a prescription antibiotic from the quinolone class of drugs (eg, ciprofloxacin) for traveler's diarrhea.
- Avoid beaches, freshwater streams, canals, and lakes because they may be

contaminated with raw sewage that can lead to skin disorders.

- Avoid driving. Motor vehicle accidents are the leading cause of death and disability in both developed and developing countries.
- Never drive under the influence of alcohol or drugs.
- Use a money belt or neck security purse to store ID cards, money, credit cards, and passports.
- Obey host country laws.
- Always make a photocopy of your passport and keep it separate from your passport. This will expedite replacement if the passport is lost or stolen.
- Always travel in groups.
- Keep abreast of the current political situation and any acts of terrorism.
- Leave expensive jewelry at home.
- Do not, under any circumstances, use illicit drugs while abroad. What may be a misdemeanor in the United States could result in two to 10 years in jail or even a death sentence in some countries.
- Drink responsibly. Excessive alcohol consumption may lead to poor decision making and leave you vulnerable to physical or sexual abuse.
- Condoms purchased in developing countries may be porous or susceptible to leakage or breakage. They may not protect against pregnancy or sexually transmitted diseases.

While Traveling

Health Promotion Teaching Project

The health promotion teaching project was developed by the authors to help learners integrate a cultural competence framework into the design of a health promotion program that targets high-risk health behaviors—among individuals, families, or communities—in the host culture. Traditional healthcare practices, shared belief systems, norms, and lifestyles are also integrated throughout the program's design by student nurses. This project should be planned prior to departure and implemented upon arrival in the host community. Directions for a health promotion teaching project and a sample presentation are provided in Appendix 7.1 and on the CD-ROM that accompanies this book.

Immersion Clinical Experiences

Time students spend interacting with individuals, families, the community, or other healthcare members can be invaluable. These sessions can be either observational or participatory in nature. Sites may include, but should not be limited to, hospitals, clinics, homes, day care centers, schools, community centers, churches, or neighborhoods.

Journal Writing

Journaling is a reflective experience that helps the student internalize experiences. The journal is designed to record the students' experiences—observational or interpersonal—while on the field study tour of another culture. Reflection is a critical behavior within the learning process. It not only enables the learner to critically examine events and assess how they relate to key course concepts, but it also engages the student in setting a direction to maximize the field experience during subsequent learning experiences. In essence, this reflective process promotes the self-directed, life-long learning that is necessary for today's professional nurse. Figure 7.3 outlines directions for writing a journal. A sample student journal is included on the CD-ROM that accompanies this book.

Short Group Debriefing Sessions

Take time periodically to check with the students while abroad to discuss their experiences and their interpretation of experiences. If students are participating in a variety of activities simultaneously, this gives them an opportunity to reconnect and learn about each other's experiences.

Take Time for Fun

Be sure to build in fun time. Be a tourist for a while and explore. Go to museums, shop, eat at a nice restaurant, see a performance, visit ruins, and take pictures. This may be the students' only opportunity to be in this country.

Figure 7.3 - Directions for Writing a Journal

Journal Writing Directions

1. Use either a composition book or a 9–by–11 inch notebook. Write your name in the notebook.
2. Date all entries.
3. Within the cultural encounter experience, reflect on all course outcomes. You may comment on two or three course outcomes per day. By the end of the field study experience, all course outcomes will have been reflected upon.
4. Consider the following questions as you comment on each course outcome:
   - What valuable insight did you gain today as a result of your experiences?
   - What helped your learning today?
   - What hindered your learning today?
   - What might you do differently next time as a result of your reflections?
   - Can you suggest strategies to enhance today's learning experience?
   - What professional nursing behavior did you observe that did (or did not) assist the client and family toward positive adaptation?
   - How did the interdisciplinary team function today to promote health and wellness behaviors with individuals and families of groups of the selected culture?
5. Submit your journal to course faculty before beginning the next day's activities. The journal will be returned to you in time for you to begin recording your next reflections.
6. If you have reflections that extend beyond the course outcomes, please share them in the journal. Learning is *not* limited to the course outcomes.

After Traveling

Picture Party

Upon returning home, host a gathering for students, so they can share pictures and swap stories. This is a good time for debriefing and bringing closure to the trip.

Bulletin Board Presentation

Have the students create a display depicting their experiences in a prominent area of the nursing school. This provides an opportunity for students to relive their experiences, bond with peers, and provoke excitement among classmates for possible future travel.

Oral Presentations

Students can compile a PowerPoint slide presentation to share their experiences at a student nurses' meeting or during a class with their peers. A sample of a student presentation is included on the CD-ROM that accompanies this book.

Publications

Students can refer to their journals to write about their experiences for the school paper or a local nursing association. Submissions for publication allow students another opportunity to sharing of their experience.

What Probably Will Happen When
Taking Students on a Short-term Study Abroad Trip

Andrea Johnson is an associate professor of professional communications, specializing in intercultural communication, at Alverno College. She has been coordinating short-term travel courses and traveling with students for many years. Her destinations have included France six times, Jamaica five times, and Costa Rica twice.

Johnson and the authors are developing an interdisciplinary travel course titled *Cultural Perspectives in Health Care and Community Education: Jamaica.* The course is an elective being offered to education, community leadership, global studies, nursing, professional communications, and psychology students.

Johnson writes that nine situations are extremely likely to occur when students are traveling for a study-abroad program.

- No matter how well you have prepared them, students will complain.
- Inevitably, two or three students will drop out. This can—and probably

will—affect the cost of the trip.

- Students who drop out will not want to follow the cancellation refund policy.
- Every time the group goes somewhere—or returns—one or two people will be late or be nowhere to be found.
- Many students will overestimate their ability to communicate in another language, deal with a crisis situation, or detect unsafe people or situations. Usually, all three will occur.
- Someone will not like the food, hotel, their roommate, the town, the television (or lack thereof), the country, the people, or you.
- Someone will need medical assistance—sometimes just a bandage, cough drop, or analgesic.
- Most students will love the experience and learn much more than you had imagined they would.
- At one point, you will probably say to yourself, "This isn't worth it." At another point, you will say, "This was definitely worth it." And you will do it again.

Summary

Professional nurses are expected to provide care that is culturally competent and many nurse leaders believe that competence is best achieved through immersion in another culture. Immersion experiences can be provided both in the home country and abroad. Short-term travel courses fit well for students who have commitments that would preclude them from engaging in a full-semester travel experience. When teaching a travel course, faculty have the opportunity to combine their devotion to teaching with their love for travel. Thorough planning prior to travel will ensure a deep and rewarding learning experience for all participants throughout the immersion experience.

Websites

 The following websites may be helpful for faculty developing a travel course. These and all websites mentioned in this chapter can be accessed from the CD-ROM accompanying this book. Simply launch your Internet browser, put the

CD-ROM in the drive, go to Chapter 7 on the CD, and click on the website address.

Traveler's Health

www.cdc.gov/travel
www.who.int/ith
www.insuremytrip.com

Government and Travel

travel.state.gov
travel.state.gov/travel_warnings.html
www.lifeandliberty.gov
travel.state.gov/student_tips_brochure.html
www.culturegram.com
www.paho.org
www.who.int/en
www.usps.com/passport

Transcultural Nursing

www.tcns.org/6/ubb.x
www.culturediversity.org
www.fons.org/networks/tcnha
www.sunyit.edu/library/html/culturedmed/bib/transcultural

Learning Activities

1. Interview a faculty at a local nursing school who has taught a travel course. Compare and contrast that teacher's experience with what is discussed in this chapter. Share your findings with a colleague.
2. Design a travel course. Identify a host country. What kinds of issues would you need to address for that host country?
3. Visit the office of a healthcare provider who specializes in travel medicine. What kinds of issues are the focus of this provider? What did you learn about safe travel that you had not previously known?

References

Alverno College International and Intercultural Center. (2002). *Travelwise! Health and safety information for study and travel abroad.* Milwaukee: Author.

Beeman, P. (1991). Nursing education, practice, and professional identity: A transcultural course in England. *Journal of Nursing Education, 30*(2), 63-67.

Bond, M. L., & Jones, M. E. (1994). Short-term cultural immersion in Mexico. *Nursing and Health Care, 15*, 249-253.

Burnard, P. (1994). Planning international nursing courses. *Nursing Standard, 8*(16), 24-25.

Campinha-Bacote, J. (1994). *The process of competence in health care: A culturally competent model of care.* Cincinnati: Transcultural C.A.R.E. Associates.

Campinha-Bacote, J. (1999). A model and instrument for addressing cultural competence in health care. *Journal of Nursing Education, 38*(5), 203-207.

Colling, J., & Wilson, T. (1998). Short-term reciprocal international academic exchange program. The United States and United Kingdom. *Journal of Nursing Education,37*(1), 34-36.

Cotroneo, M., Grunzweig, W., & Hollingsworth, A. (1986). All real living is meeting: The task of international education in a nursing curriculum. *Journal of Nursing Education, 25*(9), 384-386.

Cummings, P. H. (1998). Educational innovations. Nursing in Barbados: A fourth-year elective practice experience for nursing students and registered nurses. *Journal of Nursing Education, 37*(1), 42-44.

Frisch, N. (1990). An international nursing student exchange program: An educational experience that enhanced student cognitive development. *Journal of Nursing Education, 29*(1), 10-12.

Grant, E., & McKenna, L. (2003). International clinical placements for undergraduate students. *Journal of Clinical Nursing, 12*(4), 529-535.

Haloburdo, E. P., & Thompson, M. A. (1998). A comparison of international learning experiences for baccalaureate nursing students: Developed and developing countries. *Journal of Nursing Education, 37*(1), 13-21.

Johnson, A. (2004). Personal notes used for PCM 445 intercultural communication course. Milwaukee: Alverno College.

Kirkpatrick, M. K., & Brown, S. (1999). Efficacy of an international exchange via the Internet. *Journal of Nursing Education, 38*(6), 278-281.

Lachat, M. F., & Zerbe, M. B. (1992). Planning a baccalaureate clinical practicum abroad. International Nursing Review, 39*(2),* 53-56.

Leininger, M. (1994). Transcultural nursing education: A worldwide imperative. *Nursing and Health Care, 15*(5), 254-257.

Lindquist, G. J. (1990). Integration of international and transcultural content in nursing curricula: A process for change. *Journal of Professional Nursing, 6*(5), 272-279.

Messias, D. K. (2001). Globalization, nursing, and health for all. *Journal of Nursing Scholarship, 33*(1), 9-11.

Purnell, L. D., and Paulanka, B. J. (1998). *Transcultural health care: A culturally competent approach.* Philadelphia: F.A. Davis.

Scherubel, J. C. (2001). A global health analysis project for baccalaureate nursing students. *Journal of Professional Nursing, 17*(2), 96-100.

Spector, R. E. (2004). *Cultural diversity in health and illness* (6th ed.). Upper Saddle River, NJ: Pearson Prentice Hall.

Stevens, G. L. (1998). Experience the culture. *Journal of Nursing Education, 37*(1), 30-33.

Story, D., Frederick, A., Hoornstra, L., Krob, A., Mayer, H., Meyers, S., et al. (1996). Educational innovations. American nursing students in an English maternity setting. *Journal of Nursing Education, 35*(7), 329-331.

Styles, M. (1993). The world as classroom. *Nursing and Health Care, 14*, 507.

Walsh, L. V., & DeJoseph, J. (2003). "I saw it in a different light": International learning experiences in baccalaureate nursing education. *Journal of Nursing Education, 42*(6), 266-272.

Appendix 7.1
Student Health Promotion Teaching Project

Directions

There are two parts to this project:
1. A written health promotion plan; and
2. A persuasive speech.

Part 1: Written health promotion plan

1. Identify one high-risk health behavior from among the 10 leading causes of death and injury for the selected culture.
2. Consult references (texts or Internet) to determine what is known about the behavior and what type of individual, family, or community health promotion activities have been implemented to attempt modification of the high-risk behavior. Note their success rates, ie, the decline in risk behavior, injury, and/or death.
3. Design a health promotion program that integrates:
   - A historical perspective of previous intervention programs;
   - A cultural competence model for professional nursing practice;
   - Traditional healthcare practices, shared belief systems, norms, and lifeways of the selected culture;
   - Primary health care nursing perspectives; and
   - Communication issues in bi-cultural settings.
4. Assume that a *needs assessment* has been done and that the results of this indicated a need and a desire for your proposed program to target your selected high-risk health behavior. This initial stage in the program planning process is referred to as the *formulation phase*.
5. Use the *Healthy People 2010* objective or other appropriate model pertinent to your target behavior as your major health promotion program outcome.
6. Identify three sub-objectives or outcomes that support the major program outcome. These outcomes statements must be *behavioral, measurable*, and *observable*.
7. Conceptualize your options for solving the high-risk health behavior and consider a minimum of three solutions. Use a decision tree to demonstrate this conceptualization. (See Stanhope & Lancaster, 2000, p. 422.)

8. Detail an estimate of costs, resources, and program activities for each of the three solutions identified in step 7. List the supplies, equipment, facilities, and personnel that are needed to implement each solution.

9. Evaluate each alternative to judge the costs, benefits, and acceptability to the client, community, and provider.

10. Formulate a tentative plan to implement selected option(s).

11. Identify methods to evaluate outcomes and risk factor modification. Note the type of evaluation to be done, tools to be used to measure outcomes, who will conduct the evaluation, and at what time in the program implementation the evaluation will be conducted.

12. Submit to your teacher all steps of this health promotion program planning process in a flow sheet format. (You may want to use a computer program like Inspiration to help you design your flow chart.)

13. Include a typed reference or bibliography page.

References for this assessment include all course texts, articles, readings, and experiences. Two additional resources are suggested for review before the program is designed:

Stanhope, M., and Lancaster, J. (2000). *Community and Public Health Nursing.* (5th ed., pp. 416-437) St. Louis: Mosby.

Public Health Service. (2000, Jan.). *Healthy People 2010 Conference Edition.* Retrieved from U.S. Department of Health and Human Services website: www.health.gov/healthypeople.

Part 2: Persuasive speech

Assume the audience for your speech is composed of interdisciplinary health team members from a community in the selected culture. Like you, they wish to lower high-risk health behaviors within the community and are eagerly awaiting your ideas at this presentation. Be prepared to present this speech during the final assessment class period.

1. Prepare a five-to-seven minute speech (no more!) to persuade members of a selected culture to adopt the health promotion program you have designed for their community. In the speech, be sure to highlight the target risk behavior,

its prevalence in the community, and your rationale for selecting this focus for your health promotion plan.

2. Describe how two or three influences (eg, religious, ecological, cultural, historical, geographic, political, social, economic, or technological) have helped create the high-risk behavior. Be sure to cite the resources you used to describe the selected influences that contributed to the health concern.

3. Persuade your audience that your health plan is effectively designed to target the high-risk behavior and promote wellness for the individual, family, and community. Convince them through the use of creative and unique ideas as well as effective communication strategies that your plan will indeed make a difference.

4. Your presentation must have outcomes, an outline, and a reference page. Additional handouts are optional. All materials should be typed. Using media is a key ingredient of an effective communicator and should not be overlooked. Overheads must be professionally prepared on PowerPoint presentation software or comparable software.

5. Speech outcomes must be accurately formulated so they are behavioral, observable, and measurable. For example:

   At the conclusion of this presentation, the (audience, learner) will be able to (verbalize, demonstrate, utilize):
   - Objective 1 …
   - Objective 2 …
   - Objective 3 …

Chapter 8: Revitalizing for Success with Active Learning Approaches

Kathleen Ohman, MS, EdD, RN, CCRN

Imagine walking into a senior nursing class two weeks before spring break. The students look tired and bored! What do you do? How do you arouse their interest? As teachers, we have all been faced with a similar situation. Dr. Ohman provides answers to these questions. After reading this chapter, you may want to keep it marked for easy reference! – Linda Caputi

Introduction

Nurse educators are faced with many challenges. The nursing discipline requires that students think conceptually, reflect, question, generalize, think beyond the immediate situation, and immerse themselves in abstract and technical language (Daly & Jackson, 1999). Student nurses also must be prepared for the registered nurse role in a variety of settings. They will be expected to be knowledgeable, competent in psychomotor skills, adept at accessing and using information, and capable of clinical reasoning and higher-level thinking (Ironside, 2004; Pullen, Murray & McGee, 2003; Simpson & Courtney, 2002; Smith & Johnson, 2002). To accomplish these expectations in a short amount of time, attention must be paid to how faculty teach and how students learn.

Research suggests that the most successful learning methods are those that promote active learning (Barr & Tagg, 1995; Boggs, 1995-96; Diamond, 1998;

Educational Philosophy

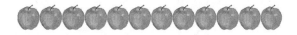

The teacher should be a designer of a supportive, creative, lively, and encouraging learning environment. Students must be encouraged to be active participants in their learning. When students are guided in critical inquiry, then challenged and held accountable for their learning, they can achieve and perform beyond their expectations. Optimism, commitment, and respect are equally important at all levels of the educational process. – Kathleen Ohman

Ironside, 2004; O'Banion, 1997; McCarthy, 1995; McKeachie, 2002; Royce, 2001; Weimer, 2002; Youngblood & Beitz, 2001). Additionally, it is more likely that content will be learned when it is attended to, remembered, and reinforced in a "fun setting" (Herrman, 2002; Karnes, 1999; Vanetzian & Corrigan, 1996). The selection of active, student-centered learning methods, however, should not be haphazard but guided by theories and frameworks of learning (Billings and Halstead, 1998). Not every method is appropriate to each situation. Care must be taken to ensure a fit between a particular active learning approach and:

- A nursing faculty's philosophical beliefs on teaching and learning;
- The evidence base for the approach selected;
- Characteristics of the learners; and
- The outcomes to be achieved during a class period.

Because student learning styles and preferences may differ, each method may have a different effect on learning outcomes for each student.

There are a number of learning theories and frameworks applicable to nursing education that can guide the selection of active learning approaches (Caputi, 2004). These include:

- Cognitive learning theory;
- Humanistic learning theory; and
- Adult learning theory.

The use of critical, feminist, and phenomenological pedagogies also have been reported to be helpful in creating more egalitarian and cooperative learning environments in nursing education (Beck, 1995; Hartrick, 1998; Heinrich, 2001; Ironside, 2003; MacLeod, 1995). The reader is referred to Norton (1998a) and Ironside (2001) for a complete discussion of these theories and pedagogies, including the roles of the faculty and student, advantages and disadvantages, and application.

The purpose of this chapter is to provide ideas to re-energize student-centered teaching to promote student learning. A few active teaching-learning methods for classroom instruction within the theoretical frameworks addressed above will be described and a few examples presented.

Arousal: Creating an Anticipatory Set

An important aspect of engaging learners in the learning process is "arousal" (de Tornyay and Thompson, 1987). Arousal is using positive emotion to capture the learners' attention. Using positive emotions avoids stimulating learners' negative emotions, such as anxiety, anger, or boredom. An arousal activity takes a minimal amount of class time and merely sets the stage for learning. Effective learning, however, extends beyond the role of faculty as entertainer. The effective faculty is a facilitator of student learning (Lowenstein & Bradshaw, 2001) and must move the learners beyond the expectation of being entertained as passive participants in the learning process.

Many examples of stimulating arousal to engage learners are reported in the literature (London, 2004; Deck, 2003; Herrman, 2002; Rowles & Brigham, 1998). Beginning class with a short reading, demonstration, humorous anecdote, or even a physical activity can engage the learners. For example, prior to initiating a discussion about assessment of a client with altered cardiac tissue perfusion, the students can be instructed to jog in place. While students are jogging, ask them to plug their noses. Then, ask them to hold their breath. The teacher should be engaged in this activity along with students to know how long to sustain the jogging. Once students are seated following the activity, discuss symptoms the students experienced after jogging. The discussion can be expanded by asking students what additional symptoms might be noted if they were experiencing altered tissue perfusion as a result of coronary artery disease and unstable angina. Physical activity is highly effective in initiating arousal.

Another example from Vizino (1998) is using an unrelated object, such as an old shoe, to stimulate thought. Participants are asked how the problem under consideration in class is like an old shoe. The author suggests providing the first connection, such as "the problem is like the old shoe because it has a sole." The use of a totally unrelated object can help students make connections between two diverse concepts (Vizino, 1998).

Think Aloud

Think aloud is a methodology in which students verbalize their thinking while they are thinking. This learning strategy encourages students to assimilate old meanings with new meanings and is an example of cognitive learning theory.

This method may be particularly helpful when guiding students in clinical or service learning experiences (Bradshaw, 2001). It can also be used in group learning situations. Think-aloud strategies are strongly supported by the work of Benner, Hooper-Kyriakidis, and Stannard (1999).

Photographs, Pictures, and Video Clips

Photographs and pictures can be used to promote critical thinking and evaluate the depth and breadth of students' knowledge (Dearman, 2003; Ulrich & Glendon, 1999). Computerized images on a variety of topics can be easily found using an Internet search engine such as Google (2004). With proper citation, these images can be printed for use as a hard copy, transparency, or PowerPoint slide. The addition of visual animations and sound, available in computerized presentation packages like PowerPoint, can be helpful in making a point, initiating a discussion, or making comparisons.

Animated computer images and video clips also can be included in presentations to promote class discussion. These enhancements can be procured from a variety of websites with the aid of a search engine. Examples of animations and video clips include those found at HeartPoint Gallery (2004), The Heart: An Online Exploration (1996), and The Noninvasive Cardiac Test Center (2004). The URLs for these websites can be accessed from the CD-ROM accompanying this book. Simply launch your Internet browser, put the CD-ROM in the drive, go to Chapter 8 on the CD, and click on the website address.

One approach to using computerized enhancements is to incorporate a video clip to help students teach and prepare clients for diagnostic tests. A video clip of an echocardiogram and a heart catheterization can be used (Echocardiogram, 2002; The Noninvasive Cardiac Test Center, 2004). After viewing the video, ask two or more students to write on the board how they would explain these tests to clients. Then other students may be asked to identify the commonalities in client preparation and note specific differences. This methodology is useful to actively engage students and promote critical thinking. The aphorism "A picture is worth a thousand words" is very relevant.

Mnemonics

A mnemonic is a visual or verbal device that enhances efficient memorization and easy access to stored memory because of its novelty or familiarity (Beitz, 1997). Though they have been denounced as low-level learning, mnemonics facilitate faster "chunking" of material into memory and create a cognitive pattern for making linkages with higher-level concepts. Nursing students need to know certain facts before they can apply and critically reflect on the information (Ulrich and Glendon, 1999). The ability to quickly retrieve critical information enhances clinical decision making, problem solving, and test taking (Case, 1994).

An example of a mnemonic for learning the names and location of cardiac auscultation points is *Auscultation Points To Monitor*. This phrase combines words with a visual image. The first letter of each word represents the valve areas to auscultate: aortic, pulmonic, tricuspid, and mitral. (A, P, T, and M). (See Figure 8.1.) The visual component is to visualize the number two on the chest starting above the right nipple line (auscultate aortic), move horizontally about 2 inches to a point left of the sternum (auscultate pulmonic), move down the left of the sternum about 4 inches (auscultate tricuspid), and extend horizontally below the left nipple about 2 inches (auscultate mitral). This approximates starting auscultation at the second intercostal space to the right then left of the sternum (aortic and pulmonic), auscultating at the fourth intercostal space to the left of the sternum (tricuspid) and finally auscultating at the left fifth intercostal space at the left midclavicular line (mitral). Anecdotal feedback from students indicates they had a hard time remembering the auscultation points until they learned this mnemonic.

Simulations

Simulations are representations of actual life events. They may be presented through media, computer software (virtual reality, computer-assisted instruction, CD-ROM), role play, case study analysis, or games that actively involve learners in applying the course content (Gaberson & Oermann, 1999; Johnson, Zerwic, & Theis, 1999; Rowles and Brigham, 1998).

Movie segments, commercials, or clips from television shows also can be shown to reinforce concepts (Herrman, 2002). For example, a segment from the television show *ER* can be used to help students learn medical and nursing

Figure 8.1 - Illustration of Mnemonic for Auscultating Heart Sounds

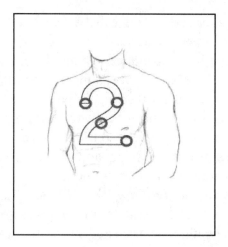

management for complications from pregnancy-induced hypertension. Faculty must obtain copyright permission to use a taped episode of a television show. Develop a handout that addresses scenes from the episode. For each scene include the following elements:

- Information about the client being viewed in the episode;
- Information about some of the actions the students will be observing; and
- Questions that relate to the medical and nursing management.

Before viewing the scenes, have students read through the handout so they are familiar with the questions. After viewing the video, discuss the questions and any additional information not covered in the video.

Interactive multimedia has been used successfully to teach basic nursing skills. A study by Jeffries, Rew, and Cramer (2002) found no significant difference in cognitive gains between one group of students taught basic nursing skills by the traditional lecture and demonstration approach and another taught through interactive CD-ROMs and interactive classroom laboratory stations. Students in the study group worked in pairs to practice the designated skills, discussed focused study questions and research-based material on the selected skill, and practiced at interactive stations facilitated by the teacher. Findings indicated the groups were similar in their ability to demonstrate the basic skills correctly in the learning laboratory. However, student satisfaction was significantly different by group ($P=0.01$), with the interactive, student-centered group more satisfied than the group experiencing the traditional teaching method.

Simulations with standardized patients (SP) also have been reported in the literature (Merrick et al, 2000; Schwind et al, 2001; Tamblyn, 1998; Yoo, 2003). SPs are individuals recruited and trained to perform in a particular client role. Yoo and Yoo (2003) studied the effect of two teaching methods on the clinical competence of nursing students enrolled in a nursing fundamentals course. One method used the traditional teaching approach with lecture and laboratory practice with a mannequin. The other method used live SP models. The study found that students in the SP group had significantly higher scores in clinical judgment, clinical skill performance, and communication than the traditional group. The consistency of findings with other studies suggests the SP methodology is more conducive to internalizing psychomotor skills than the traditional method. The SP method allows students to experience more realistic problem solving.

Concept Mapping, Mind Mapping, and Drawings

Concept mapping (mind mapping) and drawings are other learning methods supported by cognitive learning theory. Mapping is using a graphic or pictorial tool to illustrate key concepts. Such a tool can be used to show relationships between and among topics (Donald, 2002; King & Shell, 2002; Norton, 1998a). Students can use this tool independently, in small-group work, or in large-classroom situations. This methodology is useful in assisting students to think critically about the interrelatedness of new and previously learned information. Concept mapping has been used as an approach to teaching and learning about care planning in healthcare settings (Schuster, 2002). Research indicates that concept mapping improves all levels of student performance in nursing (Irvine, 1995).

Successful use of drawings as a learning method for courses in pathophysiology and healthy aging was reported by Masters and Christensen (2002). Students were asked to complete a series of drawings to depict their own conceptualization of assigned material. Reproducing textbook illustrations was prohibited. For the pathophysiology course, students completed the reading assignment and then depicted through drawings the effects of specified pathophysiology on normal anatomy and physiology. In the healthy aging course, students were required to draw overlays of changes that occur with aging and how these changes relate to pathophysiology. Christensen (2002) reported positive student and faculty responses to the project and noted that the quality of classroom discussion and student retention had improved.

Case-Based Learning

Case-based learning is a student-centered learning method in which students actively solve complex problems that mimic actual clinical practice. Case-based learning enables students to integrate theoretical knowledge and skills of clinical reasoning, critical thinking, problem solving, and interpersonal skills, and apply these to hypothetical or real-case scenarios (Ertmer & Russell, 1995). Case-based learning is supported by principles derived from cognitive theories and the caring framework.

The effectiveness of case-based learning has been studied by DeMarco, Hayward and Lynch (2002). A weekly, one-hour, small-group, case-based learning experience was included in the course "Leading and Managing in Nursing." One case-based scenario presented by the authors was a managerial situation that dealt with interpersonal and/or intraprofessional conflict, delegation decisions in a multiskilled work force, and quality improvement processes in a client situation. To complete the case, students consulted multiple sources including texts, class notes, the Internet, and professionals in the field. Students submitted formal reports describing their findings, recommendations, and rationale, and presented their papers to the group. Research findings suggest that case-based methods stimulate knowledge development from the clinical to the classroom setting and vice versa. Additionally, the study found that working with cases increased students' confidence related to class material and working successfully with others.

Problem-Based Learning

Problem-based learning originated at McMaster University in Canada in the late 1960s for medical education and is now being used in nursing education (Alexander, et al, 2002). Problems reflecting real clinical situations are designed to challenge students to probe deeply and think rigorously to determine possible solutions to the problem. A characteristic of problem-based learning is that the content for solving the problem is not presented to the students but must be identified by the group, researched by individual students, and presented to the group for discussion (Bentley, 2001). Problem-based learning promotes active learning (Alexander, et al, 2002) and may be the primary approach used in a nursing program or may be combined with other learning methods (Cannon & Schell, 2001).

Vanetzian and Corrigan (1996) presented an example of problem-based learning. Students independently completed a case study about caring for a woman with diabetes. Written guidelines were provided to encourage disciplined thinking and clinical reasoning about the facts provided in the case study. Problems and critical thinking questions were posed, which prompted reflective, thoughtful responses. Students arrived for class prepared to discuss the information and questions in the case study. Additional information was provided during class and new questions were posed for a focused discussion. Critical thinking was enhanced when students were actively preparing for the case study and inquiry was supported in the safety of the classroom environment.

Reflection

Reflection is a process of purposeful thinking to develop understanding, insight, clinical judgment, and critical thinking (Gray, 2003). Reflection incorporates principles from adult learning theory, humanism, cognitive-development theory, feminism, and phenomenology. Through focusing on past and current learning experiences, students use reflection to enhance and extend their learning. New ideas and ways of thinking are promoted through an internal dialogue with oneself self (Norton, 1998b). Techniques for reflection need to include thoughtful analysis and evaluation. Suggestions include writing assignments, journals, portfolios, reaction papers, classroom discussions, focus groups, and shared readings. As with any learning method, time for reflection needs to be built into the design of selected assignments.

Scanlan, Care, and Udod (2002) completed a qualitative study to understand more fully the meaning and use of personal reflection in teaching and how reflection contributes to the development of classroom teaching expertise. Findings from this study suggest that faculty experiences are integral to the use of reflection in teaching. Reflection is useful for faculty to make connections between the discussion content and students' experiences. The authors found that role modeling and questioning were common techniques used to help students make connections with the content. However, understanding the influence of context on reflection requires further study.

Narrative Pedagogy

Narrative pedagogy, developed by Diekelmann (2001), is a teaching-learning approach in which faculty and students publicly share and interpret stories of their experiences. Its use requires the teacher to be well-versed in the content area. However, narrative pedagogy decenters the content and encourages teachers and students to think about the meanings of the content being learned and its significance to the students' emerging practice (Ironside, 2004).

Ironside (2003) reported implementing and evaluating the use of narrative pedagogy in a one-credit introductory nursing course offered to students during their first undergraduate semester. On the first day of class students completed the College Classroom Environment Scale (CCES) to rate their anticipated perceptions of the learning environment for the course and for later data comparisons. The course began with students and faculty writing and sharing stories of caring for another person or being cared for by someone else. The process of interpreting stories allowed for exploration of the topic. Various questions were posed by the teacher. Reflection led to further exploration of the topic for the next class meeting.

Following completion of the course, students again completed the CCES to determine if there were significant differences between their perception of the learning environment and the actual experience. Qualitative data also were collected via nonstructured interviews. Students were asked to reflect on the course just completed and to describe a particular event that stood out because it reflected what it meant to be a student in the course. Students were asked to share an example of what worked or did not work in the course. The data were analyzed for themes.

Findings of the study indicated there was no statistically significant difference between the pre- and posttest scores on the CCES for 84 percent of the items. This meant there was no difference between what students anticipated and what they actually experienced. Ten of the 62 items showed a significant change, indicating the students found the learning climate worse than expected.

In some situations, however, mean scores on the semester-end CCES were directly opposite the experiences students reported during the interviews. For example, a highly significant decrease was found on the questionnaire item, "Students in this class have gotten to know each other well." Yet, in interviews, students' comments indicated that they got to know their peers well. The authors concluded that further research is needed to develop evaluation tools that are congruent with the pedagogy being used.

One possible modification to narrative pedagogy for use in an adult nursing course involves asking students to write a story about a specific topic such as head trauma, from their own or an acquaintance's experience. Because students may be reluctant to read their stories, the teacher also writes a story to help students feel comfortable with sharing their accounts. From the stories, the teacher draws themes of signs and symptoms, diagnostic measures, medical and nursing management, and psychosocial responses. The teacher can ask questions such as, "Besides the signs and symptoms you have mentioned, what else might be important to assess?" This question can be modified to address the other themes of a story. Once the discussion is completed, students compose nursing diagnoses and outcomes for their own story and write them on the board. Students then examine the nursing diagnoses to determine if the major diagnoses for a client with head trauma have been addressed. For the next class period, students are assigned to read about a research-based nursing intervention and be prepared to present the intervention to the class.

Experiential Learning

Experiential learning is another effective method to promote learning in nursing students (Glendon & Ulrich, 1997; Stevens, 1998; Tanner, 1999; Welch et al, 2001). In experiential learning, people learn from experience and build upon what they have learned through practice (Jarvis, 1999).

Welch, et al (2001), reported incorporating an experiential learning assignment into an undergraduate nursing course. Students completed a group project that focused on integrating stress theory and research. Research and monograph readings about stress and student stress were assigned and a class seminar on the findings of stress research was presented. Following these activities, individual students interviewed subjects of varying age, gender, and ethnicity. During interviews, the students were to identify stressors, symptoms, coping strategies, emotions, and a subjective sense of wellness or illness. Following the interviews, the students analyzed the data, wrote pertinent nursing diagnoses, identified research-based interventions, and selected applicable community resources.

Once students had completed the assignment, they were assigned to groups of eight or nine to analyze the group data and complete oral and poster presentations. Many students incorporated skits, games, panel discussions, videotapes, and slides into their presentations.

Student and faculty evaluations over four courses indicated this was an exceptional learning experience. Furthermore, the experiential assignment stimulated research among undergraduate nursing students. The authors reported that some nursing students in the sophomore year contacted faculty to inquire about becoming involved in research.

An experiential learning activity found to be highly effective with junior nursing students is a lived experience of an older adult. The activity has generated empathy, compassion, and knowledge about a content area. This assignment combines a writing assignment and an experiential assignment. Students write a paper that includes a client problem, two client populations who might experience this problem, and recommended assistance or adaptations for the problem. Sample problems are altered mobility, impaired communication, or altered sensation. For 24 hours, students experienced what it was like to have this problem. They were required to have the assistance of an unimpaired individual to prevent injury. Students attended classes and activities, for example, with a walker or in a wheelchair, mimicked inability to talk, wore mittens, or had pebbles in their shoes. Upon completion of the activity, students wrote about their experiences and the responses of others. Consistently students wrote about how this experience changed their attitudes toward people with a disability.

Role Play, Discussion, Debate, Use of Questioning, and Use of Materials that Present an Opposing Opinion

Role play, discussion, debate, use of questioning, and use of materials that present an opposing opinion are supported by cognitive-development theories of learning. These learning methods promote faculty-student interactions and student-student interactions where students are exposed to alternative ways of thinking, reasoning, and viewing the world. Both content and teaching-learning experiences are chosen to foster the cognitive development of the student, encouraging and even forcing students to think (Dressel and Marcus, 1998).

Table 8.1 - Explanation of Neuro-deficit Role Play

A Communication Exercise	
Nurse Role	**Client Role**
Scene 1 (five minutes)	**Scene 1 (five minutes)**
You are the nurse assigned to care for a client who has had a stroke. Following the handout provided, complete a health history and assessment of your assigned "client." During data gathering, you need to protect the safety of your client.	You are a client who has experienced a stroke. You have **one** of the following motor deficits of your choosing: arm paralysis, leg paralysis, or other paralysis. Your "nurse" will be completing a health history and assessment. During data gathering, you begin to slip in your chair and lean to one side.
Scene 2 (five minutes)	**Scene 2 (five minutes)**
Your client now has aphasia. Continue with the health assessment on your client. You need to determine the type of aphasia your client is experiencing and develop strategies to communicate so that you can finish your assessment.	The nurse needs to continue with the assessment; however, you have developed aphasia. The first color listed below that corresponds to a color of your clothing is your aphasia type: **black** is expressive aphasia, **blue** is receptive aphasia, and **other** is mixed. You need to roleplay your communication deficit and respond only when appropriate communication strategies are used by the nurse.

A 10- to 15-minute role play can be used to actively involve students in communicating with a simulated client with a deficit. Student pairs are given a piece of paper which describes a role and actions for a role. Students are not permitted to see their partner's paper. The role play is explained in Table 8.1.

Following completion of the exercise, the class should discuss the experience, emphasizing essential data for assessment, interventions to promote safety, and communication methods for the different types of aphasia.

Cooperative Learning Experiences or Collaborative Learning

In cooperative learning experiences or collaborative learning, teams of learners work on assignments and assume responsibility for group learning outcomes (Rowles & Brigham, 1998). This learning method encourages teamwork and reflective learning. Large learning assignments can be accomplished efficiently.

The Internet and group-conferencing software have been successfully used in cooperative learning experiences. Cooperative learning also has been used in nursing laboratory practice activities, such as physical assessment. Not only does cooperative learning promote the cognitive domain of knowledge development and the psychomotor domain of skill development, it promotes affective learning in which students need to demonstrate a willingness to engage in practice with peers.

Research suggests that cooperative approaches result in higher achievement and greater productivity by all students, more positive relationships among students, and greater psychological health (Johnson, Johnson, & Holubec, 1998). However, potential disadvantages of cooperative learning approaches include student resistance to frequent group assignments and unequal student participation.

Think-Pair-Share

Think-pair-share is a cooperative learning strategy that can be used in seminars or presentations. The professor poses a problem or question and students are given 60 seconds of "think time." Students then share their thoughts and responses with a peer. Pairs of students, or a random selection of students, present their responses to the class (Ulrich & Glendon, 1999). This strategy can be used to enhance rapid thinking in situations requiring immediate action.

Jigsaw

Jigsaw is another a cooperative learning strategy in which multiple groupings are used to enhance critical thinking (Ulrich & Glendon, 1999). Charania, Kausar, and Cassum (2001) report using jigsaw with a group of nursing students studying concepts related to fractures:
- Pain;
- Inflammation;
- Immobility; and
- Stress management.

Students are assigned to research one of the four concepts, and then grouped with other students who studied the same concept to discuss their findings and develop expertise in the concept. Next, the groups are rearranged so each new group has an expert on each concept. Each group member discusses and clarifies for the group the information about her or his assigned concept. Each group is asked to formulate a nursing approach to caring for a client with a fracture, integrating all four concepts. Finally, each group makes a brief presentation about their nursing approach.

The students and faculty regarded jigsaw as an enjoyable, stimulating, meaningful, and effective learning method which enhanced critical thinking and meaningfulness of the information. A few students noted insecurity because jigsaw inhibited their note-taking, which raised concerns about preparation for the examination on the topic.

Learning Communities

Learning communities are "a delivery system and a facilitating structure for the practice of collaborative learning" (Smith & MacGregor, 1998, p. 593). One model of a learning community involves linking a course or courses between different disciplines with faculty members co-planning syllabi and sharing responsibility for teaching the course. This model currently is being used between the nursing and nutrition departments for a healthy lifestyles course at the College of Saint Benedict and Saint John's University in Minnesota.

Another model of a learning community links a few class periods between different disciplines. The students are given common assignments and learning activities for a segment of a course. Other models can be more ambitiously configured with clusters of courses developed around broad interdisciplinary themes. Though the structures may vary for collaborative learning, there is a common intention of building both academic and social communities for students (Smith and MacGregor, 1998).

Service Learning

Service learning is supported by most learning theories. It has been incorporated into nursing education though it can present a challenge as most nursing curricula are credit-heavy. Service learning is directed toward a goal of social responsibility and involves work that meets actual community needs, fosters a sense of caring for others, and includes time for reflective thinking. It is different from other types of experiential learning, such as cooperative learning, internships, field practicums, and clinical experiences (Carpenter, 1999).

Examples of service learning presented in the literature include volunteering in an introductory nursing course at the local Boys and Girls Club, participating in the local American Red Cross as an extensive course component in community health, and helping outreach workers distribute HIV prevention information as a limited component in a nursing course (Harrington, 1999). Nursing students at the College of Saint Benedict and Saint John's University enroll in three, one-credit elective courses during the curriculum. One purpose of these courses is service learning. Students have served meals at homeless shelters, conducted food and clothing drives, participated in screenings, and organized community events.

Summary

Faculty face many challenges in adopting teaching-learning methods that energize students and focus on learning. Only a few of the many options available to faculty were presented in this chapter. In an era of increased educational accountability, faculty need to decide which learning methods best facilitate student learning (Boggs, 1999; Ewell, 1997; Skiba, 1997). Before any method is implemented, the learning outcomes to be achieved must be carefully and purposefully considered.

Learning Activities

1. Identify an arousal activity you can use to engage learners in a class on a topic of your choice. Use the activity and discuss with a colleague the students' response to the activity.
2. Teach a class using a PowerPoint presentation with just text and graphics. Ask students to complete an evaluation of your class addressing the teaching method. Then, teach another class with a PowerPoint presentation that uses animation, graphics, and video. Have students evaluate this class using the same criteria on the previous evaluation. Compare and contrast the students' evaluations.

3. Ask students to develop a mnemonic to help them learn a topic of their choice. Ask them to explain their mnemonic and how it helps them recall the information.

References

Alexander, J., McDaniel, G., Baldwin, M., & Money, B. (2002). Promoting, applying, and evaluating problem-based learning in the undergraduate nursing curriculum. *Nursing Education Perspectives, 33*(5), 248-253.

Barr, R., & Tagg, J. (1995). From teaching to learning—a new paradigm for undergraduate education. *Change: The Magazine of Higher Learning, 27*(6), 13-25.

Beck, S. E. (1995). Cooperative learning and feminist pedagogy: A model for classroom instruction in nursing education. *Journal of Nursing Education, 34*, 222-227.

Beitz, J. (1997). Unleashing the power of memory: The mighty mnemonic. *Nurse Educator, 22*(2), 25-29.

Bentley, G. (2001). Problem-based learning. In A. Lowenstein & M. Bradshaw (Eds.), *Fuszard's innovative teaching strategies in nursing* (3rd ed.). Gaithersburg, MD: Aspen Publishers.

Billings, D., & Halstead, J. (Eds.). (1998). *Teaching in nursing: A guide for faculty.* Philadelphia: Saunders.

Benner, P., Hooper-Kyriakidis, P., & Stannard, D. (1999). *Clinical wisdom and interventions in Critical Care: A thinking-in-action-approach.* Philadelphia: Saunders.

Boggs, G. (1995-1996). The learning paradigm. *Community College Journal, 66*(3), 24-27.

Bradshaw, M. (2001). Philosophical approaches to clinical instruction. In A. Lowenstein & M. Bradshaw (Eds.), *Fuszard's innovative teaching strategies in nursing* (3rd ed.). Gaithersburg, MD: Aspen Publishers.

Carpenter, D. (1999). The concept of service-learning. In P. Bailey, D. Carpenter & P. Harrington (Eds.), *Integrating community service into nursing education: A guide to service-learning* (pp. 1-18). New York: Springer.

Caputi, L. (2004). An overview of the educational process. In L. Caputi & L. Engelmann (Eds.), *Teaching nursing: The art and science*, Vol. 1 & 2. Glen Ellyn, IL: College of DuPage Press.

Case, B. (1994). Walking around the elephant: A critical thinking strategy for decision making. *Journal of Continuing Education in Nursing, 25*, 101-109.

Charania, N., Kausar, F., & Cassum, S. (2001). Playing jigsaw: A cooperative learning experience. *Journal of Nursing Education, 40*(9), 420-421.

Cannon, C., & Schell, K. (2001). Problem-based learning: Preparing nurses for practice. In B. Duch, S. Groh & D. Allen (Eds.), *The power of problem-based learning.* Sterling, VA: Stylus Publishing.

Daly, J., & Jackson, D. (1999). On the use of nursing theory in nurse education, nursing practice, and nursing research in Australia. *Nursing Science Quarterly, 12*, 342-345.

Dearman, C. N. (2003). Using clinical scenarios in nursing education. In M. Oermann & K. Heinrich (Eds.), *Annual review of nursing education. Vol. 1* (pp. 341-355). New York: Springer.

Deck, M. (2003). Instant teaching tools. *Journal for Nurses in Staff Development, 19*(2), 106-107.

de Tornyay, R., & Thompson, M. (1987*). Strategies for teaching nursing* (3rd ed.). New York: John Wiley & Sons.

DeMarco, R., Hayward, L., & Lynch, M. (2002). Nursing students' experiences with and strategic approaches to case-based instruction: A replication and comparison study between two disciplines. *Journal of Nursing Education, 41*(4), 165-176.

Diamond, R. (1998). *Designing & assessing courses & curricula: A practical guide.* San Francisco, CA: Jossey-Bass.

Diekelmann, N. (2001). Narrative pedagogy: Heideggerian hermeneutical analyses of lived experiences of students, teachers, and clinicians. *Advances in Nursing Science, 23*, 53-71.

Donald, J. (2002). *Learning to think: Disciplinary perspectives.* San Francisco: Jossey-Bass.

Dressel, P., & Marcus, D. (1998). Teaching styles and effects on learning. In K. Feldman & M. Paulsen (Eds.), *Teaching and learning in the college classroom.* Needham Heights, MA: Simon & Schuster.

Echocardiogram (2002). Retrieved March 1, 2004, from MayoClinic.com Heart Center website: http://www.mayoclinic.com/invoke.cfm?objectid=910C7A2F-EC20-4C27-ADF4CFFE1502B1E4&locID.

Ertmer, P., & Russell, J. (1995, July-Aug.). Using case studies to enhance instructional design education. *Educational Technology,* 23-31.

Ewell, P. (1997, Dec.). Organizing for learning: A new imperative. *American Association of Higher Education Bulletin.*

The Franklin Institute (1996). *The heart: An online exploration.* Retrieved March 1, 2004, from http://www.fi.edu/biosci2/heart.html.

Gaberson, K., & Oermann, M. (1999). *Clinical teaching strategies in nursing.* New York: Springer.

Glendon, K., & Ulrich, D. (1997). Teaching tools. Unfolding cases: An experiential learning model. *Journal of Nursing Education, 22*(4), 15-18.

Google (2004). Retrieved March 1, 2004, from http://www.google.com.

Gray, M. (2003). Beyond content: Generating critical thinking in the classroom. *Nurse Educator, 28*(3), 136-140.

Harrington, P. (1999). Integrating service-learning into the curriculum. In P. Bailey, D. Carpenter & P. Harrington (Eds.), *Integrating community service into nursing education: A guide to service-learning* (pp.19-41). New York: Springer.

Hartrick, G. (1998). A critical pedagogy for family nursing. *Journal of Nursing Education, 37*, 80-84.

HeartCenter Online (2004). *The noninvasive cardiac test center.* Retrieved March 1, 2004, from http://www.heartcenteronline.com/myheartdr/home/splash1.cfm?sp_id=129&T_Id=1132&searchterm.

HeartPoint Gallery (2000). Retrieved March 1, 2004, from HeartPoint website: http://www.heartpoint.com/gallery.html.

Heinrich, K. T. (2001). Doctoral women as passionate scholars: An exploratory inquiry of passionate dissertation scholarship. *Advances in Nursing Science, 23*, 88-103.

Herrman, J. (2002). The 60-second nurse educator: Creative strategies to inspire learning. *Nursing Education Perspectives, 23*(5), 222-227.

Irvine, L. (1995). Can concept mapping be used to promote meaningful learning in nursing education? *Journal of Advanced Nursing, 21*, 1175-1179.

Ironside, P. (2001). Creating a research base for nursing education: An interpretative review of conventional, critical, feminist, postmodern, and phenomenological pedagogies. *Advances in Nursing Science, 23*(3), 72-87.

Ironside, P. (2003). Trying something new: Implementing and evaluating narrative pedagogy using a multimethod approach. *Nursing Education Perspectives, 24*(3), 122-128.

Ironside, P. (2004). "Covering content" and teaching thinking: Deconstructing the additive curriculum. *Journal of Nursing Education, 43*(1), 5-12.

Jarvis, P. (1999). The way forward for practice education. *Nursing Education Today, 19*(4), 269-273.

Jeffries, P., Rew, S., & Cramer, J. (2002). A comparison of student-centered versus traditional methods of teaching basic nursing skills in a learning laboratory. *Nursing Education Perspective, 23*(1), 14-19.

Johnson, D., Johnson, R., & Holubec, E. (1998). *Cooperation in the classroom* (7th ed.). Edina, MN: Interaction Book Co.

Johnson, J., Zerwic, J., & Theis, S. (1999). Clinical simulation laboratory: An adjunct to clinical teaching. *Nurse Educator, 24*(5), 37-41.

Karnes, N. (1999). The learn to earn game: Increasing student participation in postclinical conference through gaming. *Nurse Educator, 24*(6), 5, 18, 27.

King, M., & Shell, R. (2002). Teaching and evaluating critical thinking with concept maps. *Nurse Educator, 27*(5), 214-216.

London, F. (2004). Using humor in the classroom. In L. Caputi & L. Engelmann (Eds.), *Teaching nursing: The art and science* (pp. 84-100). Glen Ellyn, IL: College of DuPage Press.

Lowenstein, A., & Bradshaw, M. (2001). *Fuszard's innovative teaching strategies in nursing* (3rd ed.). Gaithersburg, MD: Aspen Publishers.

MacLeod, M. L. (1995). What does it mean to be well taught? A hermeneutic analysis of the lived experiences of students and teachers in baccalaureate nursing education. *Journal of Nursing Education, 34*, 197-203.

Masters, J. A., & Christensen, M. H. (2002). What is a picture really worth? Old teaching techniques and the "new" nursing student. *Nurse Educator, 27*(1), 41, 46.

McCarthy, G. (1995). Research on teaching methods in nursing. In D.Modly, J. Fitzpatrick, P. Poletti, & R. Zanotti (Eds.), *Advancing nursing education worldwide* (pp. 45-58). New York: Springer.

McKeachie, W. (2002). *Teaching tips: Strategies, research, and theory for college and university teachers* (11th ed.). Boston: Houghton Mifflin.

Merrick, H. W., Nowacek, G., Boyer, J., & Robertson, J. (2000). Comparison of the objective structured clinical examination with the performance of third-year medical students' surgery. *The American Journal of Surgery, 179*, 286-288.

Norton, B. (1998a). From teaching to learning: Theoretical foundations. In D. Billings & J. Halstead (Eds.), *Teaching in nursing: A guide for faculty* (pp. 211-245). Philadelphia:

W. B. Saunders.

Norton, B. (1998b). Selecting learning experiences to achieve curriculum outcomes. In D. Billings, & J. Halstead (Eds.), *Teaching in nursing: A guide for faculty* (pp. 151-169). Philadelphia: W. B. Saunders.

O'Banion, T. (1997). *A learning college for the 21st century.* Phoenix: American Council on Education and The Oryx Press.

O'Connor, A. (2001). *Clinical instruction and evaluation: A teaching resource.* Sudbury, MA: Jones and Bartlett.

Oermann, M., & Gaberson, K. (1998). *Evaluation and testing in nursing education.* New York: Springer.

Pullen, R., Murray, P., & McGee, K. S. (2003). Using care groups to mentor novice nursing students. In M. Oermann & K. Heinrich (Eds.), *Annual review of nursing education. Vol. 1* (pp. 147-161). New York: Springer.

Rowles, C. & Brigham, C. (1998). Strategies to promote critical thinking and active learning. In D. Billings & J. Halstead (Eds.), *Teaching in nursing: A guide for faculty* (pp. 247-274). Philadelphia: W. B. Saunders.

Royce, D. (2001). *Teaching tips for college and university instructors.* Needham Heights, MA: Allyn & Bacon.

Scanlan, J., Care, W., & Udod, S. (2002). Unravelling the unknowns of reflection in classroom teaching. *Journal of Advanced Nursing, 38*(2), 136-143.

Schuster, P. (2002). *Concept mapping: A critical-thinking approach to care planning.* Philadelphia: F. A. Davis.

Schwind, C. J., Boehler, M., Folse, R., Dunnington, G., & Markwell, S. J. (2001). Development of physical examination skills in a third-year surgical clerkship. *The American Journal of Surgery, 181,* 338-340.

Simpson, E. & Courtney, M. (2002). Critical thinking in nursing education: Literature review. *International Journal of Nursing Practice, 8,* 89-98.

Skiba D. (1997). Transforming nursing education to celebrate learning. *Nursing & Health Care Perspectives, 18*(3), 124-9, 148.

Smith, B., & Johnson, Y. (2002). Using structured clinical preparation to stimulate reflection and foster critical thinking. *Journal of Nursing Education, 41*(4), 182-185.

Smith, B., & MacGregor, J. (1998). What is collaborative learning? In K. Feldman & M. Paulsen (Eds.), *Teaching and learning in the college classroom.* Needham Heights, MA: Simon & Schuster.

Stevens, G. (1998). Experience the culture. *Journal of Nursing Education, 37*(1), 30-33.

Tamblyn, R. (1998). Use of standardized patients in the assessment of medical practice. *Canadian Medical Association Journal, 158,* 205-207.

Tanner, C. (1999). Evidence based practice, research and critical thinking. *Journal of Nursing Education, 38*(3), 99.

Ulrich, D., & Glendon, K. (1999). *Interactive group learning: Strategies for nurse educators.* New York: Springer.

Vanetzian, E. & Corrigan, B. (1996). "Prep" for class and class activity: Key to critical thinking. *Nurse Educator, 21*(2):45-48.

Vizino, H., (1998). Old shoe stimulation. In M. Deck (Ed.), *More instant teaching tools for health educators.* St. Louis: Mosby.

Welch, J., Jeffries, P., Lyon, B., Boland, D., & Backer, J. (2001). Experiential learning: Integrating theory and research into practice. *Nurse Educator*, *26*(5), 240-243.

Weimer, M. (2002). *Learner-centered teaching*. San Francisco, CA: Jossey-Bass.

Yoo, M., & Yoo, Y. (2003). The effectiveness of standardized patients as a teaching method for nursing fundamentals. *Journal of Nursing Education, 42*(10), 444-448.

Youngblood, N., & Beitz, J. (2001). Developing critical thinking with active learning strategies. *Nurse Educator, 26*(1), 39-42.

Chapter 9: Online Clinical Discussions: An Opportunity for Reflective Thought

Glennys K. Compton, BSN, MSN, RN, ANP

Much has been written about online discussion groups. They are a very useful tool in contemporary teaching. This chapter addresses online discussions, focusing specifically on how they are used to replace face-to-face clinical postconference discussions. Finally, a means to help students and teacher stay awake and alert during this very important clinical experience! – Linda Caputi

Introduction

Time, space, and an unpredictable environment are consistent problems for most clinical nursing faculty. With research in cognitive learning indicating that college students typically can devote no more than 20 minutes of concentrated attention at a time, the complexity of establishing a classroom timeline is clear. Fatigue after a busy clinical experience most likely shortens this time further.

Nursing education programs have curricula that are well defined in order to meet:

- College and university standards;
- State licensing criteria;
- Accreditation standards, such as those from the National League for Nursing Accrediting Commission and the Commission on Collegiate Nursing Education;

Educational Philosophy

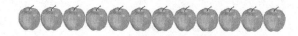

I believe that learning is the result of a successful collaboration between students and their mentor. The process used to learn is as important as the achievement. The experience of learning something new, and the experimentation and reflection on the understanding gained, are important and long lasting for students. My role is to actively modify my teaching practice to meet the needs of learners. I believe that technology-based teaching can reach out to learners' needs. – Glennys K. Compton

- Professional certification guidelines; and
- Compliance with federal regulations.

Outcomes for units and course completion are specifically and carefully designed to be appropriate to the students' progression in the curriculum, but these outcomes must be challenging enough to promote the achievement of higher-level thinking. *Amid this complexity, where does the opportunity for focused student reflection about clinical learning occur?*

The lack of adequate space for meeting in the clinical arena presents another set of issues for educators and clinical administrators. Frequently, clinical sites host numerous schools with clinical groups of various sizes working throughout a facility. Clinical timeframes for groups typically conclude at similar times and end-of-day review and presentations often are scheduled concurrently. Available rooms are at a premium in most hospitals and clinics. *Amid this complexity, where does the opportunity for focused student reflection about clinical learning occur?*

Within a short period of time, it becomes obvious to the experienced clinical teacher that students in each group perform psychomotor skills, solve problems, and employ critical thinking at varied levels. No clinical day is typical. What is carefully planned to be a manageable group of experiences for students frequently can deteriorate into a form of organized chaos. New orders are written that require medications to be researched, discussed in detail, then administered by faculty and student. Treatments appear on client care plans that must be reviewed with the staff. The student must then consult policy manuals and locate needed supplies. Often clients leave the unit for unscheduled diagnostic test procedures that, although they provide students with enriching experiences, were not part of the faculty's planned clinical day. These and a multitude of other developments can result in a clinical teacher or student arriving at a designated postclinical conference late. Additionally, canceling a clinical conference can annoy institutional room schedulers and disrupt planned student reflection experiences. *Amid this complexity, where does the opportunity for focused student reflection about clinical learning occur?*

This chapter attempts to offer a solution to this recurring question through the use of computer technology. A system is offered for postconference discussion that encourages reflective thought through the use of online discussion. This chapter also will:

- Examine the benefits of clinical reflection for nursing students provided by postclinical discussion in a web-enhanced clinical or theory course;

• Discuss the benefits and limitations of synchronous versus asynchronous web-enhanced clinical discussion formats;

• Identify potential roadblocks that may inhibit successful online clinical discussion; and

• Suggest criteria for establishing a clinical discussion in an online setting.

A Technology-Based Learning Environment

Finding the answers to this recurring question—*Amid this complexity, where does the opportunity for focused student reflection about clinical learning occur?*—calls for an approach that incorporates new learning tools, enhanced by technology, for 21st century nursing students who find technological advances stimulating. It is clear that technology will continue to be embedded in the nursing profession and in medicine as a whole.

According to McKeachie (2002), "When instructors ground their choice of technology tools in individual course goals, personal teaching philosophy, and discipline-specific values, technology tools are capable of enhancing teaching and learning" (p. 205). By changing a face-to-face, clinically based discussion into one that is web-enhanced, the clinical discussion forum is afforded the time to become reflective in nature. That is, students have time to think and reflect on the day's happenings. They are not rushed through a conference that must be held at a prescheduled time.

The effects of time constraints, the lack of adequate classroom space, and the unpredictability of opportunity for students' reflection following clinical experiences become less problematic. Additionally, extended web-enhanced discussion allows clinical students to know and appreciate one another as caregivers. By observing how their peers think and by researching answers to posted ideas, students have opportunity to grow in their ability to understand ambiguous problems or ethical issues that develop in the clinical setting or in the greater community and affect nursing. Therefore, a web-based discussion can extend and strengthen the professional interaction and support that occur within a clinical group.

Pedagogically, when the faculty is guiding discussion, students are best-served when the teacher serves as a facilitator, resource provider, or research librarian rather than as an expert dispensing knowledge (Berge, 1997). These roles remain the same for both online and in-class discussion.

Technology-based learning environments can have a positive influence on student motivation. Successfully integrating technology into clinical discussion begins with developing a pedagogical role for that technology. McKeachie (2002) points out that it is not the tool of technology that improves teaching and learning, but how the teacher integrates the tool into the curriculum and the educational setting that makes a difference. When a teacher creates a technology-enriched learning environment that gives learners tools to browse, link, compare and contrast, represent, and summarize information, the learners become engaged in a process of constructing meaning from information and experiences. Close examination of instructional and course goals makes it easier to choose appropriate technology and learning activities to support these goals.

The instructional strategies used to develop the technology-enriched learning environment should emphasize learning as part of an **activity** that is situated in an **authentic environment**. Discussion based on clinical issues is an important part of this strategy. This strategy promotes the creation of learning environments that are "more authentic, situated, interactive, project-oriented, interdisciplinary, learner-centered, and take into account the variety of student learning styles" (Berge, 1997, p. 13). When clinical discussions held in the clinical setting become sporadic and hurried, or fail to occur because of clinical emergencies, online discussions can offer a more reliable and effective mode for student reflection and discussion.

Developing Communication Skills

Developing effective communication skills should be a primary goal for the establishment of an online discussion forum. Communication in an online forum requires skills other than the verbal and listening skills used in face-to-face conference. Reading comprehension and writing skills are important communication tools for online forums, and experience using these skills will be beneficial during the students' professional careers. By combining theory-based classroom discussions in real time and postclinical discussion in virtual time, students can realize the potential of higher levels of communication skill development.

The Power of Reflection

The idea that reflection is of critical value for adult learners is well researched. Schon (1983) found student practitioners moved ahead by taking newly gained knowledge-in-action to the process of applying reflection-in-action. Vella (1994) described practical application of reflection as a process of "doing-reflecting-deciding-changing-new doing" (p.12). To facilitate this process, it is important for the teacher to prepare for discussion. "Most online educators have realized that generating good discussions online takes careful planning and structuring. Breaking large numbers of students into small groups (typically under 10), providing specific tasks (such as researching answers for set questions or finding web resources), and setting timelines for discussion are all elements that are increasingly used and adapted to the online environment to give structure and to help the learner to take an active part" (Mason, 1998). Free-for-all chat-style discussions largely have been abandoned for serious teaching purposes. Ewens (1989) argued that carefully planned discussions "elicit higher levels of reflective thinking and creative problem solving, including synthesis, application, and evaluation" (p. 27).

Information learned through active discussion generally is retained better than material learned through lecture format. Whether instruction takes place in a conventional face-to-face class or in a web-based electronic forum, promotion of a comfortable environment for communication and reflection is essential for encouraging students to speak and share their ideas (Cummings, 1998).

If discussion is so valuable, why isn't it used more in postclinical seminars and in face-to-face classroom formats? There are at least two reasons found in the literature. The first reason is that most college faculty have not learned how to develop effective discussions. The second reason is that discussion is not a time-efficient way to arrive at conclusions. In other words, discussion takes time for thought and reflection before arriving at meaningful closure. When faculty are concerned about having enough time to cover assigned topics, substantial time is not available for in-class discussion forums. Enhancing the course with a course management system (CMS)-based discussion gives students and faculty the gift of time for reflection.

Traditionally, nursing students are provided postclinical conference time to reflect on the clinical day and to promote self assessment of their clinical effectiveness as problem solvers. Some nursing programs use this time for organized learning activities that relate to specific teaching opportunities provided by the professional staff in the clinical setting. Students may or may not write weekly reflections and self assessments in journals or other written assignments. Often, students have minimal input into their clinical evaluations because the teacher first submits an evaluation of their weekly clinical performance. All these are barriers to promoting reflection.

Nonetheless, even if clinical reflection is not a formal assignment, students will reflect both privately and publicly on their experiences. It is often through informal discussion with peers—who may or may not be nursing students—that students review and reflect on their own performance, the skill level of professionals they encounter, and other events of the clinical day. However, as privacy laws are becoming more regulated, students are being told that discussion of clinical events outside of the facility is unacceptable behavior and is, in fact, illegal. Developing consistent, program-wide, supervised reflection opportunities for students is therefore more important than ever before.

As students provide client care, they need to monitor their own adherence to safety and skill standards as well as the effectiveness of their therapeutic communication. "Self monitoring is reflection in the midst of action and enables students to make changes spontaneously as a result of doing the kind of thinking on their feet that includes observing and judging" (Loacker, 2000, p. 6). Cowan (1998) distinguished analytical reflection—"How **should** I do it?"—from evaluative reflection—"How well **can** I do it?" or "Should I do it better?" (p.17). The more self assessment is used, the more it becomes a habit and criteria become internalized. Self monitoring develops as an ongoing process for improving performance. Online discussion can foster reflection, which in turn can lead students to self monitor when they provide nursing care.

Benefits for the Clinical Faculty

Depending on the flow of the clinical day, the absence of a mandatory end-of-clinic conference can be freeing for both students and clinical faculty. For example, if the teacher needs to spend additional time on the unit with a student, students who have completed their care may report off and leave the unit to attend other classes, fulfill personal commitments, or just rest after a hectic day. Meanwhile, the teacher is able to remain with students who are completing their work. When a clinical day has been especially hectic, the teacher can use this time to complete a final review of student-client dyads and to recheck student documentation. Using this postclinical, on-site time to document students' performances for their developmental evaluation also can be a positive consequence of moving clinical conferences online.

Time Commitment

It is important to note that online clinical postconference discussions will require more than the one hour of time that faculty typically spends conducting the traditional postconference. Students should be made aware of the hours and days the faculty will not respond to messages; for example, between 4 PM on Friday and 8 AM on Monday. This type of teaching can become absorbing and time consuming, and nursing faculty need to be cognizant of the time commitment.

Issues to Address When Establishing an Online Clinical Discussion

When deciding to establish online clinical discussion, the complexity may initially seem to be beyond the average teacher's expertise. Participating in a professional organization that includes online discussion or enrolling in an online course that includes discussion format are ways to gain understanding and ideas related to this use of technology. Most colleges and universities provide information technology assistance to faculty or workshops for novice users of CMS. Although online discussion is only one useful aspect of course management software, more features can be incorporated into a course gradually as the teacher's comfort zone grows. For example, announcement boards, syllabi resources, CD-formatted texts, quiz and test centers, email capabilities, and areas to store and post grades are all available with online course management software.

The role of the teacher in online discussion depends on the purpose, audience, and forum. Online discussion as a way to promote reflection and critical thinking in a clinical course uses the model that Salmon (2000) defines as content plus support. Salmon describes a five-step model:

1. Technical issues are addressed and students are welcomed by orientation activities (the access and motivation phase).
2. Online socialization is encouraged.
3. Participants begin to focus on information exchange.

4. Discussion is facilitated to support student knowledge construction.
5. Reflection occurs as participants take on responsibility for the discussion.

A clinical discussion format emphasizes the higher stages of the model, specifically in step 3 through step 5.

The clinical teacher must decide whether to use an asynchronous or synchronous discussion format. In **asynchronous** discussions students respond to messages posted on a bulletin board at a time convenient to them. **Synchronous** discussions are held in real time with all members logged on concurrently. When using this option as a substitute for face-to-face discussions, it is important to notify students in advance that they will be required to be online at specified times. Failure to alert students in advance about the use of synchronous online discussions can cause resentment. Rarely do students appreciate the benefit of weekly online synchronous discussion if they feel it is more desirable to attend in person and have a live discussion.

Synchronous conferences are sometimes stressful for students who feel they lack the keyboarding or grammatical skills needed for the quick turnaround time of live discussion. In the asynchronous format, students who are more reticent have an opportunity to participate in a more relaxed and confident manner. They can take time to check references, ponder their responses, and edit their comments. Students with more dominant verbal abilities may be surprised at the high level of critical thinking their quiet classmates are able to employ in online discussions. Struggling students often gain new understanding from reading the analysis of complex clinical issues posted by students who are more advanced or better critical thinkers. For faculty, using asynchronous online discussion allows them to respond to students more thoughtfully than they may be able to on the fly in class.

Getting Started

The learning curve for students beginning online interaction is not as steep as it was in the past. Most students have had some experience using the web, either in another course or for personal use. Most have shopped or conducted research online. However, hardware and software may still cause concerns.

Hardware and Software Concerns

Basic components of online discussion are content delivery, communication, and evaluation. Content delivery is enhanced or hindered by equipment available to students and by the CMS available to the course designer. Not all technology tools are the same. Not all students have high-speed Internet access, reliable computer equipment, or a good understanding of computer technology. Web-based CMS programs provide tools that allow the teacher to create and manage course websites. Web-based CMS programs include space for a course syllabus, a calendar, course announcements, assignments, online discussions, and group work such as quizzes or tests.

Table 9.1 provides a brief listing of CMS programs. Purchased packages provide support services and do not promote outside advertising. Free packages do not have these advantages. However, free software can be useful if the school has not purchased a CMS program or the teacher prefers the design of one of the free software programs.

Table 9.1 - CMS Programs

Type	Example	Instructional Use
Commercial	Blackboard	Presenting and integrating information
	WebCT	
Online Free Use	TopClass	Interacting and collaborating
	Virtual U	
	Ucompass Educator	
	Web-Course in a Box	
	UM Course Tools	

As consideration is given for adopting technology into clinical course content, students' technology abilities play an important role in decision making. Data from national studies confirm that all Americans are gaining greater access to technology. Internet access is now available in 99 percent of colleges and 95 percent of public high schools. However, Internet usage continues to reflect a digital divide among income, age, and racial groups (McKeachie, 2002, p. 211). Therefore, it is important that faculty avoid making assumptions about students' ability to use the Internet. Conducting a brief, confidential survey at the beginning of the course can help determine if students are familiar with the applications they will be expected to use. During a brief in-class orientation, students should be given a list of resources for technology support.

Using the Software

Both the teacher and the students will require some time to familiarize themselves with the CMS package. Scheduling a group orientation to introduce the online software is important because it prevents the need for numerous individual tutoring sessions. Providing students with printed basic information, such as the course URL, and a comprehensive practical guide decreases the time needed to access the course website and the potential for frustration among students. Holding a session to demonstrate the use of the forum and allow students to gain hands-on experience using their new identification codes and passwords can be a positive way for the group to begin. Asking students to introduce themselves online ensures they establish a connection with the other members of the course. Through the CMS facilitator management options, the teacher can monitor when students are logging into the course site.

Guidelines for Positive Postings

Students should always use online etiquette. McIsaac, Blocher, Mahes, and Vrasidas (1999) recommend that teachers distribute a handout that explains "say-writing and netiquette." For example, words in **ALL CAPS** are equivalent to yelling or scolding. A **:)**, which can be created with a colon and a right parenthesis, connotes a friendly tone.

The handout should provide students with additional tips for posting messages. Ideas include (adapted from Denman, 1999):
- Think of each assignment as a dialogue and not an essay.
- Focus on one single idea and limit your message to one paragraph.
- Think about the assignment before you read other responses or post your message.
- In your response, you can turn your thoughts into a question or play devil's advocate. This is especially helpful if you are the first person to post a response.
- Avoid writing an answer that gives an airtight response and ignores other

possible answers.
- Once you have posted, check to see if anyone responds and continue the dialogue.

Response Time

For faculty and students alike, logging on and responding to comments in a timely manner is important because students tend to expect quick responses to their comments and concerns. Students need to know their site is being monitored and that a question posted to the teacher will receive a response within 24 to 48 hours. Clearly posting teacher availability for virtual office hours on the discussion board is helpful to students. The teacher should be available online for an hour a day, two or three days a week, especially when a class does not meet face-to-face on a weekly basis.

Email, a part of most CMS programs, allows students to send confidential questions or responses directly to their teacher or peers. The teacher can send group emails to all students through the CMS website with one easy click. Faculty should use caution when a message is intended for only one student so it is not inadvertently sent to the entire group.

Grading Student Discussions

While it would be ideal if all students participated merely for the sake of their learning, teachers can ensure student participation by grading online discussions. If discussions are not graded, students will see the sessions as less important and, for a variety of reasons, will choose not to participate (Harasim, Hiltz, Teles & Turoff, 1995). CMS programs make it easy to track student log-in statistics. Creating the expectation of participation is important and the requirements—for example, an acceptable length for discussion responses—must be clearly communicated to students. For example, guidelines might include:
- Entries should contain 500 to 750 words each week;
- Students must enter one or two messages each week; and
- Short, socially oriented messages are valued, but the postconference discussion topic must be addressed in each entry.

Qualitative evaluation of postings is possible but it requires more effort by the teacher. Connections between group members can often develop through socially oriented comments. These help build trust within the group.

What Makes The Discussion Click?

Developing **open-ended** questions for students that provoke thoughtful responses is a key element for creating effective online discussions. Questions serve a variety of purposes. Teachers can design questions to expand on points, check perceptions, obtain information, start conversations, and obtain specific illustrations from outside resources.

Care must be taken to phrase questions so they are not offensive. This can be especially difficult when facial expressions that typically provide feedback to a teacher are unavailable online. It is difficult to predict when a question may trigger deep feelings for a student. Poorly phrased questions may:

- Offend participants who may feel they are being interrogated or treated in a condescending manner;
- Encourage answers that are socially acceptable rather than honest; and
- Decrease critical thinking rather than encourage and promote it.

In most classroom settings, total anonymity is not guaranteed for students. In some online settings, students may use codes and discussion cohorts may never meet face to face. Teachers can identify the student log-ins being used, but may not know who is actually at the keyboard. Unfortunately, cheating occurs online just as it does in the face-to-face setting; it merely takes on a different form.

The benefit of online discussion may not be clear to students who have not had prior experience with the format, and students who have participated may have experienced discussions that did not stimulate critical thinking. Making the online discussion forum mandatory can be an effective way to encourage students to log on and participate. Having students evaluate the effectiveness of the discussion midway through the course can steer participants and the teacher in directions that are more effective or may validate that the group discussion is providing meaningful insight. Discussion does not need to end when the bell rings at the end of class or the clock says that students must leave the clinical site. "A discussion can go on indefinitely, or as long as two individuals are willing to devote the time to a continuing dialogue" (Cummings, 1998).

Making the Most of an Online Discussion Forum

Assessing how discussion is currently used in the face-to-face classroom and clinical arenas is an important step when planning online discussions. Think about the following:

- If face-to-face discussions last less than 10 minutes, what is impeding additional discussion?
- Will moving discussions to an online forum with CMS provide a benefit?
- Can some lecture material be provided online to open classroom time for discussion or group interaction?
- What percentage of students is actively engaging in regular discussion?
- Is participation in class discussion a part of the course grade?
- What is to be achieved by the end of the discussion forum?

Effective discussion of any type requires careful preparation by the teacher. The faculty must understand the purpose of asking the questions. Following are some guidelines:

- Plan discussions so they complement what is happening in the rest of the course and are not perceived as tangential and unimportant.
- Determine how a question under consideration fits within the development or assessment of students' understanding of the topic.
- Plan activities that have specific objectives, can generate students' purposeful responses, and add meaning.
- Focus on points that are considered crucial to clinical understanding in the specialty area and reinforce learning.
- Plan discussions that are based on the literature and assigned reading topics; then move into content students want to explore.
- After a few weeks of the course, ask participants to suggest clinical topics for discussion. This can be stimulating for both students and faculty. Frequently, students are puzzled by discussion topics or have read about medical developments they would like to discuss in more detail. Providing a forum for these questions can be meaningful to students and can take advantage of the benefits of the out-of-the-clinical timeframe format. Not all questions can be discussed in an online forum but immediate discussion is generated as students pose topics. Some of the topics may warrant in-depth exploration in an asynchronous discussion.

The Teacher's Role

Step back and let the students discuss without saying too much. Serve as a facilitator. Create a safe environment that is learning-friendly and promotes improved communication skills. Create an expectation of participation and encourage interaction with other participants. Recognize students' contributions, especially those that demonstrate critical thinking. Provide students with time to think and recognize that their silence may be their thinking time. Do not rush to fill the silence.

Teacher Participation

Minimal teacher input during online discussion allows for more in-depth student involvement. As soon as the teacher comments, students tend to interpret this as authoritative. The discussion can easily develop into a student-to-faculty dialogue instead of a student-to-student dialogue. "A teacher who answers everything will decrease the opportunities for student participation and the discussion will become teacher-centered rather than student-centered" (Harasim, Hiltz, Teles & Turoff, 1995, p. 177). It is important to let participants know the teacher is reading the discussion board regularly and is following the discussion closely. Building on the online discussion forum by referring to specific points, as well as grading or crediting participation, conveys to students that the teacher is committed to the virtual discussion component of the course. Encouraging and recognizing students' participation in a positive way leads to more effective learning.

Examples

So, where do you start with an online clinical discussion? The teacher typically posts a summary of an event that occurred during the clinical day. Students are then invited to discuss that event. Following are examples of situations posted by faculty that have stimulated student discussion.

1. You have just overheard three of your peers in the cafeteria discussing their clinical day. One student is describing her client's unusual situation in detail and the others appear to be enjoying the story of her misadventures with

this client's dressing change. What should you do? On what are you basing your decision?

2. It is important for professional nurses to read and listen to media reports to learn what clients are hearing related to healthcare issues. Nurses have the added responsibility of paying attention to the professional literature to assure nursing practice is current. Two recent examples include studies that prove that nurses and others can spread infection to vulnerable populations through bacteria imbedded in the loose edges of artificial nails and the severe acute respiratory syndrome (SARS) epidemic that has made worldwide news. What is your responsibility when you note a nursing assistant in the nursery wearing artificial nails? Many of those who died in Hong Kong and China were nurses and other healthcare providers. How do you think epidemics like SARS will affect you as a healthcare professional?

3. Both the public and medical professionals are constantly bombarded by the media's coverage of new and exciting, cutting-edge medical discoveries. Occasionally, the fact that their findings are preliminary will be honestly stated by those conducting the study. What have you found lately that you think we should be aware of? Are you skeptical about what you've read or does the research seem to be coming from a reputable source and to be potentially exciting for consumers and/or professionals in medicine and nursing?

4. Life after graduation is on your minds. How will you make good decisions about your career as a nurse regarding salary, benefits, hours, safe learning experiences, and opportunities for promotion? What can you do for yourselves and what do you want to see the college do to help you make good choices?

5. When a client is having problems with relationships or is experiencing a health crisis, it is important for the nurse to assess that client's coping resources. Some clients have broad networks of family or friends that provide encouragement or help. A few will never reach out and admit they are in need. Still others will find their own unique ways to manage interpersonal problems. Pets often provide people with a way to feel less isolated and express relatedness. Expressive media such as art, music, or writings may help a person resolve upsetting experiences. Identify a popular song, work of art, or novel that gave meaning to you when you were coping with a loss or crisis. How did this help you?

6. Ella is an 86-year-old woman who was admitted to the unit with congestive

heart failure (CHF). She is crying when you enter her room and asks you to leave her alone and let her die in peace. You assess that she is oriented X3. From reading her history, you know that she has been admitted six times in the past year for similar CHF episodes. She is listed as a full code. Ella has a court-appointed guardian and lives in a nursing home in a nearby suburb. What do you think you should do to assist her in an ethical way?

7. We've discussed in class how difficult it is to get help for mental illness either as a client or as a family member of someone who is acutely mentally ill. However, when healthcare professionals hear intention of suicide or the implied threat of suicide, healthcare professionals are compelled to provide help often when it isn't wanted by the client. In your opinion, is committing suicide a right that people should have? Is there sometimes a **good** reason for a person to commit such an act?

8. James is a 54-year-old man who has a long history of drug and alcohol abuse. He was admitted to the emergency room and intensive care unit with bleeding esophageal varices. His doctor has just discussed a liver transplant with him and he and his wife are very interested in the idea. You know from reading his history that he was drunk when he was admitted to the emergency room. How will you approach him when he asks you for more information about the proposed transplant? Upon what will you base your understanding, your attitudes, and your communication?

Summary

Clinical instruction in all its aspects is becoming more challenging, due to short hospital stays, complex client conditions, and the nursing shortage. Online clinical discussions provide a venue for reflective thought outside the hectic, hurried clinical environment.

Learning Activities

1. Interview a nursing faculty who conducts online clinical conferences. What does the teacher view as the positive and negative aspects of this format?
2. Think about a typical clinical day with students. What client situations would offer fertile critical thinking discussions? Would these discussions be possible

using an online format?

3. Visit the websites of several vendors listed in Table 9.1. Compare and contrast their CMS programs. Which program would best suit your needs if you were to adopt online clinical discussions? Why?

References

Berge, Z. (1997). Computer conferencing and the online classroom. *International Journal of Educational Telecommunications, 3*(1). 3-21.

Brammer, L., & MacDonald, G. (2003). *The helping relationship: Process and skills.* Boston: Allyn and Bacon.

Chan, A. (1998). *Facilitating reflection and action through research.* Retrieved March 2004 from: http://www.getdiversity.com/articles-publications/facilitating-reflect&action-thru-research.html.

Cowan, J. (1998). *On becoming an innovative university teacher: Reflection in action.* Buckingham, UK: Society for Research into Higher Education and University Press.

Cummings, J. A. (1998). *Promoting student interaction in the virtual college classroom.* Retrieved March 2004 from Indiana Higher Education Telecommunication System website: http://www.ihets.org/progserv/education/distance/faculty_papers/1998/indiana2.html.

Denman, M. (1999). Word & world (handout for students at Stanford University). In Ameritech Faculty Development Technology Program (2000).

Ewens, W. (1989). Teaching using discussion. In R. A. Neff & M. Weimer (Eds.). *Classroom communication: Collected readings for effective discussion and questioning* (pp. 27-30). Madison, WI: Magna Publications.

Harasim, L., Hiltz, S. R., Teles, L., & Turoff, M. (1995). *Learning networks: A field guide to teaching and learning online.* Cambridge, MA: The MIT Press.

Loacker, G. (Ed.). (2000). *Self assessment at Alverno College.* Milwaukee: Alverno College Institute.

Mason, R. (1998, October). Models of online courses. *ALN Magazine, 3*(3). Retrieved March 2004 from: http://www.aln.org/publications/magazine/v2n2/mason.asp.

McKeachie, W. (2002). *McKeachie's teaching tips* (11th ed.). Boston: Houghton Mifflin.

Neff, R. A., & Weimer, M. (1989). *Classroom communication: Collected readings for effective discussion and questioning.* Madison, WI: Magna Publications.

Salmon, G. (2000). *E-moderating: The key to teaching and learning online.* London: Kogan Page.

Schon, D.A. (1983). *The reflective practitioner.* New York: Basic Books.

Vella, J. (1994). *Learning to listen, learning to teach.* San Francisco: Jossey-Bass.

Chapter 10: Reflective Writing: A New Approach in Clinical Assessment

Catherine A. Andrews, MS, PhD, RN

Instructing, assessing, and evaluating students in the clinical experience are, at best, difficult tasks, even for the most experienced faculty. Most teachers would welcome new approaches. This chapter presents a very innovative approach to carrying out these educational functions. Although it may take time to become skillful applying this approach, it is well worth the effort. I, for one, will be using it immediately! – Linda Caputi

Introduction

From the day the clinical faculty walks into a hospital, nursing home, clinic, or community healthcare setting with students, the process of clinical assessment is underway. For teachers, assessing students in the clinical setting is fraught with excitement, trepidation, and tremendous responsibility. However, this aspect of a clinical faculty's role is also tremendously rewarding and satisfying, for it affords the opportunity to witness nursing students' ever-evolving thinking. Clinical faculty are in the pivotal place where concepts heard in classrooms come to life and unfold right before students' eyes. This chapter covers the concept of clinical assessment in a nontraditional yet exciting way.

Educational Philosophy

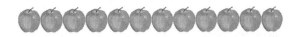

I strive to call students to educational experiences in ways that actively engage them with me as their partner in learning. Together we create a place where we analyze and interpret situations by exploring multiple possibilities. The practice of reflecting centers my teaching, enabling me to presence myself with students by attending to the characteristics that make them unique individuals. By unveiling what experiences mean, we learn together, knowing and connecting with each other in a caring community. – Catherine A. Andrews

The Practice of Assessment

According to Webster's New World Dictionary (1994), the term **assess** has two roots. In the old French, **assesser** means "to impose a tax or set a rate." The Latin root, **assessus**, has a similarly authoritative tone, with its definition "to sit beside, as to assist in the office of judge." Thus, **to assess** means to be with or accompany, and connotes that the outcome of this practice is a decision or judgment with significant implications. When assessing students in clinical courses, the faculty is called to accompany them and to use the information gleaned from being with them as a means for assigning a grade—either pass or fail, or a letter from A to F.

The processes of assessment and evaluation, although difficult to differentiate, do call for different ways of relating with students. In clinical settings, the teacher guides and assists students as they learn the practice of nursing. That is, nursing faculty often provide students with information when they ask questions, offer suggestions on how to approach situations, and so on. Clinical faculty are valuable resources to students. As faculty work with students, they also gather information about the students, determining how they think about situations. Evaluation calls for the faculty to determine if students have achieved predetermined outcomes, which are often stated as course objectives. In the structure of any academic course, there are expectations that a teacher has and goals that must be accomplished to obtain a satisfactory grade. Thus, students are accompanied in ways that enable the teacher to gather information that assists and substantiates the final evaluation. Simply stated, assessment means gathering information and evaluation means judging students.

When accompanying students, the teacher seeks to connect with them in meaningful ways. That is, interactions are purposeful with a focus on learning how to think and act like a nurse. As the teacher and students work together, they create connections that can enhance or impede assessment. It is important that the clinical teacher use a number of activities that foster assessing and connecting with students in a variety of ways. Connections are created in one-on-one conversations, in group discussions, and in written documentation in the form of clinical assignments. Each contact that is made between the teacher and student becomes part of a dialogue that contributes to the dynamic and ongoing assessment process.

The focus of clinical courses is learning in the practice setting; however, the clinical teacher soon learns there are many additional concerns that must be addressed in clinical settings. The milieu of the unit that is created by the specific client care setting—whether it is an acute care or rehabilitation unit—along with policies and procedures, care delivery systems, and norms, dramatically affects the learning environment in a clinical course. Clinical faculty must likewise attend to curricular goals and course objectives applied to this particular setting. The context of the clinical setting, course content, and sequence in the curriculum—at the beginning or end of the student's development—dramatically influence clinical assessment.

How does the teacher with a group of as many as 12 students go about the work of assessment? How can teachers capture each student's thinking and learning as they witness knowledge and skill acquisition? Are there approaches that will assist teachers to keep dialogue flowing, current, and open, leading toward making connections that empower students to learn? And most important, are there meaningful ways for the teacher to accompany **this** particular group of students in **this** setting as their eyes are opened to nursing practice?

Tracking Learning: The What

Underlying each clinical experience is the ultimate goal of learning to think and practice as a nurse. The clinical teacher pays close attention to certain situations, seeking to determine how students are learning the practices of nurses. Likewise, students perform and act in ways that reveal their understanding of nursing, which is often tenuous, incomplete, and changing. It must be remembered that when students and teachers engage in clinical courses together, each person approaches the situation from a unique perspective. Because students progress in their learning, it is important to track their changes.

A variety of tools (Gaberson & Oermann, 1999) have a long tradition in nursing education and are useful ways for faculty to track students' learning in clinical settings. The skill performance checklist can be used to record students' psychomotor skill acquisition. The teacher also can record anecdotal notes that describe the students' behaviors as they participate in care as another way to monitor each student's progress. Written assignments such as nursing care plans, interpersonal process recordings, and teaching plans are additional forms of documentation that have great utility for verifying how students interpret and apply concepts learned in classroom courses. Additionally, clinical logs or journals that encourage students to express their thoughts and feelings as they care for clients provide another useful instrument for assessing students. All of these have merit because they provide valuable information regarding students' understanding of course content—that is, the **what** of students' learning— particularly acquisition of theoretical knowledge and mastery of skills.

Tracking Learning: The How

Mere application of information and accurate performance of psychomotor skills are not sufficient to practice nursing. Critical thinking, or as nurses refer to it, clinical judgment, clinical reasoning, or clinical decision making, must also be developed (Alfaro-LeFevre, 2004; Benner, Tanner & Chesla, 1996) and assessed. This kind of thinking encompasses a broad range of skills that includes, but is not limited to interpretation, analysis, evaluation, inference, explanation, and self-regulation. Therefore, as a clinical teacher, it is equally important to understand not only **what** students are learning, but **how** they are learning the different dimensions of nursing and nursing care, and **how** they are experiencing learning to practice nursing. To do this, it is vital that the clinical teacher have a glimpse of students' thinking as it occurs. By being able to capture thoughts and interpretations as they happen, the teacher is afforded very useful information about not only the content that influences the student's thinking, but also how it is experienced and understood. Additionally, critical thinking skills only can be developed within the context of situations, because the context determines the appropriate actions to take. Thus, unveiling and addressing the context that surrounds situations is important when guiding students in clinical settings.

Narrative Pedagogy: Merging the What and How in Learning

Diekelmann (1991; 1993; 2001; 2004) has studied nursing education for many years. Through her research on the lived experiences of students, teachers, and clinicians, Diekelmann has developed narrative pedagogy, which is an interpretive phenomenological approach to teaching and learning. Narrative pedagogy calls out the interpretive aspect of reflection with others through seeking the meaning of situations. This pedagogy illuminates the common practices that occur in nursing education, rather than emphasizing skill mastery and knowledge acquisition. This is not to say that students do not learn skills or content when enacting narrative pedagogy, because learning skills and acquiring knowledge are common practices of teaching and learning in nursing education. Narrative pedagogy seeks to overcome the individualism, isolation, competition, and teacher-centeredness that prevail in conventional pedagogies such as outcomes- or competency-based education (Andrews et al, 2001). When enacting narrative pedagogy, teachers and students gather together as a community of learners using stories to relate their experiences and discuss and interpret them together. They explore the meanings and significance of the recounted situations, often coming to think in new ways. When using narrative pedagogy, the teacher accompanies students by calling them to examine, explore, and deconstruct clinical experiences to unveil the thinking, meaning, and learning that occurs **during** the clinical situation.

Influenced by Diekelmann, the author has instituted learning activities that are shaped by narrative pedagogy. In the remainder of this chapter, one of these activities is described and examined in detail. Samples of students' and a teacher's written work are provided with an accompanying interpretation that illuminates the utility of this activity. This exercise is extremely engaging, enlightening, and useful, because it affords the clinical teacher a view of each student's thoughts, feelings, and concerns as they emerge. It provides the teacher with insights about the **what**—the content—each student attends to as well as **how** the situation is experienced and interpreted—their thinking. Thus, the teacher is able to assess learning as it occurs within a clinical context while accompanying students in a way that engenders community.

Postclinical Conferencing: The Call to Reflection and Dialogue

Postclinical conferences typically occur at the end of the clinical shift and can serve many functions. They provide a forum for discussing clinical activities that occurred during the shift. Having the teacher and students analyze clinical situations together allows cooperative learning and problem solving to occur. This is often a time when students debrief, expressing their feelings and receiving mutual support from each other (Gaberson & Oermann, 1999; Stokes, 1998). Postclinical conferences encourage open dialogue and give students the freedom to express their feelings. However, if the teacher asks a hard question or corrects a student, the experience can become oppressive and the discussion may become stilted and restrained.

It is common practice to reserve time for these discussions at the end of the clinical shift, no matter where the clinical experience takes place. Both the students and their teacher come to these gatherings with many feelings and somewhat scattered thoughts. Each may be dealing with pressing issues and sorting through questions such as, "Did I forget anything?" and, "Should I have told someone about...?" Or, thoughts may center on feelings, such as, "I'm glad this is over. It didn't go as well as I'd planned," or, "I feel so good because...." On the other hand, students are often weary after experiencing the anxiety and excitement of the clinical day and may feel too tired to think straight. Dealing with these varied mindsets is a challenge because each person's thoughts and feelings easily could become a topic of conversation. However, it is most often the case that students look to the teacher to initiate and facilitate the discussion. This expectation can easily lead to a teacher-centered dialogue because the teacher's leading remarks and the questions that ensue most likely will determine the topics and the flow of the discussion.

One way to ease the transition between being active on the clinical unit and being passive in conference is to start with a period of reflection or active thinking. Beginning a conversation by reflecting together makes the discussion more egalitarian because the teacher no longer determines the focus of the dialogue. Narratives for discussion are generated during the first part of the clinical conference using a list of thought-provoking statements (see Figure 10.1) that can be distributed to students at the beginning of the course or kept by one person in the group. Once everyone has gathered for the postconference, these statements are addressed. Either one person can volunteer to select a phrase for response by each student or each student can choose a phrase and write a response.

Phrases that generate engaged discussions are ones that call forth situations that stand out in the student's memory as meaningful because they evoke wonder, surprise, admiration, dissonance, or discomfort. Responses should be conversational rather than scholarly. Every response and style of writing is accepted. This creates an informal, nonthreatening, warm, and open environment.

For several minutes each individual in the group—including the teacher—reflects on the chosen phrase and then begins writing a response. During this quiet time, the participants engage in reflective thinking. Dewey defines reflective thinking as "turning a subject over in the mind and giving it serious and consecutive consideration" (1933, p. 3). With this approach, one is taken from the present moment and called to relive what has occurred, but from a very different and purposeful perspective. Schon (1983) asserts that to learn from

168

Figure 10.1 - Postconference Phrases

Today I worried about...

Today I felt the happiest when...

My greatest fear today was...

Today the thing I liked the most was...

Today I wondered about...

If I could have changed something today it would be...

Today the thing I saw nurses do that I admired the most was...

Today I felt the saddest when...

On our last day together, the thing I'll remember the most is...

Write two paragraphs about anything you'd like.

experience, professionals need to both reflect in action and reflect on action. Because nurses practice in clinical situations that are often ill-defined and unstructured, reflecting on them provides an excellent avenue to capture the learning that occurs from experiences. By stepping back and thinking about a situation after it occurred, as well as recalling their thinking while they were in the situation, students come to understand how they can learn from experience. Additionally, when students are given the time to reflect, different thinking skills, such as self-awareness, description, critical analysis, synthesis, and evaluation, emerge (Atkins & Murphy, 1996). Further, when students can reflect together, the context that surrounds clinical judgments is illuminated. By interpreting clinical situations aloud, students and teachers engage in community reflexive scholarship (Diekelmann, 2001). They examine the nature of experiences, unveiling the nuances from which the nurses' situational thinking arises (Ironside, 1999).

Following five to 10 minutes of contemplative writing, each member of the clinical group reads his or her written thoughts aloud. Engaging students in this way overcomes isolation and competition because each individual's voice is heard, accepted, and acknowledged. Personal thoughts are described and can be amplified or challenged through the ensuing dialogue. When individuals share their thoughts audibly and publicly, new possibilities for interpretation emerge and new understandings unfold. Commonalities between experiences help students realize they are more alike than they are different, which discourages isolation and individualism. This camaraderie engenders community and enriches subsequent clinical experiences. The assessment process is enhanced as the teacher listens to **what** students are attending to—the content—and **how** they are learning—experiencing and interpreting situations.

Samples of Students' Thoughts

The following are excerpts of stories that were written by junior nursing students during a clinical rotation on a postsurgical unit. The discussion that follows each excerpt offers one way to interpret and use the student's thoughts for assessment and proposes ways to interpret the passage to develop and call out critical thinking.

Jill's Story: Changes in Thinking

On this day, participants responded to the phrase, "Today I wondered about…." Jill wrote:

Today I wondered about how I would relate to my client. Since he has advanced Parkinson's, he has a hard time talking. I was worried about feeding him dinner. I knew that I had to talk to him, so that he didn't feel as awkward. At first it was really weird, but then I realized that maybe he couldn't speak all that well, but maybe his mind was still working. I told him about how nice the weather was and how summer is on its way. Though he didn't respond vocally, he did open his eyes. As the night went on, he became more receptive to me. After we changed his Depends and repositioned him, I sat down and asked him how he was doing and if he was in pain. While I was talking to him, I touched his hand, which was on the side rail. He reached over with his other hand and touched mine. So, in conclusion, I wonder if he is as demented as everyone thinks or if he simply can't speak well.

In this passage, Jill recounts her consternation regarding the challenges she faced when caring for a gentleman who had a speech impairment. She expresses her initial discomfort by saying, "it was really weird" but follows with a description that shows how she came to view the situation from a different perspective. Remembering that the mind is separate from the vocal chords, she notices that even though her client does not speak, he responds and thus communicates to her with his eyes. As the shift progresses, Jill picks up other subtle cues that prompt her to say, "he became more receptive to me." She, likewise, uses nonverbal communication in the form of touch, and notices how he responds to her. Jill concludes her wonderings by revealing a change in her thinking. She overturns her earlier assumptions, coming to wonder if dementia is at the root of her client's speech impairment, as others seemingly led her to believe, or if the Parkinson's alone is keeping him from speaking.

Assessment: Gathering Information

Hearing this poignant narrative, a clinical teacher is immediately apprised of the many dimensions of nursing that Jill is attending to as a beginning nursing student. She reports parts of the dinner conversation, revealing that she socializes with her client as he eats. Jill conveys how she problem solves, because when one avenue of communication is compromised, she chooses another to demonstrate her concern and compassion. Additionally, Jill's account describes the nursing interventions she carried out, specifically feeding, repositioning, and keeping her client dry.

Each of these notations reveals what Jill is doing, but in this account, one also learns how Jill experienced and interpreted the interactions she had with her client. These thoughts are not usually visible to clinical faculty and can only be inferred during the brief interactions when student and teacher are together. This brief excerpt makes visible not only **what** stood out for Jill, but also **how** she comes to new understandings. She moves from feeling "weird" to being "touched," not only in the physical sense, but also in a compassionate way.

In addition to gathering information that helps the teacher assess Jill's progress, a narrative like this may generate a discussion about a variety of topics germane to nursing practice. For example, cognitive information may be discussed by someone asking for more specifics about nonverbal communication, such as,

"How did you know that your client was more receptive to you?" A student could also ask about Parkinson's disease, seeking to learn more about its manifestations. Jill's answer would provide information about the observations she made as she describes the signs and symptoms she noticed. In this case, Jill's wondering led her to also think about the term **demented**. What does this term mean to Jill? Is it the same thing as having a speech impediment? This excerpt might spark a discussion about the similarities and differences of dealing with clients with physical disabilities. For example, someone might offer a comment such as, "Jill's experience reminds me of the time I took care of someone who was visually impaired." Calling out other narratives reveals commonalities between situations often experienced in nursing; links are created between and among students, breaking down barriers while fostering affinity and camaraderie.

In an attempt to unveil **how** students are learning, there are other avenues that could just as easily be explored. Teachers can help students explore and identify self-evident assumptions that often are not recognized when the student is in the moment. Jill starts her narrative by mentioning the phenomenon of relating. Although the topic is addressed in classroom courses, how often do teachers explore with students **how** to relate with clients in clinical situations? Because verbal communication is one way of relating, but not one that Jill can use with her client, she seems stymied and even states, "at first it was really weird." How does Jill get through that? What does it mean for Jill and for her client to not be able to communicate verbally? What does it look like to be receptive? How does it feel? In clinical situations, there is a **context** that surrounds each incident that calls for thinking and acting in different ways. Using narrative pedagogy reveals these nuances, and excerpts like this bring them to life. Jill's comments reveal how she comes to interpret and witness nonverbal communication from a very personal and intimate perspective.

Sean's Story: Expressing Myriad Thoughts

Because each person elects to write about his or her concern as it surfaces, this assignment encourages variety and complete freedom of expression and responses may be very different from each other. Prompted by the same phrase, Sean wrote the following:

Today I wondered about making judgments on advancing my client's diet. I also wondered what surgery did he really have since the Kardex didn't match what the chart said. I also wondered why my client who had laparoscopic surgery would stay here for three days. I wondered what will I write my care plan about!

Rather than centering on one aspect of care, in his concise narrative, Sean describes a variety of issues that are pressing for him. The tone of Sean's narrative suggests that there are several aspects of his clinical shift that are perplexing and somewhat problematic. He is concerned with nutrition, but also with issues of documentation. Each area is a consideration for the nurse and the listener is reminded of the many decisions that face nurses and nursing students, often in a very brief time. Also embedded in Sean's wondering response are the worries and fears that he has about his care plan, an issue that is specific to him in his role as a nursing student.

Assessment: Gathering Information

Although Sean does not describe the specific judgments made regarding advancing a client's diet, his comment alone suggests that he knows there are several factors to consider. Was he wondering about specific signs indicating that he should advance the diet or were his thoughts centered on expressed needs identified by the client and not evidenced in the diet the client was receiving? Noting that the documentation in the chart regarding the client's operative procedure did not match what was found on the Kardex, Sean recognizes the potential for disparity among hospital records. Sean mentions this as a "wondering" point, because it was obviously a cause for concern. What should guide Sean, as the nurse caring for the client: the Kardex or the chart? Sean's statement regarding a three-day postoperative stay following laparoscopic surgery suggests a conflict in what he understands to be normal following this type of surgery. Lastly, in addition to all of the above clinical issues that Sean is dealing with, he has to write a care plan applying what is unfolding in the clinical setting.

Sean's Story: A Call to Explore Together

Sean's thoughts, like Jill's, reveal a variety of talking points for the group to consider. Sean's comments provide additional insights that are very beneficial to the clinical teacher who is formatively assessing Sean's thinking and interpretation of course content. Clinical faculty commonly assess student progress and thinking by the questions students ask and by those that are left unasked. For instance, Sean's wonderings tell the teacher that he understands the general course of a laparoscopic surgical procedure. He also understands that diet post surgery was an important issue to clarify. A student who was less prepared may not have known to question a diet.

Exploration of the factors that nurses entertain when they advance a client's diet is one possible avenue of discussion. Sean's mention of the mismatch in information between the Kardex and the chart could lead to a group discussion of possible reasons for this incongruity, addressing the normal flow of communication and reasons why there may be disruption, and an exploration of legal aspects of documentation. A discussion about laparoscopic surgery would be equally relevant. Although this surgery usually indicates minimal hospitalization, this is not always the case. Given the client's history and current state of health, the group might ponder reasons for the prolonged hospitalization.

Additionally, although clinical faculty are aware that incongruity of information between documents is a fairly common phenomenon, witnessing the discord and consternation that results when this happens to students can be very enlightening. The teacher gains a deep appreciation of how this seemingly incidental disharmony can influence clinical preparation. Sean also voices concern about a course expectation—the care plan. Hearing this, the teacher is made aware of another struggle facing Sean—and perhaps the other students. By voicing his concern aloud, Sean created a forum for all of the students to express their concerns about the assignment. An opportunity is created for the group to think together about Sean's client and the care-planning process. The teacher is given a very specific way to assist students and accompany them through this thinking process.

Additional Examples

Additional examples of students' using reflective writing are contained in Appendix 10.1. These examples use four difference phrases taken from Figure 10.1:

- Today I felt the happiest when…;
- Today, the thing I saw the nurse do and admired the most was…;
- Today I worried about…; and
- If I could have changed something today, it would be….

Several students addressed each of these phrases. Following each student's response, the author analyzes the response, suggesting assessment information in the student's response and possible topics for discussion.

The Teacher's Thoughts

As clinical teachers attend to nursing students in clinical courses, the dilemmas the students face are not often visible. When enacting narrative pedagogy, the teacher completes the assignment with the students. Responding to the same prompt, the teacher wrote:

Today I wondered about the real meaning of the "H" in BPH [benign prostatic hypertrophy]. When I was reading Krista's client's chart with her, I noticed that in one place the term hyperplasia was used and in another place hypertrophy was used. This caused me to wonder what the difference is between these two words. So while all of you were helping your clients with dinner, I looked up both words in the medical dictionary. The term hypertrophy *means an enlargement or overgrowth of the existing cells, while* hyperplasia *means an increase in the volume of a tissue or organ caused by the formation and growth of new normal cells. This caused me to wonder if each condition is treated by having a TURP [trans-urethral resection of the prostate], which I also discovered is true. I love it when I learn something new!*

From a brief encounter with a client's chart, the teacher's curiosity was aroused. Although she unquestionably had translated the term hypertrophy, she noticed that another term could just as easily be substituted for the "H" in BPH. This puzzlement caused her to investigate further, leading to a new discovery and an understanding that broadened her knowledge base.

Giving Messages

Although the teacher's narrative cannot be used to assess students, per se, it does gather students with their teacher in an productive community, because students witness nursing practice through their teacher-as-nurse's eyes. Sharing this incident with students gives several messages. Although some might say this is a triviality, the teacher's wonderings match those of beginning students who often notice details missed by practicing nurses. Not only does the teacher help clarify the difference between two frequently used medical terms that students will encounter during their careers, she also verifies that there is a tremendous amount of information to be learned in health care and one cannot ever   know   it all. The teacher follows through with her inquisitiveness, revealing that one should pursue those inklings when uncertain. By making time to do this, the teacher also elucidates the practice of learning while on the clinical unit, reminding students of resources while pointing out how they should be used. Although students are often told that nursing calls for professionals to be life-long learners, in this short notation, the teacher demonstrates how this concept applies in the practice setting. In this instance, students see the teacher as learner.

Possibilities for Discussion

Like the students' excerpts, a narrative like this can initiate a discussion that might follow several paths. Are there other words that are equally perplexing to group members? Because there are a multitude of abbreviations and medical terms to master in clinical courses, group members may share their experiences when trying to learn new words. What resources do they use? Which ones are most helpful and why? Or, the group may want to explore the signs and symptoms of each condition named. Are they the same or different? How is the TURP performed? How is Krista's client responding post-operatively? Additionally, the group may mention time management as a concern. The teacher made time to look up the word. Given the demands of busy shifts, do nurses routinely do this? This short excerpt can also lead to a discussion about continuing education and its role in nurse's lives.

Summary

Clinical assessment is a dynamic and active process that demands diligent and deliberate attention. Clinical faculty are challenged to connect with students whose approaches to thinking, reasoning, and learning are very diverse. Engaging students in activities that not only reveal their thinking but also simultaneously encourage them to meaningfully express themselves is very desirable. An interpretive phenomenological approach, such as the reflective writing assignment described here, is one way to augment clinical assessment tools that have a long history in clinical education. This narrative approach not only captures students' thinking, but also provides a unique way to further develop the embodied and situational thinking that characterizes nursing practice.

What is most appealing about this approach is the inexhaustible possibilities for discussion it creates. Topics and avenues for exploration are seemingly limitless. Discussions flow from actual situations that are recent and relevant to every group member. Theoretical dimensions of nursing merge with actual client care situations and in dynamic clinical settings. This assignment fits every clinical setting and can be incorporated into any type of nursing program. Exploring situations from multiple perspectives generates new understandings while simultaneously creating new partnerships among students and teachers. Clinical assessment is enriched, becoming a practice that is even more exciting, engaging, and rewarding.

Learning Activities

1. During a postconference session, direct students to address one of the phrases listed in Figure 10.1 and submit their responses to you. Analyze these writings for assessment information in the students' responses and identify possible topics for discussion. Discuss your findings during the next postconference session.
2. Use the following exercise with students. After students have completed the exercise, compare and contrast this approach with other approaches you have used in your class.
    Objective: Attempt to bridge nursing practice with theoretical frameworks (in this case, organizational models).
    Instructions to students
    -   As you reflect on the ideas proposed in the assigned readings, recall an experience in which organization played a part in patient care.
    -   Select a model you think was being used.
    -   What are the benefits of this approach?
    -   What are the drawbacks?
3. Use the following exercise with students. After students have completed the exercise, compare and contrast this approach with other approaches you have

used in your class.

Objective: Foster application of material and promote critical thinking, using this exercise that calls for analysis (in this case, of communication).

Instructions to students

Before we begin our discussion, take a few minutes to think about a time that stands out for you when communication broke down. This can be a time related to a nursing class, a clinical situation, or your personal life. When you've completed your description, analyze it with respect to the ideas forwarded in your text by asking:

- What went wrong?
- Which factors affected communication to create the problem?
- Which technique could have helped the situation?

4. Use the following exercise with students. After students have completed the exercise, compare and contrast this approach with other approaches you have used in your class.

Objective: This assignment can be used in a trends and issues or leadership course with undergraduate nursing students.

Instructions to students

As you read the textbook chapters for today's assignment, write your comments on the following:

- What are some of the major factors that currently influence healthcare delivery in the United States?
- How have changes in the healthcare delivery system impacted nursing? (Include both positive and negative outcomes.)
- Is the ability to receive health care an individual's **right** (ie, should it be available to everyone) or is it a **privilege** (ie, should it be only for those who can afford it)?
- As a soon-to-be graduate nurse, why are these two topics important to you?

References

Alfaro-LeFevre, R. (2004). *Critical thinking and clinical judgment: A practical approach* (3rd edition). St. Louis: Saunders

Andrews, C. A., Ironside, P. M., Nosek, C., Sims, S. L., Swenson, M. M., Yeomans, C., et al. (2001). Enacting narrative pedagogy: The lived experiences of students and teachers *Nursing and Health Care Perspectives, 22,* 252-259.

Atkins, S. & Murphy, K. (1996). Reflection: A review of the literature. *Journal of Advanced Nursing,18,* 1188-1192.

Benner, P., Tanner, C., & Chesla, C. (1996). *Expertise in nursing practice: Caring, clinical judgment and ethics.* New York: Springer Publishing.

Dewey, J. (1933). *How we think: A restatement of the relation of reflective thinking to the educative process.* Boston: Heath.

Diekelmann, N. L. (1991). The emancipatory power of the narrative. *Curriculum revolution: Community building and activism.* New York: The National League for Nursing Press, 41-62.

Diekelmann, N. L. (1993). Behavioral pedagogy: A Heideggerian hermeneutical analysis of the lived experiences of students and teachers in baccalaureate nursing education. *Journal of Nursing Education, 32,* 245-250.

Diekelmann, N. L. (2001). Narrative pedagogy: Heideggerian hermeneutical analyses of the lived experiences of students, teachers and clinicians. *Advances in Nursing Science, 23*(3), 53-71.

Diekelmann, N. L., & Diekelmann, J. (in press). *Schooling learning teaching: Toward a narrative pedagogy.* Madison, WI: University of Wisconsin Press.

Gaberson, K., & Oermann, M. (1999). *Clinical teaching strategies in nursing.* New York: Springer Publishing.

Ironside, P. (1999) Thinking in nursing education: A student's experience learning to think. *Nursing and Health Care Perspectives, 20,* 238-242.

Schon, D. (1983). *The reflective practitioner: How professionals think in action.* New York: Basic Books.

Stokes, L. (1998). Teaching in the clinical setting. In D. M. Billings & J. A. Halstead (Eds.), *Teaching in nursing* (pp. 281-297). Philadelphia: Saunders.

Webster's New World Dictionary. (1994). New York: Prentice Hall.

Appendix 10.1 -
Guidelines for Using Reflective Writing for Assessment and Dialogue

Once each student has written a response to one of the phrases used to stimulate postconference discussion (see Figure 10.1), the teacher can use the narratives to assess students' learning and facilitate a conversation that can flow in a variety of directions. The students' narratives alert the teacher to what captures their attention and what is meaningful to them. Topics of interest arise in ways that are timely and relevant to a particular group of students.

Clinical courses typically are coupled with theory courses that address client conditions, diagnostic tests, nursing assessments, and interventions. By discussing specific topics as they are witnessed and described in narratives, the teacher can reinforce and enhance classroom content to foster meaningful learning.

In the clinical setting, faculty also guide students to perform in ways that foster sound **nursing practices**. Mindful of these, the clinical faculty can pick up cues from the students' descriptions of how they perform these practices by listening to the behaviors they mention in their narratives.

Communication is another dimension of nursing that develops in the clinical setting. Students learn how to converse in different ways with a variety of individuals, including clients, nurses, and other healthcare professionals. Each type of communication calls for particular responses and as students describe specific incidents, the teacher is afforded opportunities to explore further.

Furthermore, as students progress in clinical courses, they find themselves in emotional situations. These experiences call for processing and interpretation because of the great impact they have on **personal development**. By attending to this aspect of clinical learning, the teacher advances the growth of professional norms and values.

Application of course content, nursing practices, communication, and personal development are just a few examples of themes that can be explored in depth using a short narrative. This information is useful both for assessing students' understanding and as a springboard to further dialogue.

The following passages are excerpts of undergraduate students' responses to four of the phrases from Figure 10.1. Brief analyses of assessment information and suggestions for promoting discussion are proposed. Each of the following narratives could be explicated in different ways, depending on the setting and the student's place in the nursing program. The interpretations that follow are framed in the context of interacting with undergraduate students in a medical-surgical clinical nursing course.

Topic 1: Today I felt the happiest when...

Student 1

Today, I felt the happiest when I caught an error in the IV flow rate. The flow rate was set at 50 cc/hr on 0.45% NS along with 50 cc/hr of TPN. I remembered when I did my research that the total IV flow rate was supposed to be at 125 cc/ hr. I discussed this with the nurse and I corrected the flow rate with her. She thanked me for bringing this to her attention. I see myself developing the critical thinking skills necessary to be a nurse more and more. What I once thought to be impossible is now mine for the taking.

Assessment information

This student is:
1. Properly gathering specific information about the client's IV fluids (content);
2. Relaying important information to the primary nurse (communication);
3. Reflecting on her practice and seeing change (personal development); and
4. Gaining confidence in her evolving abilities (personal development).

Possible topics and questions for discussion

1. Fluid and electrolytes
    a. What are the differences between TPN and IV solutions?
    b. Why would a client be getting a combination of fluids like this?
2. Communication
    a. How and when did you approach the nurse about this?
    b. Her response was positive. What if it was not? What would you do?
3. Critical thinking
    a. What does critical thinking mean to you?
    b. How do you recognize critical thinking in the nurses you see on this unit?
4. Personal growth

    a. How are you different than you were at the beginning of this course?

    b. How will this new understanding affect you in the future?

Student 2

Today I was happy when my nurse Eric [on the night shift], and Evelyn [the nurse on the day shift], talked to me about my client and listened to my reporting of my client's vitals. He made me feel like I was actually part of the healthcare team.

Assessment information

This student is:

1. Attaining important baseline data (nursing practice);
2. Reporting information appropriately (communication); and
3. Gaining a positive feeling in the role of student nurse (personal development).

Possible topics and questions for discussion

1. Baseline information
    a. Why is it important that each nurse collect baseline information?
    b. What could happen if the nurse didn't get this information?
2. Reporting information
    a. How do you decide what to report and what not to report?
    b. Is there a proper time to report information to your primary nurse?
3. Personal feelings
    a. How did this interaction differ from others you've had with respect to feeling part of the healthcare team?
    b. What are some other things nurses could do to help you feel part of the team?

Student 3

I was happiest when I saw that my client was in good spirits. I had had clients who didn't feel very good the past few weeks and it was really nice to be able to talk to my client about other issues than pain. She has a positive attitude and likes to chat. It made me happy to be there for my client in a way that was more friendly and emotional than medical and problem solving.

Assessment information

This student is:
1. Observing the effect of pain on conversations (content);
2. Picking up cues that are generating client-centered conversations (communication);
3. Noticing psychosocial responses to hospitalization (content); and
4. Discerning that there are different ways of "being" with clients (personal development).

Possible topics and questions for discussion

1. Pain
   a. What tells you that your client is in pain?
   b. Should this be your primary concern all the time?
2. Client-centered conversations
   a. Should all conversations be client-centered?
   b. Have you ever changed the topic of conversation? What happened?
3. Psychosocial responses
   a. What tells you that a client has a positive attitude?
   b. What can the nurse do when a client has a negative attitude?
4. Different ways of being
   a. Shouldn't the nurse always be "friendly" and "emotional"?
   b. Can a nurse be **too** friendly or **too** emotional?

Topic 2: Today, the thing I saw the nurse do that I admired the most was…

Student 1

The way Roberta talked to her client and the attitude she exuded. She was very chipper and was even able to subtly joke with her client. She also jokes around quite a bit but remains professional. I think that humor is an amazing thing and does amazing things to the body and a person. I believe that it takes a strong compassionate person (nurse!) to be so positive and cheery all the time and have the ability to joke with her client and still be professional.

Assessment information

This student is:
1. Noting the ways nurses communicate (communication);
2. Comparing joking with professional characteristics (content);
3. Recognizing that humor has positive effects (content); and
4. Defining characteristics that he/she believes a nurse should have (content).

Possible topics and questions for discussion

1. Ways of communicating with clients
    a. What are other ways you have seen nurses communicate?
    b. What approach do you think you use the most?
2. Professionalism
    a. What does it mean to you to communicate professionally?
    b. Were you surprised to see the nurse joke with her client?
3. Humor
    a. Can you describe some effects of humor on the body?
    b. In what ways do these benefit a hospitalized person?
4. Nurse characteristics
    a. What does it mean to you to be strong? Compassionate?
    b. Does a nurse have to be "positive and cheery" all the time?

Student 2

Even though my nurse was extremely busy throughout the night she took time to answer my questions and guide me if I needed it. She was also wonderful with my client. She spoke to her in a comforting voice and took the time again out of her busy night to hold hands with my client and just talk to her informally.

Assessment information

This student is:

1. Noticing how busy nurses are (nursing practice);
2. Communicating with the nurse through questions (communication); and
3. Observing the nuances of verbal and nonverbal communication (content).

Possible topics and questions for discussion

1. Nurses' work
   a. Which tasks do you think consume the majority of a hospital nurse's time?
   b. Why is it admirable that the nurse take time for a student? Isn't this part of a professional's role?
2. Questions
   a. What kinds of questions are appropriate to ask the primary nurse?
   b. What do you do when you can't find your primary nurse?
3. Nonverbal communication
   a. Have you seen nurses use touch very often?
   b. Why do you think this is a powerful communication tool?

Student 3

I don't know if I admire what I saw, but I'm glad I got a chance to see what I did. One of the [night] nurses came into work tonight very tired and her shift had just begun. While she was organizing her clients' records and plans of care, she noticed that some of them were going to be difficult clients. She is a pretty vocal lady and she complained out loud about how bad a night it was going to be. Then she noticed one of her clients didn't have transfer orders. She called the floor [from where the client had been transferred] and was blunt with the person she spoke with. I understand why it's frustrating, but I felt she shouldn't have been so rude.

Assessment information

This student is:
1. Observing organizational skills of nurses (nursing practice);
2. Noticing that nurses "label" clients (communication); and
3. Listening to statements nurses make (communication).

Possible topics and questions for discussion

1. Organizational skills
    a. What tools do nurses use to plan the care they give?
    b. What information do you think the nurse was paying attention to?
2. Client labels
    a. How would you describe a "difficult" client?
    b. Do you think a nurse should care for this kind of client differently?
3. Dealing with frustration
    a. Are there proper ways to communicate when the nurse is frustrated?
    b. What are some things you've done when you're in a situation that is frustrating?

Topic 3: Today I worried about…

Student 1

Today I worried about caring for a male client. Since I have only cared for women thus far, I was concerned with how I would relate to a man. I am still worried about changing his colostomy bag. I am going to have Annette [a primary nurse] help me, and this will ease my anxiety a bit.

Assessment information

This student is:
1. Concerned about gender and its impact on relationships (communication);
2. Recognizing limitations (personal development); and
3. Identifying resources and planning to use them (nursing practice).

Possible topics and questions for discussion

1. Caring for someone of a different gender
    a. How do you think gender affects professional relationships?
    b. Did you use a different approach than you use with women? Why or why not?
2. Limitations
    a. How do you know when to ask for help?

      b. Do you think there are times when you should be able to figure things out by yourself?

3. Resources

      a. Are there other resources in hospitals who can assist the individual who has an ostomy?

      b. In what ways have you seen other healthcare professionals assist staff nurses?

Student 2

Today I was worried about the restlessness and emotional instability of my client. When prepping for clinical, I was overwhelmed with the number of past medical diagnoses, mainly depression, anxiety, and addiction to OxyContin. As I was gathering his chart information last night, the nurse was grateful that I was going to be in his room. Similarly, as I was on the floor prior to clinical, my client was in great distress and massively confused. He refused to use his call light and did not understand the function of the foley.

Assessment information

This student is:
1. Anticipating unpleasant behaviors from her client (nursing practice);
2. Recognizing that psychiatric conditions impact nursing care (content);
3. Observing that the nursing staff are receptive to students (communication); and
4. Noticing signs of confusion (content).

Possible topics and questions for discussion

1. Problematic behaviors

      a. What can the nurse do when a client is restless?

      b. When should the nurse call the physician for restraints?

2. Nursing care

      a. What adaptations in care do psychiatric conditions call for in the hospital?

      b. Which approaches have you noticed are most helpful?

3. Teamwork

     a. In what ways are you feeling a part of the unit staff?

     b. How have you been able to help your primary nurse?

4. Documentation

     a. How will you document your client's confusion in the nurse's notes?

     b. In what other ways can confusion be manifested in hospitalized clients?

Student 3

Trying to keep things on schedule, especially with my client having surgery today. I know there is a lot to monitor and record and I was nervous I would forget something and I did! But my client and my nurse were understanding and helped me out a lot. I'm glad that my teacher was there when I was hanging my IV because I probably wouldn't have noticed or known how to get the air out of the tubing. But I think most of my worries seemed worse in my head than in reality.

Assessment information

This student is:

1. Recognizing the flow of postoperative care (nursing practice);

2. Monitoring intravenous fluids (content); and

3. Sorting through possibilities and consequences (personal development).

Possible topics and questions for discussion

1. Organizational skills

     a. What kinds of things were you mindful of keeping on schedule?

     b. What things can interfere with the nurse's schedule?

2. Intravenous therapy

     a. Why is it dangerous to have air in the tubing?

     b. What did the teacher do to eliminate the air?

3. Reflecting on practice

     a. Can worries be helpful to nurses?

     b. Do you always act on your worries?

Topic 4: If I could have changed something today, it would be...

Student 1

If I could have changed something today, it would be my actions when I noticed my client's company had brought her a chocolate cupcake. I knew she was diabetic and on a strict calorie diet, but did not take the action of telling the RN. The RN came in and noticed this herself.

Assessment information

This student is:
1. Observing a breakdown in adherence to diet (content);
2. Not communicating information in a timely manner (communication); and
3. Aware of her mistake (personal development).

Possible topics and questions for discussion

1. Diet restrictions
   a. Why is it important for a hospitalized client to adhere to a prescribed diet?
   b. How is healing affected by an alteration in glucose levels?
2. Reporting information
   a. What do you think prevented you from reporting this information?
   b. How could this breach in communication affect future interactions with that particular nurse?
3. Making mistakes
   a. What is the best action to take when you recognize you've made a mistake?
   b. What did you learn from this experience?

Student 2

If I could have changed something today it would be that I would have explored my client's relationship with her daughter differently. I felt like I could have helped her to express her feelings by listening or saying, "How often do you see your daughter?" Instead, I said, "It must be nice to have her here," putting words into her mouth.

Assessment information

This student is:
1. Attending to psychosocial dimensions of nursing (content);
2. Recognizing effects of comments (personal development); and
3. Strategizing other approaches that might be more beneficial (communication).

Possible topics and questions for discussion

1. Family support
    a. What are some cues nurses use to identify family support?
    b. Why is family support important for nurses to assess?
2. Personal knowing
    a. What told you that your response was not ideal?
    b. How will you avoid doing the same thing again?
3. Therapeutic communication
    a. Why is it not a good idea to "put words into people's mouths"?
    b. Why do you think your second comment was better than your first one?

Student 3

If I could have changed something today, it would be the fact that I just noticed at 6:30 PM that my client had the wrong IV bag. I had checked all of the tubes for no kinks and that all machines (IV pumps, PCA, epidural) were working properly and set at the right dosage. I also checked to make sure the bag wasn't empty or how much fluid was left, but I should have noticed at 4:00 PM! I'm just glad that I noticed because my nurse did not.

Assessment information

This student is:
1. Recognizing the breadth of details that are involved when monitoring IVs (content);

2. Aware of her error (personal development); and
3. Communicating appropriately with the primary nurse (communication).

Possible topics and questions for discussion

1. Therapy
   a. What are implications of hanging the wrong IV solution?
   b. What actions should the nurse take?
2. Mastering organization
   a. How could this mistake have been avoided?
   b. How does the nurse remember details like this?
3. Sharing responsibilities
   a. When you began your shift, how did you convey to the primary nurse which areas you would be accountable for?
   b. What are some possible implications of this event on future relationships with nursing students?

Focus on Students

Unit **3**

Chapter 11: Online Tutoring to Foster Student Success
Donita T. Ruggiero, BSN, MN, RN

Chapter 12: Teaching Nursing Students with Disabilities
Donna Carol Maheady, MS, EdD, RN, CPNP

Chapter 13: The National Council Licensure Examinations
Anne Wendt, MSN, PhD, RN

Chapter 11: Online Tutoring to Foster Student Success

Donita T. Ruggiero, BSN, MN, RN

Nursing faculty are a very dedicated group of professionals who are accustomed to working very hard. However, faculty have many responsibilities—advising, committee work, curriculum development, research, publishing—the list goes on and on. Sometimes faculty become frustrated because there is just not enough time to devote to the focus of the educational process—the student—and helping the student succeed. What can we do when we run out of time? This chapter presents a solution: the computer as tutor—one of the original uses for the personal computer conceived by the first developers of nursing education software. It is an idea whose time has come. – Linda Caputi

Educational Philosophy

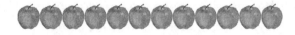

Students have a right to receive—and we as educators have the duty to provide—the highest quality educational experience possible within our capabilities and resources. The educator has to grab student motivation and create meaningful educational experiences that promote student success. Because students learn in different ways, the educator must be artful enough to create a variety of learning situations. My greatest achievement as a teacher is when students who enter the first-semester nursing course with little knowledge of nursing theory and skills are then able to complete the semester integrating new knowledge and skills into the care of a patient in the clinical setting. – Donita T. Ruggiero

Introduction

The content of nursing education curricula has increased in complexity and difficulty over the last decade. Ofori and Charlton (2002) report that academic failure remains the most commonly cited reason for attrition in nursing programs. Students need a support system that can help them succeed in their coursework. A personal tutor system has been suggested as a way to help students pass nursing courses. However, clear guidelines that operationalize this notion of a personal tutor have yet to be developed (Gidman, 2001). With the popularity of personal computers and web-based instruction, an online tutoring tool may be an extremely efficient and effective method for providing tutoring help for students.

An Online Tutoring Program

Online tutoring as a tool to improve student retention is a new concept in nursing education. Prior to the author's development of an online tutoring program, a review of the literature was conducted. No such programs were found. However, the literature has a plethora of articles on student retention programs (Brady & Sherrod, 2003; Klisch, 2000; Lockie & Burke, 1999; Shelton, 2003; Symes, Tart, Travis & Toombs, 2002). Examples of nursing student retention programs include peer tutoring, supplemental instruction, academic counseling, and other organized programs. The majority of nursing student retention programs require the student to be physically present on campus to participate.

Many nursing students are considered adult learners. These students have had one or more jobs prior to admission to the nursing program and will continue to work while completing course requirements. Students often have family obligations and other responsibilities that require much time, attention, and emotion. These obligations are often obstacles to academic assistance because they prevent the student from being on campus to participate in organized retention programs.

Online tutoring can be used to provide the student an opportunity to participate in an organized retention program without being physically present in the classroom. The online tutoring program provides flexibility because it can be accessed any time of the day or night, or during the weekend. Students can access the program from any computer with Internet access.

Goals of Online Tutoring

After the teacher identifies the need for academic support and the possible solution of an online tutoring program, the program's goals are established. The goals of an online tutoring program are to:
- Develop a student retention program available at times convenient for students and outside of the classroom setting;
- Enhance students' use of computer technology;
- Increase the availability of faculty to students outside the classroom setting; and
- Improve student retention.

Software to Support an Online Course

Software that faculty can use as a platform for an online tutoring program may already be in place on the college system. Widely used programs like Blackboard and WebCT make it easy to develop content for online tutoring and manage a tutoring program. Features of these software programs allow teachers to:
- Post announcements, assignments, and other materials;
- Create tests using a variety of test-item formats;
- Utilize a variety of methods of communication, including discussion boards, chat rooms, and group and individual email; and
- Post grades.

Each of the programs has its own learning curve, but most colleges using the software provide training for faculty. Fortunately, the software becomes easier to use as the faculty gain experience developing instructional modules. After initial training, additional learning time may be required as new versions of the software become available.

Developing the Online Tutoring Program

The department should designate one faculty member as the coordinator for the online tutoring program. The coordinator is responsible for working with faculty to develop modules, input materials into the software, and perform ongoing maintenance of the program.

Tutorials are organized by dividing the various topics of the course into modules. Modules can also be developed that address note taking, study skills, and test anxiety. Figure 11.1 lists modules for an online tutoring in a fundamentals of nursing course.

Figure 11.1 - Modules in an Online Tutoring Program

Adaptation
This module contains information on the general concept of adaptation. There is a terminology matching section, an exercise to assist you in learning the aspects of levels of adaptation, and a quiz.

Body Fluid Balance
In this module, you'll learn terminology regarding fluid balance, distinguish between types of fluids, and take a quiz to test your knowledge of fluid balance.

Nutrition
Modules on nutrition and nutritional assessment have been posted. They include a matching exercise to learn terminology along with Name That Nutrient! Take quizzes on these topics to test your knowledge!

Pain
Check your knowledge of pain terminology. Answers will be posted October 25. After you've studied and completed the above exercise, take the quiz.

Legal/Ethical
Match your legal and ethical knowledge. Look at situations you as a nurse may face and decide if the issue is legal or ethical. Also, determine how you, as the nurse, would handle the situation. After studying the content and completing the above exercises, take the quiz to test your legal and ethical knowledge.

Immobility
Learn terminology associated with immobility. The case study will illustrate the effects of immobility on a client. As a nurse, you will plan care for this client. The immobility quiz contains sample test questions.

A course module contains content taught in the classroom, but in a different format. It may provide further explanation or a simpler version of the content presented in class. Or, the module may present the material in a new or different approach to give students additional perspective on the topic. If online tutoring is optional for students, teachers should not include new content because some students may choose not to use the program.

Exercises that allow the student to apply the material taught in lecture are valuable aspects of online modules. Examples include terminology matching and word games such as crossword puzzles.

Case studies demonstrating the application of material taught in lecture are especially valuable. "A case study is a teaching tool designed to simulate a client situation. It allows students to practice making decisions, explore alternate types of thinking, learn about treatment modalities, and evaluate results of their decisions without causing harm to a real client. Case studies can also foster critical thinking, collaboration, and competence" (Purtee, Ulloth & Caputi, 2004, p. 307). Five steps are used to develop a case study (DeYoung, 2003):

1. Develop objectives.
2. Select a situation.
3. Develop the characters.
4. Develop the discussion questions.
5. Provide group discussion.

In an online setting, a discussion board can be used for the group discussion (step 5). Students can post their answers and learn from each other, which encourages collaboration.

Application exercises should be posted the day of the lecture. Students may be given several days to complete the exercise before the answers are posted. Students should be informed they will obtain the maximum benefit from online tutoring only if they complete each exercise before viewing the answers. Students come to understand that learning comes not from getting the right answer, but in the thought process used to arrive at an answer. Memorizing the answers for should be discouraged. Figure 11.2 contains examples of practice items that can be used for a module on skin and wound care.

Organizing a Module

There are opposing viewpoints regarding whether or not to develop modules on every lecture or topic taught in a course. For guidance consider how often online tutoring is used throughout the curriculum. If it is part of every course,

Figure 11.2 - Content in an Online Tutoring Module

Skin Integrity Terminology Matching
Match your knowledge of terms related to skin integrity. Check back on November 2; answers will be posted then.

Skin Integrity Terminology Matching Answers
Complete the above exercise, then check your answers here!

Dress That Wound!
You are the nurse caring for clients with these wounds. What type of dressing would you use? Formulate your answers. Check back on November 2 for suggestions.

Dress That Wound Answers!
Check here for suggested answers on how a nurse would dress these wounds.

Web Links
Go to web links and check out the AHCPR website. On this site are the pressure ulcer prevention and treatment clinical practice guidelines.

Show Me Your Wound!
Go to websites and click on the link to Show Me Your Wound!

Skin Integrity
Click the link above to take quiz.

then it would be feasible to develop modules on every topic. However, if online tutoring is used in one particular course but not throughout the curriculum, its use should be limited to no more than two-thirds of the topics taught in the course. This restriction allows students to remain independent in their study when reviewing topics not covered online. This also prevents students from becoming overly dependent on online tutoring.

Beginning the module with a terminology exercise helps students determine their knowledge of the language associated with a given topic. This may be accomplished with a terminology matching exercise, crossword puzzle, or other word game.

Since nursing is a practice discipline in which the nurse must apply classroom learning to actual client situations, faculty are encouraged to develop exercises that require the student to apply knowledge to a client situation. For example, a student may be presented with scenarios describing specific clients, each with a wound. The student must determine which type of wound care and dressing would be used for each client. Because these exercises focus on application, students are asked to attend lecture and complete the reading assignments for the class prior to accessing these types of exercises.

Finally, the module concludes with sample test questions. These questions help students determine their level of knowledge on a particular topic.

Sample Test Questions

Feedback from students reveals that one of the most valuable aspects of online tutoring is the sample test questions included at the end of each module. These sample test questions are similar to, but not exactly the same as, questions used on the course test. The sample test questions can be used as a gauge to measure students' knowledge of the topic and their ability to apply that knowledge.

Test questions can be in multiple choice, ordering, fill in the blank, matching, and other formats. It is sometimes particularly helpful to include items patterned after the traditional NCLEX multiple choice questions as well as the new alternative item types.

The student takes the quiz and immediately receives a score. Rationales for both correct and incorrect answers are included to enhance learning and understanding of course content (Morrison, 2004). Refer to Figure 11.3 for sample test questions used in an online tutoring program.

Links to Websites

One major advantage of an online tutoring program is that faculty may link students to websites that can add substantially to their learning experience. These websites include official governmental sites, nursing specific sites, or faculty developed sites. Following are several websites currently used in an online tutoring program. These URLs can easily be launched from the CD accompanying this book. Simply launch your Internet browser, put the CD-ROM in the drive, go to Chapter 11 on the CD, and click on the website address.

- **Medical Abbreviations/Drug Database**
  www.medilexicon.com
  Use this website to search for the meaning of medical abbreviations and information on medications.

Figure 11.3 - Sample Test Questions Used in an Online Tutoring Module

Question: The client is concerned about his grandchildren at home when he is hospitalized next week. He's unsure as to how they'll be cared for and by whom. He tells the clinic nurse he feels tense and nervous. The client is experiencing what stage of anxiety?

Answer: A. Mild

      ✓ B. Moderate

      C. Severe

      D. Fear

Feedback: B is the correct answer. Feelings of tension and nervousness are symptoms of moderate anxiety. Fear is incorrect because the event is in the future: Who will care for the grandchildren when he is in the hospital next week? He's unsure. Fear is definite.

Question: Which of the following statements would the nurse use to assess the effectiveness of coping strategies?

Answer: A. Describe the stress in your life.

      B. How long have you had this stress?

      C. What have you used to handle the stress?

      ✓ D. How has this been working for you?

Feedback: D is the correct answer. Asking how this has worked for the client is a question to gather data regarding the effectiveness of coping strategies. Answer A will elicit data regarding the presence of stress. B will elicit data regarding the duration of stress. C will elicit data regarding what coping strategies the client uses.

Question: The client has just experienced a stressful event. The event is stressful to the entire body and the General Adaptation Syndrome is initiated. In the Alarm Reaction Stage:

Answer: A. Blood sugar is depleted.

      B. Pupils constrict.

      C. Hormone levels stabilize.

      ✓ D. Fight or flight response occurs.

Feedback: D is the correct answer. In the Alarm Reaction Stage of the GAS, blood sugar (A) levels increase for energy. Pupils (B) dilate to enhance visual perception. Hormone levels (C) rise to increase blood volume.

- **Progressive Muscle Relaxation**
  caps.unc.edu/4audios.htm
  Do you have test anxiety? Learn progressive muscle relaxation. This website provides information about how practicing progressive muscle relaxation can help combat test anxiety.
- **APA Publication Manual Crib Sheet**
  www.kotesol.org/pubs/submissions/apa-crib.html
  Focuses on how to cite print sources (eg, articles, books) and online materials.

Communication

Good teaching encourages frequent contact between students and faculty (Chickering & Gamson, 1987). The communication capabilities of online teaching are valuable in meeting this goal. Most software used for online teaching provides discussion, chat, and email capability. On the discussion board, the student or teacher can initiate a discussion forum, and all enrolled students may post messages to the discussion board. The chat room can be used at times to facilitate synchronous discussion. Email provides yet another channel for communication; students may email the teacher individually, or the entire class as a group. Students report that this communication is valuable not only for discussing the online tutoring module, but also for sharing messages and schedules with the entire class. The teacher can also use email to expedite messages to the class.

Faculty Issues

As with all aspects of the educational process, developing an online tutoring program involves issues that require special consideration. This section covers some of these issues.

Content Development

Who should develop the content for the modules used in an online tutoring program? The logical answer is the faculty who teach the various course topics. Because these faculty have the expertise required to develop the content and exercises, it takes less time to develop a module. A faculty who does not typically teach a particular topic would need more time to develop a module than a teacher who is very familiar with the content.

Time: Development, Maintenance, and Student Support

The time it takes to develop each module varies. It is reasonable to expect to spend 10 to 15 hours per hour of classroom lecture material. The total time required to develop an entire online tutoring program depends on the number of modules included in the program. Factors that influence the time required for development include:

- The creativity required to develop challenging activities;
- The number of exercises and test questions included; and
- The faculty's knowledge about the content.

Levels of creativity vary among faculty. Faculty may choose to work together to combine talents in both concrete and conceptual thinking to develop highly creative learning activities. Generally, a more creative module requires more time for development.

Time is also needed to maintain the online tutoring program once it has been developed. Each time the course is offered, the content must be reviewed to ensure it is current and reflects the lessons taught in the course. If the teacher, textbook, or content changes, it may be necessary to modify the content of the online modules.

Providing technical support for students also can be time consuming. Students may have difficulty accessing and using the online modules if they are unfamiliar with the program software. Faculty must spend time assisting these students.

At the beginning of each course, faculty may spend several hours enrolling students and instructing them in the use of the online tutoring program. This time may be reduced if the school has an established procedure with computer support staff who take on some of these enrollment and software orientation tasks.

Faculty Support

Faculty support is essential to the success of the online tutoring program. Faculty must believe that online tutoring is a sound educational practice that enhances student learning. It is important to encourage all faculty—even those who choose not to develop the modules themselves—to take ownership of the program. This buy-in is important so students using the program receive encouragement from all faculty.

It is understandable that not all faculty may be interested in this approach. However, if the nursing program has made a commitment to provide students the opportunity to learn from an online tutoring program, then all faculty should facilitate the students' success with this program. Faculty who are not directly involved in creating the modules may wish to help those who are by sharing content expertise, reviewing the modules, and providing feedback on the modules, exercises, and test items. The faculty developing the tutorial must be assured that test questions posted on the online course do not duplicate those used on the classroom tests. Faculty working together can provide the best assurance that this does not happen.

Ownership

The issue of ownership of the material developed for online tutoring should be clearly addressed prior to the program's development. Commonly, if faculty develop a course as part of their work responsibilities, on college time, and using college equipment and resources, then the college owns the materials. However, if faculty develop the material without compensation from the college, on their own time, and using their own computer and resources, then the faculty own the material. Language addressing ownership of materials may be part of a faculty contract or college board policy. If not, it is important for the faculty and college board to be in agreement about who owns the materials.

Student Issues

Faculty must consider whether each student has the computer skills necessary for the course and whether each student has access to a computer. With the advent of distance education and online classes, how do you determine if a student has the basic computer skills to navigate an online course? Computer literacy is an issue schools across the country are addressing; at many schools, a computer literacy course is part of the core curriculum. The same issue applies to students in an online tutoring program.

The question of computer literacy may be addressed as part of a needs assessment to determine if an online tutoring program would be used by students. The program may conduct an interest survey to ask students:

1. Would you use an online tutoring program for this course if one were available?
2. Do you have a computer with Internet access at home?
3. Would you use a computer to access an online tutoring program from home, school computer lab, school library, public library, or another location?
4. Would you use the following components of an online tutoring program?
   - Content modules
   - Practice items
   - Critical thinking exercises
   - Sample test questions
   - Discussion board
   - Chat room
   - Email

Faculty must also consider the type of computer equipment and Internet access the students use. As a general rule, faculty should write the course for the lowest common denominator; that is, assume that students have slow computers and dial-up Internet access. Technology that is not readily available for common home use should not be incorporated. For example, faculty may want to include a multimedia PowerPoint presentation in the online program. However, multimedia programs like PowerPoint create large files that may take considerable time to download on a computer with a slow processor and a dial-up Internet connection, so it might be better to avoid PowerPoint documents in this setting. Students using a dial-up connection for their Internet access also will have difficulty viewing streaming videos posted by faculty.

Cost of an Online Tutoring Program

Funding an online tutoring program may be challenging. Students may be required to register for the program or the school may offer the program as an academic support for no additional fee. The program, however, will require certain expenditures. Money may be needed for:

- Software to develop the program;
- Faculty salaries; and
- Hard copy of module content.

Software

Faculty aspiring to develop an online tutoring program should investigate what software is already being used at their institutions; purchasing new software might not be necessary if the nursing school can tap into existing resources. Software such as Blackboard and WebCT are platforms commonly used by colleges for online course offerings.

Faculty Salaries

Development of an online tutoring program can be very time intensive, and faculty must be compensated for their efforts. This compensation may be in the form of additional salary, a lighter teaching load, or release time. Many institutions have established protocols regarding faculty compensation for developing web-based courses. These guidelines may be applied to an online tutoring program.

Hard Copy of Module Content

One cost the college must consider prior to initiating the program is the cost of printing. Many students learn best when they can review materials in hard-copy format. Therefore, they may want to have a paper copy of all of the materials in the online tutoring program. If the student attempts to print pages upon pages of online course material using college equipment, there must be some mechanism for dealing with these costs.

The school can handle printing costs in several ways. First, the school can absorb the cost of paper and printer cartridges into its budget. Second, students may be charged for each page printed. One way to manage students' printing charges is to institute a debit card system. The students—or the school, using a student technology fee—can load funds onto a debit card each semester. Students can then use the debit card to pay for printing throughout the semester. Other possible approaches are charging each student a technology fee, in addition to other course fees, to defray the cost of printing; or selling hard copies of the course material through the college bookstore.

Evaluation: Does the Online Tutoring Program Work?

Evaluation is necessary to determine if the goals of the online tutoring program have been met. Evaluation methods should be identified prior to the initiation of the program. Measurement can use both qualitative and quantitative methods.

Qualitative Evaluation

At the end of each course, students can be surveyed to determine qualitative data. Figure 11.4 shows an end-of-term survey.

Quantitative Evaluation

To prevent bias, the method to collect quantitative data should be determined prior to initiating the program. If the goal is student retention, percentages of students successfully completing the course can be compared with previous classes. However, many other factors can affect student retention in a particular term. Comparing grades on the same test with those in the class the previous term is another method that can be used; however, test content should be identical for each class for the comparison to be valid.

Perhaps the best method for collecting the most significant quantitative data about the effectiveness of an online tutoring program is to compare the test scores of students using online tutoring with the scores of students not using the tutoring program. This method can be used only if there are a sufficient number of students in the class who are not using online tutoring. One variable that may influence the comparison of these two groups of students is that the students using the online tutoring program are self-selected. Students with a high grade-point average, who typically use every available resource, may be the students choosing to use the online tutoring program. One way to control for this variable is to compare the admission test scores of the two groups and determine if there is a statistical difference between the groups.

Summary

Online tutoring is one method to improve student success. This method can be very effective when customized to a particular course. Students can be guided

Figure 11.4 - End-of-Term Survey

1. I utilized online tutoring this semester.   __Yes __No
        If no, reason for not using: _____

2. Overall, I found online tutoring helpful.   __Yes __No

3. Online tutoring helped me to: (check all that apply)
        ___ clarify content I was unclear about after lecture.
        ___ reinforce content taught in lecture.
        ___ increase communication and availability of instruction outside the
              classroom setting.
        ___ distinguish between content I understood and content I needed to
              study further.
        ___ prepare for actual test questions.
        ___ other: _____

    Other:

4. Areas of online tutoring I found helpful were:
        ___ content modules in course documents
        ___ discussion board
        ___ quizzes in modules
        ___ websites

5. Comments:

to engage in critical thinking by using custom designed exercises. Perhaps one of the biggest advantages of an online tutoring program is that it is a student retention strategy that provides flexibility and convenience for nursing students who typically have very little free time.

Learning Activities

1. Design a module for a subject you teach. Include creative exercises, website links, a case study, and sample test questions.
2. Develop an initial interest survey to determine student interest in an online tutoring program, and which topic areas students would like included in the program.
3. Formulate a tool to measure qualitative data after the initiation of online tutoring. Discuss the method you would use to collect this data.

References

Brady, M. S., & Sherrod, D. R. (2003). Retaining men in nursing programs designed for women. *Journal of Nursing Education, 42*(4), 159-162.

Chickering, A. W., & Gamson, Z. F. (1987). Seven principles for good practice in undergraduate education. *AAHE Bulletin, 39*(7), 3-7.

DeYoung, S. (2003). *Teaching strategies for nurse educators*. Upper Saddle River, NJ: Prentice Hall.

Gidman, J. (2001). The role of the personal tutor: A literature review. *Nurse Education Today, 21*(5), 359-365.

Klish, M. (2000). Retention strategies for ESL nursing students. *Journal of Multicultural Nursing & Health, 6*(1), 21-29.

Lockie, N. M., & Burke, L. J. (1999). Partnership in learning for utmost success (PLUS): Evaluation of a retention program for at-risk nursing students. *Journal of Nursing Education, 38*(4), 188-192.

Morrison, S. (2004). Test construction and analysis: Can I do it? In L. Caputi & L. Engelmann (Eds.), *Teaching nursing: The art and science, Vol. 1 & 2.* Glen Ellyn, IL: College of DuPage Press.

Ofori, R., & Charlton, J. P. (2002). A path model of factors influencing the academic performance of nursing students. *Journal of Advanced Nursing, 38*(5), 507-515.

Purtee, M., Ulloth, J., & Caputi, L. (2004). Developing and using case studies. In L. Caputi & L. Engelmann (Eds.), *Teaching nursing: The art and science, Vol. 1 & 2.* Glen Ellyn, IL: College of DuPage Press.

Shelton, E. N. (2003). Faculty support and student retention. *Journal of Nursing Education, 42*(2), 68-76.

Symes, L., Tart, Kravis, L., & Toombs, M. S. (2002). Developing and retaining expert learners: The student success program. *Nurse Educator, 27*(5), 227-231.

Chapter 12: Teaching Nursing Students with Disabilities

Donna Carol Maheady, MS, EdD, RN, CPNP

The current nursing student population is more diverse than ever, and that diversity includes students with a range of disabilities. This area of educational policy is evolving and changes will continue as the Americans with Disabilities Act provides guidance for a variety of situations. Dr. Maheady offers some basic advice for teaching nursing students with disabilities. — Linda Caputi

Introduction

If it hasn't happened yet, it is only a matter of time before you learn that you have a student with a disability in your lecture class or clinical group. A positive attitude from you, the teacher, will be the foundation to help this student achieve success in the program. Reflecting on your personal views about disability is vital prior to working with a student with a disability. An attitude that celebrates the abilities that everyone can bring to nursing will shine on your student's performance and promote harmony within the group.

Students with disabilities may have learning disabilities, hearing or vision loss, mobility limitations, chronic physical illness, or mental illness (Chickadonz, Beach & Fox 1983; Creamer, 2003; Eliason, 1992; Huyer, 2003; Kolanko, 2003; Maheady, 1999; Pischke-Winn, Andreoli & Halstead, 2003; Styrcula, 2003;

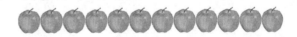

Educational Philosophy

My philosophy is focused on inclusion and has evolved from my advocacy work for people with disabilities. I believe that all nursing students have the potential to learn and that nursing education programs need to provide equal access to students with disabilities. Inclusion of students with disabilities benefits patients, educators, nurses, and other students. Providing accommodations for students with disabilities enhances the teaching-learning experience for everyone. Nursing educators should welcome students with disabilities to the nursing students' table. — Donna Carol Maheady

Watkins, 2002). It is important to be mindful of the fact that students with disabilities can have valuable skills such as sign language and lip reading, and may have empathy and insight from their personal experiences.

Persaud and Leedom (2002) found that faculty had a significant effect on a student's ability to succeed in a nursing program. Learning and working with people with disabilities benefits nursing education and practice in many ways. Students with disabilities often have remarkable compensatory abilities. As an example, the following passage reminds us of the remarkable abilities and potential embedded within our senses.

When describing his experience as a medical student in India, Dr. Ramachandran recalled professors who instructed students about how to identify disease by just smelling the patient—the unmistakable, sweetish nail polish breath of diabetic ketosis; the freshly baked bread odor of typhoid fever; the newly plucked chicken feather aroma of rubella; the foul smell of a lung abscess; and the ammonia-like Windex odor of a patient in liver failure; and insistence on our diagnosing Parkinson's disease with our eyes closed—by simply listening to the patients' footsteps (Ramachandran & Blakeslee, 1999).

This chapter presents practical information and teaching strategies that will benefit **all** students. It includes a review of admission and retention standards, people-first language, universal instructional design, and reasonable accommodations. Inclusion-building activities are presented along with learning activities for nursing educators. Case examples address accommodations that may need to be considered for a nursing student with hearing loss, learning disability, Crohn's disease, spinal cord injury, and mental illness. An example of an Individualized Nursing Education Program is included along with current and future resources for nursing students with disabilities and for faculty.

Terminology: People-First Language

Over the years, the politically correct language surrounding disability issues has changed. People with cognitive deficits have moved from being called "retarded" to being called "mentally challenged." The word "handicapped," acceptable in the past, is now discouraged and is often referred to as the "h"

210

word. "Disability" is the most generally accepted term, not "handicap." Descriptive terms change and we all have a responsibility to stay current. Referring to people with disabilities using people-first language is most important. As educators, we should refer to a student with a disability as a student first. Students with disabilities should never be referred to as the "deaf student" or the "wheelchair student." A more appropriate description would be a nursing student who is deaf (or has a hearing loss), or a student who uses a wheelchair. Above all, students are students first.

Admission and Retention in Schools of Nursing

The exact number of students with disabilities applying to nursing programs or retained in programs is difficult to ascertain. With the passage of laws that protect the rights of persons with disabilities and the general change in attitude toward people with disabilities, the numbers should continue to increase.

Magilvy and Mitchell (1995) surveyed baccalaureate nursing (BSN) and associate degree nursing (ADN) programs in an attempt to describe the extent to which nursing programs admit and graduate students with disabilities. They found that most of the schools surveyed had contact with students with visual, hearing, or mobility impairments, as well as learning disabilities and mental or chronic illnesses. Learning disabilities and mental impairment were cited most frequently. Schools also report having experiences with students with other disabilities including paralysis, chronic illness, back injuries, and scoliosis (Bueche & Haxton,1983; Chickadonz, Beach & Fox, 1983; Maheady, 1999; Maheady 2003).

Watson (1995) surveyed 247 BSN programs to determine their responses to applicants with disabilities. This survey revealed that almost half of the nursing programs studied admitted students with disabilities. The most prevalent disabilities were dyslexia and other learning disabilities.

Admission and retention policies differ among nursing programs. Decisions regarding admission of students with disabilities into nursing programs typically have been made on a case-by-case basis. Therefore, inconsistencies in admission policies are found. For example, a nursing student who uses a wheelchair was admitted to a large state university in the southern United States. In the same year, a nursing student with a chronic illness was denied admission to an ADN program in a western state.

Sowers and Smith (2002) found that including physical attributes as admission standards results in students who cannot hear, see, or speak being excluded from nursing programs. These authors recommend that admission criteria focus on essential functions and technical standards of specific behaviors that nursing students are expected to perform. For example, an essential function may be "detecting a heart murmur." A student who is hard of hearing may be able to detect a heart murmur using an amplified stethoscope and a deaf student may use a stethoscope that provides visual output. These students cannot "hear," but they can perform the essential function with a reasonable accommodation.

Institutions can make the adjustment from physical attributes to essential functions and technical standards. For example, the University of Oklahoma College of Nursing developed guidelines based on the technical skills necessary to perform cardiopulmonary resuscitation (CPR). These guidelines included:

- Visual acuity to identify cyanosis;
- Hearing ability to understand normal speech without viewing the speaker's face;
- Physical ability to perform CPR;
- Speaking ability to question clients about their condition; and
- Manual dexterity to draw up solution in a syringe (Weatherby & Moran, 1989).

Davis, Bowlin, Hazzard and Futch (1992) reported that the Southern Council on Collegiate Education for Nursing developed core performance standards to assist nursing educators in developing proactive responses to support students covered by the Americans with Disabilities Act. The core performance standards for admission and progression addressed the following issues:

- Critical thinking;
- Interpersonal communication;
- Mobility;
- Motor skills;
- Hearing;
- Visual acuity; and
- Tactile ability.

Educators often cite safety concerns as a reason for denying admission to a student with a disability. Sowers and Smith (2002) report that there is no data to suggest that healthcare professionals with disabilities pose any greater safety risk to clients than healthcare professionals without disabilities. Good nurses, good nursing students, and good educators recognize their limitations and know when to ask for help. Knowing what you can do and what you cannot do is fundamental to nursing practice. Client safety is fundamental to nursing practice. These facts do not change because a student has a disability; it may mean, however, that the end is reached in a nontraditional way.

Disability Awareness Activities

Prior to the start of each academic year, it may be helpful for faculty to participate in a disability awareness in-service program. Often, the campus disability services office or counseling center may be able to lead such a program. All colleges and universities that receive federal funds must provide equal access to the consumer of the services. Some entity on campus is responsible for providing academic accommodations for students with disabilities. It may be the disability services office, counseling center, or human resources office. Students, faculty, and staff also should be made aware of campus resources for people with disabilities. Areas covered in an in-service program might include:
- Services offered by the disability service office;
- Legal entitlements of students with disabilities; and
- Information about incoming students with disabilities.

The in-service program may also include simulation activities that allow people an opportunity to "experience" a disability. Be aware that views vary on the benefit of simulation-type activities for people without disabilities. One belief is that exercises like using a wheelchair or wearing a blindfold do little to help a person understand the disabilities. The exercises are thought to be damaging and reinforce negative stereotypes. Another view is that simulation activities can be beneficial. It is best for faculty to work in consultation with the institution's disability services staff. Simulation activities may include:
- Using a wheelchair;
- Wearing dark glasses;
- Wearing headphones;
- Listening to a taped simulation of a person with schizophrenia hearing auditory hallucinations; and
- Taking an oral spelling test while wearing headphones.

If deemed appropriate, faculty should consider including these types of activities for students as well as for faculty.

Disclosure

Nursing educators need to be aware that not all students with disabilities will disclose their disability. They are scared silent. Reasons students do not disclose a disability include:
- Fear of rejection or dismissal from the program;
- Students' lack of awareness that they have a disability;
- Awareness that something is wrong, but lack of a formal diagnosis;
- Personal reasons, such as desire for privacy;
- Negative past experiences; and
- Naïvete relative to the extent their disability will influence their work as a nursing student (Maheady, 1999).

Faculty need to be vigilant in identifying these students. Some behaviors that may indicate a disability include:
- Lip reading;
- Difficulty hearing blood pressures;
- Difficulty reading charts; and
- Incongruence between a student's performance on written examinations and application to practice.

A trusting, positive relationship with a teacher can promote disclosure. Once a disability is identified, reasonable accommodations can be taken to benefit the student and—with safer nursing practice—benefit the client.

A nursing program is under no obligation to seek out students with disabilities to determine if they need additional support. It is the student's responsibility to offer the information. Of course, an atmosphere of acceptance increases the likelihood of early disclosure of a disability.

Universal Instructional Design

In prior decades universal design focused on accessibility to buildings and physical spaces. Ramps were installed and handicapped parking spaces provided. The notion of universal design has broadened and is now used in the design of instruction as well as spaces. The idea is that the needs of people with disabilities should encourage an instructional design that is flexible and supports diversity among learners. When instruction is designed following universal instructional design (UID) principles, it meets the needs of **all** students by providing an accessible and flexible learning environment (University of Guelph, 2004).

The Center for Applied Special Technology at Brown University (2004) emphasizes that UID is the "design of instructional materials and activities that allow learning goals to be achieved by individuals with wide differences in their abilities to see, hear, speak, move, read, write, understand English, attend, organize, engage, and remember." The University of Guelph's Teaching Support Services lists seven principles of UID:

1. Be accessible and fair.
2. Provide flexibility in use, participation, and presentation.
3. Be straightforward and consistent.
4. Be explicitly present and readily perceived.
5. Provide a supportive learning environment.
6. Minimize unnecessary physical effort or requirements.
7. Ensure a learning space that accommodates both students and instructional methods.

Palmer (2003) recommends the use of the principals of UID for three reasons:

*   It is simply the right thing to do.
*   There is a legal argument.
*   There is a strong economic argument.

Palmer (2003) cites the example of a student with a hearing loss attending class in a large lecture hall. The professor asks the students to form small discussion groups. This student with a hearing loss is marginalized because he cannot hear within the auditory chaos. Other marginalized students in this class include a student who uses a wheelchair who is seated in the back of the room and a student with a learning disability who works best when provided time to formulate ideas. By applying UID principles, the professor might assign questions for consideration in advance of the class, provide an asynchronous electronic forum for student contributions, use class time to debrief, and then give students time to write a reflective paper. This type of instructional design addresses the needs of this very diverse group of students.

Accommodations

From the previous discussion it is clear that making accommodations for students with disabilities is advantageous for all students. These accommodations enhance teaching, decrease barriers, and make learning more accessible for all students in the class. Educators have long been aware that students learn and process information in different ways. There are visual, sensory, auditory, and tactile learners. This knowledge is expanded to include the fact that students can also demonstrate knowledge in different ways.

Keep in mind that an accommodation only ensures access; it is not a guarantee of success. The Rehabilitation Act and the Americans with Disabilities Act were meant to "level the playing field" (Matt, 2003). The case law continues to evolve. Documentation from the student must indicate evidence that the disability substantially limits a major life activity, such as learning. The mandate to provide reasonable accommodations does not extend to adjustments that would "fundamentally alter" the nature of the course, or course requirements. There is no law against a student asking, but asking does not automatically mean the request is a reasonable accommodation. Some schools may not have the required financial resources to accommodate the disability.

Keep in mind that the laws are a floor, not a ceiling, and they do not prohibit the institution—or the faculty—from doing **more** for a student with a disability if it is appropriate. Educators can make a student's life better, even if the law does not require it. Through accommodations and extra effort, we can build relationships, foster goodwill, and provide value-added programs that exceed the norm.

Individualized Nursing Education Programs

Students with disabilities who are educated in public schools benefit from individualized education programs under the provisions of the Individuals with Disabilities Education Act, formerly called PL 94-142 or the Education for all

Handicapped Children Act of 1975. This provision can be applied to nursing students with disabilities.

Accommodations may be simple or complex and can range from an alternate examination format or time extension to a scribe or sign language interpreter. Accommodations for a disability are not "one size fits all." An effective individualized program requires teamwork and cooperation to promote the student's success. An individualized nursing education program can serve as a practical guide that describes the student's needs, identifies who is responsible for what, and promotes accountability (Maheady, 2003).

The student, faculty, and a representative from the institution's office of students with disabilities should meet as often as needed to assess the student's abilities, limitations, and needed accommodations. All information must be kept confidential, and all participants should receive a copy of the program.

Every nursing student with a disability will have different needs and circumstances. Examples of the of accommodations that might be included in an individualized nursing student's program are listed in Figure 12.1.

Developing an individualized program involves more than equipment and personnel.

Additional information that should be included in the program includes:

- Current performance (GPA and SAT scores, letters of recommendation, observations and assessments from nursing faculty);
- Letter from the student's physician;
- Annual goals and short-term objectives;
- Related services (supplementary aids, services, modifications to the program eg, tutor, note taker, textbooks recorded on audiotape, computer assisted real-time transcription [CART], sign language, or oral interpreter);
- Technological devices, including voice recognition software and assistive listening devices;
- Testing (additional time, oral or alternative format, use of a calculator or computer);
- Dates and places (when services will be provided and where);
- Transition services, including preparation for the National Council Licensing Examination (NCLEX), employment counseling, preceptorship programs; and
- Measuring progress through midterm and final evaluations.

An individualized assessment and program is imperative. Appendix 12.1 provides an example of an individualized nursing program focused on meeting the needs of one student with a disability.

Figure 12.1 - Types of Accommodations

- Amplified stethoscope to assess heart and lung sounds
- Stethoscope with visual output to visualize heart and lung sounds
- Pocket talker (device that amplifies sound in a one-on-one interaction)
- Telecommunication devices (TDDs or TTYs)
- Computer assisted real-time transcription (CART) services
- Note taker
- Captioned films and training videos
- Assistive listening systems frequency modulated (FM)
- Digital blood pressure monitors
- Digital thermometers
- Face-to-face report in place of taped report
- Amplified telephone
- Lowered desk to accommodate a wheelchair
- Regularly scheduled breaks
- Sign language interpreter
- Audiotaped lectures
- Extended time for examinations
- Visual enlarger
- Large-print books and materials
- Scribe (person who serves as a person's hands if their disability makes it difficult for them to write, or perform tasks)
- Dragon speak (utility that turns speech into text when using a computer)

The following story demonstrates how accommodations in one area of nursing education proved detrimental in another.

A nursing student had been allowed extended time for all her exams due to a documented learning disability. She is now in a clinical course learning to give injections. She is assigned a preoperative client. She draws up the preoperative medication, walks to the client's room, prepares the client, inserts the needle, and freezes. The student was alarmed to discover that she did not have an extended time for performing this procedure.

This example demonstrates why it is important for an individualized plan to look at the total picture.

Case Examples

This section presents a number of short case examples. Following each example, suggestions for teaching strategies are offered.

Case Example: Nursing Student with Hearing Loss

Maria is a junior-level student in a baccalaureate nursing program. She has a documented profound hearing loss. She reads lips and uses sign language. She has disclosed her disability and the disability services office is providing a sign language interpreter to attend classroom and clinical experiences with her. How can you as faculty help Maria meet the objectives of the lecture course you teach? The following suggestions may be helpful:

- Allow the student to sit in the front of the classroom and tape lectures if desired.
- Face the class, enunciate well, speak at a moderate pace, and avoid covering your mouth.
- Avoid standing in front of windows or other light sources.
- Provide handouts of material presented and list new vocabulary terms on the blackboard, overhead, or other projection system.
- Provide announcements, test dates, or schedule changes on paper, chalkboard, overhead, or other projection system.
- Wear a transmitter used with an assistive listening device if needed.
- Speak to the student, not the interpreter.
- Provide scripts of movies or videos shown in class.

During lecture classes, the student's listening can be assisted with the use of personal and group frequency modulated (FM) systems, loop systems, infrared systems, and hardwire systems. These systems utilize a transmitter worn by the professor and a receiver worn by the student.

It is also important to be sure students are included in group activities. To facilitate inclusion assign students to small groups by drawing numbers from a hat. This decreases the potential the student with a disability will feel left out or be picked last by classmates.

Clinical experiences present additional challenges to a successful outcome for this student. The following are some suggestions to promote success:

- Inform the charge nurse, clients, and appropriate staff members about the student's hearing loss.
- Provide the student with handouts of information presented verbally to the clinical group.
- Encourage the student to purchase a special amplified and/or electronic stethoscope.
- Establish a mutually agreed upon system of communication between you, the faculty, and the student.
- Facilitate client, staff, and peer acceptance. Serve as an acceptance bridge.
- Talk directly to the student, not the sign language interpreter.
- Provide ongoing assessments of the student's hearing related to clinical skills —blood pressure, heart and lung sounds, monitors, alarms, clients' calls for help.
- Encourage the student to practice using "99," an examination technique used to elicit vocal or tactile palpable vibrations through the bronchopulmonary system to the chest wall, as part of respiratory assessment.
- Instruct the student to place all monitors in clear view to facilitate "seeing" a beeping monitor.
- Assess the student's need for an amplified telephone in the clinical area.
- Ask all students to speak from the front of the room instead of using a roundtable format for postconferences.

There is a wide range of stethoscopes available for people with hearing loss. One is pictured in Figure 12.2. (More information about that specific device is available at the Cardionics website, www.cardionics.com.) There are "headphone styles," amplified and electronic stethoscopes, and patch cords for people with cochlear implants. Cardionics, Welch Allyn, and 3M Littman are some of the companies that manufacture special stethoscopes. In addition, a software program called Pocket Monitor records, displays, and plays back physiologic sounds.

The software, available from Cardionics can be installed on a personal digital assistant (PDA). Because of the wide range of products available, an audiologist should be consulted regarding the most appropriate stethoscope for a particular student's needs.

Figure 12.2 - Special Stethoscope

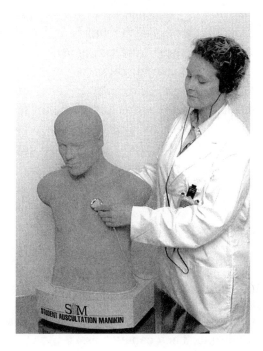

Case Example: Student with a Learning Disability

John is a first-year student in an associate degree nursing program. He has a documented learning disability with difficulty reading and spelling words—particularly medical terms. Helping this student be successful may involve the following:

- Referral to the office for students with disabilities and the local association for students with learning disabilities, where staff members will be able to recommend resources and learning strategies;
- Recommendations for studying, such as reading charts in a particular order, highlighting in different colors, or using flashcards;

- Accommodations such as the use of a Franklin speller or software, eg, Dragon Naturally Speaking;
- Books on tape; and
- Permission to tape lectures.

Butler (2000) suggests some creative devices for remembering how to spell medical terms. These suggestions may be helpful to all nursing students. For example:

- **Asthma.** Think of the first letters of the words in the sentence *Ann Seems To Have Many Attacks*. Imagine Ann having asthma attacks.
- **Coronary.** Deliberately pronounce the different parts of the word cor/on/ary. Coronary contains the letters **ron**. Think of poor Ron with coronary problems.
- **Pneumo.** Take each letter of the word and make up a silly sentence with words beginning with those letters; link the sentence to a picture in your mind. *Please Never Ever Use My Oboe.* Imagine filling your lungs to blow into an oboe.
- **Psycho.** *Please Say You Can Help Out.*

Study Buddy

A study buddy also may be helpful for this student. Some schools provide study buddies through the office of students with disabilities. A buddy may meet individually with eight to 10 students once a week during the term, helping students adhere to a schedule for completing projects and assignments on time or with minimal extended time. They can also assist by:

- Ensuring the students allow enough study time for exams and required reading;
- Helping the students schedule time during the week for leisure activities, workouts at the gym, sleep, and rest between classes; and
- Identifying other ways the students can make things work.

The buddy keeps students on target with their weekly schedule. A WatchMinder also may be helpful for a student who has problems with time management (see www.watchminder.com). Using a vibration system like that of the common pager, the device privately alerts the wearer when it is time for a particular task. It comes with 75 preprogrammed messages including reminders to get to class, talk to the teacher, pay attention, turn in an assignment, relax, get help, study, or check email.

The product website can easily be launched from the CD accompanying this book. Simply launch your Internet browser, put the CD-ROM in the drive, go to Chapter 12 on the CD, and click on the website address.

Case Example: Student with Crohn's Disease

Helen is a senior in a baccalaureate nursing program. She has documented Crohn's disease. She is receiving accommodations because of frequent clinical absences due to hospitalizations. Faculty allow her to make up the clinical time and submit papers later than other students. One day, another nursing student confronts Helen in the restroom and says, "You get away with murder around here. No matter how much time you are absent you still end up with an A in the course. The rest of us can't miss a minute without a penalty!" Helen reports this incident to you. How might you respond to this situation?

The best way to avoid situations like this is to be proactive and institute a zero-tolerance policy for harassment of any student, including those with disabilities. With a written policy in place, this matter can be addressed as unprofessional behavior under the professional conduct code.

Nursing students and faculty need to be aware that educational institutions have a responsibility to ensure equal educational opportunities for all students, including those with disabilities. This is a legal mandate under the Rehabilitation Act of 1973 and the Americans with Disabilities Act of 1990. The laws are enforced by the Office for Civil Rights. Harassing conduct can take different forms, such as:

- Verbal, eg, name calling;
- Nonverbal, eg, written statements; and
- Physical threats or humiliation.

Students and faculty must recognize that students demonstrate learning in different ways or, in this case, different time frames, but that does not mean that the standards have been lowered. Faculty can help students with disabilities to deal with these kinds of behaviors. These students can be encouraged to role play and rehearse responses to possible negative comments or situations.

Case Example: A Student Who Uses a Wheelchair in a Clinical Course

Michelle suffered a spinal cord injury from a skiing accident. Her lifelong passion was to become a nurse. She has been admitted to your nursing program. How can you help this student achieve success in an acute care setting?

Michelle's individual nursing education program might include many supports and accommodations. First, Michelle's abilities and limitations should be comprehensively assessed; then, the following may be recommended:

- Inform appropriate staff of the student's disability prior to the beginning of the clinical rotation.
- Tour the facility with the student before the rotation starts. Introduce the student to staff members.
- Identify accessible hospital units with accessible client rooms.
- Assign the student to clients with adjustable IV poles.
- Collaborate with staff members and the student to establish a plan of action if a client needs CPR.
- Assign student "buddies" or arrange for an intermediary to assist the student with client care—lifting, turning, bathing, and treatments.
- Provide a communication device, such as a cell phone or walkie-talkie, to help the student stay in touch with the teacher.
- Request that the student practice positioning a client with a transfer sheet in the nursing lab.
- Ask the student to use the seat belt on her wheelchair.
- Request that the student practice performing wound care, catheterization, and treatments on a mannequin in a bed set at varying heights.
- Encourage the student to carry extra gloves to wear after touching the wheels on the wheelchair.

A student using a wheelchair must make adaptations to the way client care is typically performed. For example, a dressing change might include these steps:

Set up for dressing change, wash hands, glove, wheel to client, remove gloves, and replace with a new pair. Do not touch wheelchair.

Another example relates to emptying a bedpan. Encourage the student to practice emptying a bedpan by placing a chux on her lap and slowly carrying the bedpan to the hopper.

Provide a diverse range of opportunities for students to demonstrate nursing skills. Diverse approaches may include hands-on whenever possible but also verbal and written assignments, developing diagrams, and completing computer simulations. Ask the student to talk through a procedure step by step. Let the student be the guide as someone else carries out the actions. Assign the student to direct CPR as another student member of the clinical group performs the steps.

To ensure inclusion of this student into the group, rotate student "buddies" every clinical day. Assign students to give a brief presentation during postconference. Students may choose to present a skill they feel confident in performing. Michelle may volunteer to present teaching clients transfer skills or self-catheterization. Another interesting skill that Michelle might present is how a nurse in a wheelchair must organize and arrange equipment to be within reach when changing a dressing.

Case Example: A Student with Mental Illness

Bianca is a junior level student in a nursing program. She has been diagnosed with a mental illness. Her physician reports she is undergoing psychotherapy and is taking medication regularly. She has difficulty taking examinations in a large classroom because she is easily distracted. Bianca also has difficulty completing examinations in the established time frame. Her physician states her reading comprehension is compromised. Accommodations suggested by her physician include a quiet room and extended time to complete exams.

How can you as faculty assist this student to be successful on examinations? Referral to the office of students with disabilities is the first step. Documentation from her physician, including multi-axial DSM-IV Diagnosis, medications, therapeutic interventions, and prognosis should be required. The following would then be suggested:

- Allow her to take her examinations in a quiet room in the office of students with disabilities or the campus testing center.
- Permit the student to have additional time to complete examinations.
- Recognize and anticipate periods of academic inactivity—stopouts versus dropouts.
- Refer the student to the school's counseling center if indicated.
- Refer the student to the local mental health organization.

The NCLEX

Nursing students need to plan ahead if they need accommodations to take the NCLEX examination. In compliance with the Americans with Disabilities Act (1990), state boards of nursing provide reasonable accommodation for applicants with disabilities that may affect their ability to take the NCLEX.

Applicants need to contact their state board of nursing **early** to learn the procedure for requesting accommodations. Policies and procedures vary from state to state. In most states, the board of nursing members review applications for accommodations. Decisions are made on a case-by-case basis. Timing is important because these decisions are made during the state board of nursing meetings, which may occur monthly or less often.

In most instances, the state board of nursing asks the applicant to supply a letter verifying diagnosis from an appropriate medical professional or professional evaluator to confirm the disability and provide information about the type of accommodation required. The board usually asks for a letter from the nursing program that indicates what modifications, if any, were granted by the program.

Accommodations that might be requested by an applicant include:
- Additional time to take the test;
- Adjustable-height table;
- Enlarged keyboard;
- Sign language interpreter;
- Modifiable colors for item text and background;
- Adjustable swivel arm for keyboard; and
- Screen magnification software.

Future Resources

The future promises to provide more and improved technology to assist people with disabilities. An example of a product under development is a clear face mask for people who read lips (Carroll, 2002). Figure 12.3 shows a wheelchair-accessible examination table currently available from Hausmann Industries, Inc. Greater availability and reduction in the cost of this type of equipment will assist nurses in practice areas in the future.

Figure 12.3 - Wheelchair-accessible ADA Exam Table

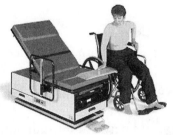

Hausmann Industries, Inc.

Summary

Disability is part of life and part of our practice as nurses and educators. Nurses are experts in helping clients rebuild their lives following a disability and experienced in writing care plans, critical pathways, and care maps to direct the process. Nursing educators can do the same for students with disabilities.

Students with disabilities can enrich the nursing profession through their experience living with disabilities. They add value to health care. An open mind and positive attitude do much to dispel the myth that every nurse has to have a strong back, perfect vision, and excellent hearing. With appropriate support and reasonable accommodations, nursing students with disabilities can be successful without compromising client safety. When you receive your next application or request for an accommodation from a student with a disability instead of thinking "No way," think "Why not?" Through your students you, other nurses, and clients will be taught!

Resources

Following are URLs that contain a wealth of information on students with disabilities. Please visit these websites to further your perspective on this topic.

These URLs can be easily launched from the CD accompanying this book. Simply launch your internet browser, put the CD-ROM in the drive, go to Chapter 12 on the CD, and then click on the website address.

227

- **Association on Higher Education and Disability**
  www.ahead.org
  An international organization of professionals committed to full participation in higher education for persons with disabilities.

- **Association of Medical Professionals with Hearing Losses**
  www.amphl.org
  Information, advocacy, and network for individuals with hearing loss who are interested in working in healthcare.

- **Association of Nurses in AIDS Care (ANAC)**
  www.anacnet.org
  ANAC has a newsletter and committee for HIV-positive nurses and students.

- **Boston University Center for Psychiatric Rehabilitation**
  www.bu.edu/cpr/reasaccom
  This online resource offers employers and educators guidance on reasonable accommodation for people with psychiatric disabilities.

- **ExceptionalNurse.com**
  www.exceptionalnurse.com
  ExceptionalNurse.com is a nonprofit resource network for nursing students and nurses with disabilities. It provides links to disability-related organizations, technology, equipment, financial aid, employment opportunities, legal resources, mentors, and research.

- **HEATH Resource Center, American Council on Education**
  www.heath.gwu.edu
  HEATH is a national clearinghouse on postsecondary education for individuals with disabilities.

- **National Library Service for the Blind and Physically Handicapped, Library of Congress**
  www.loc.gov/nls

This service provides free recorded and braille reading materials to persons with visual or physical impairments that prevent the reading of standard print. Contact the reference section.

- **Office for Civil Rights (ORC), U.S. Department of Education**
  www.ed.gov/ocr
  OCR can answer questions related to Section 504 of the Rehabilitation Act of 1973.

- **Oregon Health Sciences University, The Health Sciences Faculty Education Project**
  www.healthsciencefaculty.org
  This project helps faculty provide effective instruction for students with disabilities in healthcare professions.

- **PEPNet**
  www.pepnet.org
  PEPNet helps postsecondary institutions attract and serve individuals who are deaf or hard of hearing.

- **Western University of Health Sciences**
  www.westernu.edu/xp/edu/cdihp/about.xml
  The Center for Disabilities and the Health Professions was established in response to the concerns of the disabled community.

Learning Activities

1. Design an individualized nursing education program with reasonable accommodations for a nursing student whose right arm is six inches long. She is having difficulty putting on sterile gloves.

2. A student with cerebral palsy affecting her left side is having difficulty starting an IV due to decreased function in her left hand. She learned to compensate by using her strongest finger, her thumb, to stabilize the IV bag against a table. How could learning about the student's ability to overcome this challenge benefit other nursing students, clients, nursing educators, and nurses?

3. Write a personal reflection paper on the following: Imagine that you become disabled and are unable to practice nursing as you did in the past. What accommodations would you expect from your employer and fellow colleagues? Put this paper in a safe place. Read it again if you ever become disabled or are confronted with making accommodations for a nursing colleague or nursing student.

4. Discuss the concept of "reasonable accommodations." What might happen if a school cannot afford such accommodations?

References

Americans with Disabilities Act (1990). Public Law, No. 101-336, 42 U.S.C. 12101.

Bueche, M. N., & Haxton, D. (1983). The student with a hearing loss: coping strategies. *Nurse Educator, 8*(4), 7-11.

Brown University. *What is universal instructional design?* Retrieved Jan. 20, 2004, from www.brown.edu/administration/dean_of_the_college/uid/html/what_uid.shtml.

Butler, S. (2000). *Common medical words with spelling tips.* Retrieved Jan. 6, 2004, from Anglia Polytechnic University website: http://www.shef.ac.uk/~md1djw/hcpdisability/dyslexia/papers/medspelltips.pdf.

Carroll, S. (2002, Winter). Progress with clear face mask project. *Journal of the Association of Medical Professionals with Hearing Losses, 1*(1). Retrieved Feb. 2, 2004, from http://www.amphl.org/jamphl/fall2002/cordwellcarroll.html.

Chickadonz, H. H., Beach, E. K., & Fox, J. A. (1983). Educating a deaf nursing student. *Nursing Health Care, 4,* 327-333.

Creamer, B. (2003). Wheelchair fails to deter paraplegic from nurse's life. *Honolulu Advertiser.* Retrieved Feb. 2, 2004, from http://the.honoluluadvertiser.com/article/2003/dec/28/ln/ln10a.html.

Davis, L., Bowlin, L., Hazzard, M., & Futch, L. (1992). *Red alert: The Americans with Disabilities Act implications for nursing education.* Recommendations of a Task Force to the Board of Directors of the Southern Council on Collegiate Education for Nursing.

Education for All Handicapped Children Act (1975), 20 U.S.C. 1400 et seq.

Eliason, M. (1992). Nursing students with learning disabilities: Appropriate accommodations. *Journal of Nursing Education, 31*(8), 375-376.

Huyer, S. (2003). The gift of ADD. *Advance for Nurse Practitioners, 11*(4), 92.

Individuals with Disabilities Education Act (1990), 20 U.S.S. 1400 et seq.

Kolanko, K. (2003.) A collective case study of nursing students with learning disabilities. *Nursing Education Perspectives, 24*(5), 251–256.

Magilvy, J. L., & Mitchell, A. C. (1995) Education of nurses with special needs. *Journal of Nursing Education, 34*(1), 31-36.

Maheady, D. (1999). Jumping through hoops, walking on eggshells: The experiences of nursing students with disabilities. *Journal of Nursing Education, 38*(4), 162-170.

Maheady, D. (2003). *Nursing Students with Disabilities Change the Course*. River Edge, New Jersey: Exceptional Parent Press.

Matt, S. B. (2003, May 1). Reasonable accommodation: What does the law really require? *Journal of the Association of Medical Professional with Hearing Losses, 1*. Retrieved Feb. 3, 2004, from http://www.amphl.org/protected/summer2003/matt2003.html.

Palmer, J. (2003, Nov. 20). Not just the law; but 'the right thing.' *The Forum, 1*(1), 7. Retrieved Feb. 12, 2004, from http://www.thedisabilitiesforum.com/theforum112003.pdf.

Persaud, D., & Leedom, C. L. (2002). The American with Disabilities Act: Effect on student admission and retention practices in California nursing schools. *Journal of Nursing Education, 41*(8), 349-352.

Rehabilitation Act (1973). P.L. 93-112, Title 5, Section 504, 87 Stat.355 29 VSC Section 794.

Ramachandran, V. S. & Blakeslee, S. (1999). *Phantoms in the brain: Probing the mysteries of the human mind*. New York: Harper Collins.

Pischke-Winn, K., Andreoli, K., & Halstead, L. (2003) *Students with disabilities: Nursing education and practice*. Retrieved Feb. 12, 2004 from Rush University website: http://www.rushu.rush.edu/nursing/studisable.html.

Sowers, J., & Smith, M. (2002). Disability as difference. *Journal of Nursing Education, 41*(8), 331- 332.

Styrcula, L. (2003). Disabled, not incapable: Students with disabilities can become nurses, too. *Nursing Spectrum*. Retrieved Jan. 6, 2004, from http://www.nursingspectrum.com.

University of Guelph. (n.d.). *Our statement of universal instructional design principles*. Retrieved Jan. 20, 2004, from http://www.tss.uoguelph.ca/uid/uidprinciples.html.

Watkins, M. (2002). Disabled nursing students overcome challenges. *Nursing Spectrum*. Retrieved Feb. 9, 2004, from http://community.nursingspectrum.com/magazinearticles/article.cfm?AID=7550.

Watson, G. (1995). Nursing students with disabilities: A survey of baccalaureate nursing programs. *Journal of Professional Nursing, 11*(3), 147-153.

Weatherby, F., & Moran, M. (1989, July/Aug.). Admission criteria for handicapped students. *Nursing Outlook, 37*(4), 179-181.

Appendix 12.1
Example of an Individualized Nursing Education Program

Name: Jeanne   **Date:** August 2004

Disability: Student had a back injury and surgery on her spine. She has a weight lifting restriction of no more than 3 to 5 pounds per physician's order. She has no hearing in her left ear.

Current Performance: A junior in the baccalaureate nursing program, she is a returning student. She was admitted one year ago, and then withdrew for medical reasons. Her grade point average is 3.6. Faculty clinical evaluations of the student are excellent.

Impact on Academic Program: Student's back injury and physician's restriction of lifting no more than 3 to 5 pounds may impact clinical nursing courses, particularly objectives/nursing skills related to lifting clients, bathing clients, making beds, and performing cardiopulmonary resuscitation (CPR). Student's hearing loss may impact clinical nursing courses, particularly objectives related to nursing skills such as listening to blood pressures and heart sounds; auscultating lungs; hearing monitors, alarms, clients' calls for help, telephones, and taped reports.

Student's back injury and hearing loss may impact participation in lecture courses. This student may need front-row seating, permission to stand during lectures, taped lectures, handouts, note taker, and an assistive listening device. The office for students with disabilities may need to provide a remote control opener for heavy doors that are not automatic, note taker, assistive listening device. Because her last nursing course was one year ago, office of students with disabilities also might need to provide a tutor.

Assessments: Assessments by nursing faculty included evaluation of the student's ability to lift clients, make beds, bend down, and perform CPR. The student was found to use appropriate body mechanics, but would not be able to move heavy clients in bed given her weight lifting restrictions. It would be difficult for her to perform CPR without injuring herself.

The student's hearing was evaluated, specifically her ability to hear blood pressures and breath and heart sounds. Tapes of lung and heart sounds and a double-sided stethoscope were used. The student did not hear heart and lung sounds appropriately and was unable to hear blood pressure with a regular stethoscope. The student states she can hear material presented in lecture courses if she is allowed to sit in the front of the classroom. She states that she does not need a note taker or assistive listening device at the present time. She does not use sign language. A letter from her physician documenting her limitations and hearing loss is on file.

Assistive Technology: The student agrees to purchase a special stethoscope. She will consider using an assistive listening device in lectures if front row seating is ineffective.

Short-term Goal: Student will maintain an average grade of C or better at midterm in all nursing courses. Course work will include examinations, papers, projects, and demonstrations of clinical skills. Clinical courses will include a written evaluation by the faculty and signed by the student.

Annual Goal: Student will receive a final passing grade of C or better in all nursing courses. Coursework will include examinations, papers, projects, and demonstrations of clinical skills. Clinical courses will include a written evaluation by the faculty member, signed by the student. The student will meet all university requirements.

Accommodations, Supports, and Related Services—Faculty Advisor Responsibilities

- Refer student to campus office of students with disabilities
- Refer student to campus financial aid office
- Refer student to state vocational rehabilitation program to explore eligibility for benefits and possible funding sources for special stethoscope
- Refer student to vendors for special stethoscopes, back supports (with physician's order), and rolling suitcase for books
- Refer student to local deaf services/hearing loss organization

Clinical Courses: Objectives related to nursing skills: listening to heart sounds, breath sounds, blood pressures, alarms, monitors, clients' calls for help.

Student Responsibilities (related to hearing loss)

- Report hearing loss to clinical faculty before clinical experience begins
- Purchase special stethoscope
- Bring special stethoscope to all clinical experiences
- Report hearing loss to primary or charge nurse on unit of hospital or healthcare agency
- Request verbal report on assigned client(s) if report is taped
- Position all client monitors in clear view
- Inform assigned client(s) about hearing loss
- Monitor assigned client every 10 to 15 minutes, or more often if needed
- Assess blood pressure with special stethoscope and digital blood pressure machine when available
- Ask faculty or primary nurse to verify student assessments of client's heart and lung sounds and blood pressure
- Schedule time with lab faculty to practice use of "99" when assessing a client's lungs

Student Responsibilities (related to back injury)

- Purchase back support (with physician recommendation)
- Bring back support to all clinical experiences
- Purchase rolling suitcase to transport books and equipment
- Schedule appointment with lab faculty to practice body mechanics
- Report weight lifting restriction to primary or charge nurse
- Collaborate with primary or charge nurse regarding limitations, establish a plan of action if CPR must be performed
- Work with assigned buddy or intermediary, or ask for help when indicated, eg, turning clients, bathing clients, making beds

Faculty Responsibilities (clinical courses)

- Inform hospital/clinic charge nurse and appropriate staff members about student's hearing loss and weight lifting restriction

234

- Provide student with handouts of information presented verbally to the clinical group
- Assign student to work with a student "buddy" (moving clients, baths); rotate students each day
- Establish a mutually agreed upon system of communication between the faculty and the student
- Facilitate client, staff, and peer acceptance; serve as an acceptance bridge
- Provide ongoing assessments of student's hearing related to clinical skills (blood pressures, heart and lung sounds, monitors, alarms, clients' calls for help)
- Assess student's need for an amplified telephone on hospital units, clinics or homecare agencies
- Ask students to speak from the front of the room instead of holding roundtable discussions during postconferences

Faculty Responsibilities (lecture courses)

- Allow student to sit in the front of the classroom
- Allow student to stand during lecture if needed
- Allow student to tape lectures
- Provide handouts of material presented
- Enunciate words carefully and talk at a moderate pace
- Face the class and use audiovisual aids
- List new vocabulary or medical terms on the chalkboard or overhead
- Provide announcements, test dates, or changes in schedule on paper, chalkboard, or overhead
- Provide scripts or captioning of films and videos
- Wear transmitter for assistive listening device if needed

Testing Modifications

- Student may need an adjustable-height table

Office of Students with Disabilities

- Provide student with note taker for lecture courses for fall and spring semesters, if needed

- Provide student with remote control for heavy non-automatic door on the main campus for fall and spring semesters
- Provide student with a tutor if needed

Transition Needs

- A special stethoscope will be purchased by the student
- Student may need an adjustable-height table when taking the NCLEX
- Information regarding requests for NCLEX accommodations has been given to the student.

Evaluation of Program

This Individualized Nursing Education Program will be reevaluated at the end of the fall semester or earlier if indicated. The student or a faculty may request a reevaluation at anytime.

Signed by:

Student_____

Faculty _____

Dean or Director _____

Office of Students with Disabilities _____

Date_____

Chapter 13: The National Council Licensure Examinations

Anne Wendt, MSN, PhD, RN

For some faculty, the National Council Licensure Examination (NCLEX®) is a nemesis, something to fear. After all, NCLEX scores indirectly reflect upon us as teachers. However, this perspective is counterproductive. The best approach is to understand as much as possible about this examination and to work cooperatively with the National Council of State Boards of Nursing. After all, their goal is our goal: producing competent practitioners who are prepared to provide quality client care. – Linda Caputi

Introduction

The National Council Licensure Examinations, the NCLEX-RN® and NCLEX-PN®, are used by all boards of nursing to assist in making licensure decisions. Licensure examinations are developed to determine whether or not candidates have adequate knowledge, skills, and abilities to perform important occupational activities safely and effectively (AERA, APA, NCME, 1992; Wang, 2003). Licensure examinations for healthcare professionals should ensure that the practitioner has the essential competencies to practice in order to protect the health, safety, and welfare of the public (Schmitt, 1995). Skills that may be important to job success, but are not directly related to protecting the public, should not be included on a licensure examination (AERA, APA, NCME, 1992). Determining appropriate content for any examination, and especially a high-stakes examination like the nursing licensing examination, is a critical aspect of establishing its validity (Kane, 2002).[1]

Educational Philosophy

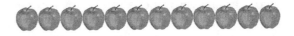

Teaching is an active process with the student and teacher as participants. The teacher provides educational activities to assist the student in attaining knowledge, skills, and attitudes that lead to a change in thinking and behavior. – Anne Wendt, MSN, PhD, RN

Background

An authoritative source on criteria for evaluating tests is the *Standards for Educational and Psychological Testing* (*Standards*) developed by the American Educational Research Association, American Psychological Association, and National Council on Measurement in Education (1992). This influential document provides criteria for evaluating tests. According to the *Standards*, some form of job or practice analysis should provide the basis for defining the content domain of an examination (AERA, APA, NCME, 1992). The National Council of State Boards of Nursing (NCSBN), which is the nursing regulatory organization responsible for developing the NCLEX examinations, collects data from practicing nurses for its analysis. Indeed, more than 4,000 entry-level nurses are surveyed regarding the frequency with which they perform a large number of nursing activities and the importance of the activities in terms of client safety. NCSBN conducts practice analysis studies every three years to ensure that the test plans reflect current nursing practice. The results of the practice analysis, along with expert opinion and feedback from all member boards of nursing, are used to help develop a test plan.

Developing a test plan based on the legal scope of practice for entry-level nurses and collecting empirical data from entry-level nurses are two very important steps for ensuring the validity of the NCLEX. Figure 13.1 outlines additional steps that are taken to provide evidence that the examination is valid.

As Figure 13.1 illustrates, ensuring the examination's validity is a lengthy process with many checks and balances. This rigorous process helps provide evidence that the examination is psychometrically sound and legally defensible. After the test plan is developed, item development sessions are held. Item writers who represent different types of nursing education programs and have the necessary expertise are selected to attend item writing sessions at NCSBN's test service office in Chicago, Illinois. After receiving an in-depth orientation, item writers receive ongoing feedback as they develop the examination items in specified content areas. The item writers must provide a rationale and references (from a list of acceptable references) for the correct answer and to rule out incorrect answer options. Next, an independent panel of nurses who work in clinical practice with entry-level nurses is selected to review the items. This panel of nurses verifies that there is only one correct—or best—answer, that the item reflects current practice, and is appropriate for entry-level nurses.

Figure 13.1 - The NCLEX Process

The process of creating the NCLEX involves a number of steps to ensure the examination's validity and reliability and the test's ability to distinguish competent candidates from those who are not competent to practice nursing safely and effectively. These steps include:

- Job analysis
- Test plan development
- Item writing
- Item review
- Editorial review
- Sensitivity review
- Member board review
- Pretesting
- Examination committee review
- Examination administration

Then several steps take place to ensure that the examination items are fair, flawless, and within the legal scope of nursing practice. Each step is conducted by separate and independent individuals and groups. One of the last steps is inserting the new questions—as ungraded items—on actual NCLEX exams to gather statistical information about the items. Only those items which candidates validate as appropriate, by their responses to the items, (ie, those items that meet statistical criteria) are used on the examination. Thus, the process used to develop the NCLEX examination items is quite comprehensive and is often used as an exemplar in the testing industry.

Test Plan Standards

According to the *Standards*, a test plan for a licensure examination should clearly explicate the content domains being evaluated by the examination. A test plan or blueprint is the document used to describe the content domains being evaluated. The test plan should be of sufficient breadth and depth to describe the practice domain to the candidate preparing to take the examination. There should be a close link between the examination content and the job content identified on the practice analysis (AERA, APA, NCME, 1992); this can be established through accurate and consistent coding of the examination items to the test plan and ultimately to the practice analysis activity statements. A great deal of time and effort is spent to ensure consistency in item coding. This ensures that examinations meet the content domain specifications outlined in the test plan as well as the job-related knowledge, skills, and abilities from the practice analysis. The test plan helps the candidate preparing to take the examination by identifying the appropriate content. Additionally, the test plan provides direction for item writers and serves as a blueprint for assembling the large item pools from which individual examination questions are selected.

According to the *Standards* and the *National Organization for Competency Assurance (NOCA) Certification Handbook* (Browning & Bugbee, 1996)—another seminal reference—there are some general requirements for test plans to be consistent with industry standards:

- A clear statement of the purpose of the test;
- A definition of the target population of candidates;
- A content outline;
- The length of the test in terms of items and time;
- The appropriate cognitive level of items;
- The item types; and
- The delivery mechanism and scoring procedures.

Purpose of the Test

A clear statement of the purpose of the test can be found on page 2 of the 2004 NCLEX-RN Test Plan and page 1 of the 2002 NCLEX-PN Test Plan. The purpose of the NCLEX is to identify those candidates who are minimally competent to practice nursing safely and effectively. In other words, the purpose of the examination is not to place candidates on a continuum from **least** to **most able**. Rather, it is to separate those who are competent to practice from those who are not.

Candidate Population

The candidate population comprises those individuals who are deemed eligible to take the examination by their boards of nursing. Each board of nursing determines the requirements for candidates to be eligible to take the examination.

The primary requirement usually is graduation from an accredited nursing program. Once the candidate is deemed eligible, the candidate can register to take the test. Most boards of nursing allow a candidate to test once every 45 days.

Content Outline

According to the *NOCA Certification Handbook* (Browning & Bugbee, 1996), the content domain of a test plan should clearly explain the content to be covered in order to facilitate candidates' preparation for the examination and test writers' development of examination items.

2004 NCLEX-RN Test Plan

According to the 2004 NCLEX-RN Test Plan, the examination content is based on **client needs** (see Appendix 13.1). This content outline was selected because it provides a universal structure that is easily understood by all candidates and does not adhere to one particular nursing theory. The content outline is not over-specified, so new content can be incorporated without necessitating a change in the test plan, but it is specific enough to provide direction for candidates preparing to take the examination and item writers developing new items. As can be seen, the test plan consists of one dimension—all of the examinations major content areas are related to this one dimension. The client needs include:

- Safe effective care environment;
- Health promotion and maintenance;
- Psychosocial integrity; and
- Physiological integrity.

In contrast, the 1995 NCLEX-RN Test Plan was based on two dimensions—client needs and phases of the nursing process.

The greatest percentage of test items are allocated to two content areas, safe effective care environment and physiological integrity. Thus, these categories are further divided into subcategories (Figure 13.2), including management of care, and basic care and comfort, so there is not one category or subcategory that is overly large or small. This allows for the item selection algorithm to be maximized and allows for some reliability in the reports generated for the candidates who fail the examination.

Figure 13.2 - Distribution of Content on the 2004 NCLEX-RN Test Plan

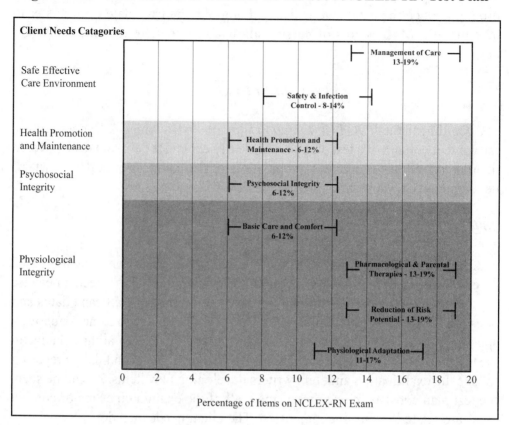

As shown in Figure 13.2, the physiological integrity category is divided into four subcategories:

- Basic care and comfort, to which 6 percent to 12 percent of the items are allocated;
- Pharmacological and parenteral therapies (13 percent to 19 percent);
- Reduction of risk potential (13 percent to 19 percent); and
- Physiological adaptation (11 percent to 17 percent).

The next largest category is safe effective care environment, which is further divided into management of care (13 percent to 19 percent of test items) and safety and infection control (8 percent to 14 percent).

The categories of health promotion and maintenance and psychosocial integrity comprise 6 percent to 12 percent each of the test items. An overall review of the test plan structure reveals that most of the content appears to be related to the physical needs of the client, with managing the healthcare environment the second major area. However, this assessment could be somewhat misleading when determining how these test plan categories relate to the competencies needed for the various nursing practice specialties. That is, there is no one-to-one correspondence between the test plan category of psychosocial integrity and the competencies required for nurses in the field of psychiatric and mental health nursing. Content related to psychiatric nursing can be found in all of the test plan categories. Similarly, content related to pediatric nursing can be found in all test plan categories.

All NCLEX content categories reflect client needs across the lifespan and in a variety of settings. In addition, certain processes are integrated into all areas of the test plans. These processes are:

- Nursing process and, for the NCLEX-PN test plan, clinical problem-solving;
- Caring;
- Communication and documentation; and
- Teaching and learning.

The concepts of cultural awareness and self-care are also integrated into the PN test plan, while the 2004 RN test plan distributed these concepts to specific test plan categories: cultural awareness to the psychosocial integrity category, and self-care to the health promotion and maintenance category. This integration of the processes means that content related to documentation can be found in all test plan categories, depending on the concept that is being documented. For example, client confidentiality documentation could be in management of care; documentation about fall prevention could be in safety and infection control; and medication administration documentation could be in pharmacological and parenteral therapies. It is the specific content of the item that determines how the item is categorized.

2002 NCLEX-PN Test Plan

The overall structure of the 2002 NCLEX-PN Test Plan (see Appendix 13.2) is similar to the RN test plan in that the framework is organized around client needs. As illustrated in Figure 13.3, a majority of the examination items are allocated to the physiological integrity needs of the client. In the safe effective care environment category, coordinated care has 6 percent to 12 percent of the items and safety and infection control has 7 percent to 13 percent of the items. In the health promotion and maintenance category, the subcategories of growth

Figure 13.3 - Distribution Content on the NCLEX-PN Exam

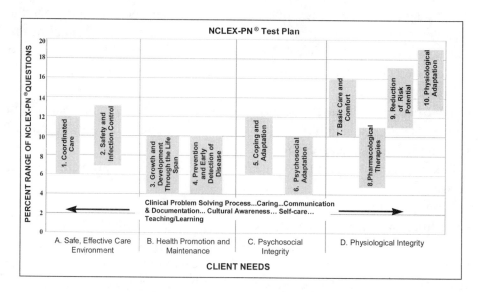

and development through the life span and prevention and early detection of disease have 4 percent to 10 percent of the items. The category of psychosocial integrity consists of coping and adaptation, with 6 percent to 12 percent of the items, and psychosocial adaptation, with 4 percent to 10 percent of the items. Changes to the NCLEX-PN Test Plan are being considered by NCSBN's delegate assembly and could be implemented in 2005.

It should be noted that for the 2002 NCLEX-PN Test Plan each of the Client Needs categories have subcategories. Items on each LPN/VN candidate's examination are selected on the basis of the subcategories. Also noteworthy is that the coordinated care and pharmacological therapies subcategories on the PN test plan are different from the management of care and pharmacological and Parenteral Therapies subcategories on the RN test plan because the scope of practice between the LPN/VN and the RN are markedly different. In general, the scope of practice for registered nurses and licensed practical/vocational nurses are different and the differences vary depending upon which jurisdiction the nurse is licensed and practicing.

Number of Test Items

The length of the NCLEX examinations is variable. The examinations are administered to candidates using computerized adaptive testing (CAT). Thus, is it not possible to state the number of items each candidate will receive because the number of items varies based on the candidate's ability and measurement precision. However, there are a minimum and maximum number of items that can be administered to each candidate. For the NCLEX-RN, candidates answer between 75 and 265 items, of which 15 are pretest or unscored items. For the NCLEX-PN, candidates must answer between 85 and 205 items, of which 25 are pretest or unscored items. Both tests have a minimum of 60 operational or scored items. This allows for sufficient opportunity in all test plan content domains for candidates to demonstrate their competence. It should be noted, however, that NCLEX results are reported as pass/fail on the total examination, so candidates can compensate for areas of relative weakness in one category of the test plan by answering items correctly in other categories of the test plan. Candidates do not need to pass a particular content area of the test plan to achieve a passing result.

Length of Time

From 1994 to 2004, there was a five-hour time limit for the NCLEX testing, including the introduction, tutorial, and rest breaks. In 2004 the time limit for the NCLEX-RN was increased to six hours. Among the most important reasons were the increased passing standard and the use of alternate item types.[2] While the alternate items themselves may not take more time than standard multiple-choice items, the tutorial to prepare candidates to answer the alternate items does take longer. To ensure that candidates have ample time to demonstrate their competence, the time limit was increased. The time allocated for the NCLEX-PN is not expected to change.

The NCLEX is a variable-length CAT. The length of the examination is determined by the candidate's responses. Once 60 operational items have been taken, testing ends when the candidate's performance is determined to be above or below the passing standard with 95 percent certainty; therefore candidates will take different amounts of time to complete the examination. Of course, the examination will stop when the maximum number of operational items (250 for NCLEX-RN and 180 for NCLEX-PN) has been taken or when the maximum time limit has been reached. A passing or failing score is not related to the number of items answered: A candidate with a relatively short examination may pass or fail, and a candidate with a long examination may pass or fail.

Cognitive Level

Since the practice of nursing requires the application of knowledge, skills, and abilities, the majority of items on the examination are written at the application or higher levels of cognitive ability using Bloom's taxonomy and revised taxonomy (Bloom, 1956; Anderson and Krathwohl, 2001). These higher-level items require more complex thought processing and problem solving. Just as in nursing practice, many of the items in the NCLEX-RN examination address complex client problems and situations. For example, if a test item addresses a pediatric client with mental illness being prepared for a medical procedure, the candidate must consider all relevant factors to answer the item correctly.

Item Types

A variety of item types are used on the NCLEX examinations. As has been shown, items go through an extensive review process before they can be used as operational items on the examination. Most items are four-option, multiple-choice items. Other types of item formats used on the NCLEX examinations may include, but are not limited to:

- Multiple response items that require a candidate to select one or more responses (see Figure 13.4);
- Fill-in-the-blank calculation items requiring the candidate to perform a calculation (see Figure 13.5);
- Ordered-response items requiring the candidate to put responses in a specific order (see Figure 13.6); and
- Hot-spot items that ask a candidate to identify an area on a picture or graphic (see Figure 13.7).

Figure 13.4 - Multiple Response Item

The nurse is caring for a client who has a wound infected with methicili-resistant Staphyococcus aureus (MRSA). Which of the following infection control precautions should the nurse implement?

Select all that apply.

☑ 1. Wear a protective gown when entering the client's room.

☐ 2. Put on a particulate respirator mask when administering to the client.

☑ 3. Wear gloves when delivering the client's meal tray.

☐ 4. Ask the client's visitors to wear a surgical mask when in the client's room.

☐ 5. Wear sterile gloves when removing the client's wound dressing.

☑ 6. Put on a face shield before irrigating the client's wound.

Figure 13.5 - Fill-in-the-Blank Calculation Item

The nurse is monitoring the dietary intake and output of a client. The nurse observes that the client has consumed 8 ounces of apple juice, one hamburger on a bun, one-half cup of green beans, 8 ounces of tea, and one cup of ice cream. How many milliliters should the nurse record for the client's intake?

_____ Milliliters

Figure 13.6 - Ordered-Response Item

The nurse is caring for a client with an acute exacerbation of Crohn's disease. In what order would the nurse perform an abdominal assessment? Prioritize the nursing actions by typing the number of the *first* action the nurse should take, followed by subsequent actions, in the answer space provided.

1	Test for rebound tenderness
2	Percussion
3	Auscultation
4	Palpation
5	Inspection

Figure 13.7 - Hot-Spot Item

The nurse is performing a cardiac assessment. Click on the area where the nurse should ausculate the mitral valve at its *loudest*

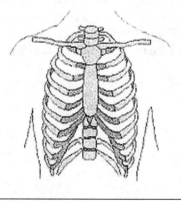

Any of the item formats, including standard multiple-choice items, may include charts, tables, or graphic images. Regardless of the item format, all items are scored as right or wrong using the Rasch measurement model (Rasch, 1956; Wright and Mok, 2000). Furthermore, all items undergo the same rigorous development process and must meet the same statistical criteria to become operational or scored items.

Delivery Mechanism and Scoring Procedures

A CAT methodology is used to administer the NCLEX examinations. The NCLEX examinations are different than a traditional pencil and paper examination because CAT is used. In traditional examinations, the level of difficulty is the same for all students because the same test items are used for every candidate. Because the examination is the same for all students, the percent of items answered correctly can be used as an indicator of the student's ability. One disadvantage of this approach is that it is inefficient. It requires high-ability students to answer all the easy items.

Because the NCLEX examination uses CAT, targeting items to the candidate's ability, the examination can produce more stable results using fewer test items. Although everyone's first item is relatively easy, subsequent items are better targeted because the system re-estimates a candidate's ability after every answer is submitted. Using the candidate's current ability estimate, the program searches the item bank for an item that has a degree of difficulty appropriate for that ability. After the candidate answers this item, the computer re-estimates the candidate's ability and selects the next item using the same procedure. This process continues until it is clear (with 95 percent certainty) that the candidate's ability is above or below the passing standard. Because the computer presents all candidates with items suited to their ability, both passers and failers tend to answer approximately 50 percent of the items correctly. Thus, the candidate's ability estimate is based upon both the percentage of items answered correctly— approximately 50 percent in most cases—and the difficulty of the items that were administered.

Reliability and Decision Consistency

Information about the reliability of a licensure examination should be available to stakeholders. For the NCLEX, decision consistency is used as an index of reliability because the decisions about a candidate's competence is reported as a pass-fail decision. The decision consistency for the NCLEX examination is approximately 0.90 for each quarter of administration.[3]

Summary

Determining important entry-level nursing competencies and using a rigorous process for developing a test plan and examination are key aspects of establishing the validity of the NCLEX-RN and NCLEX-PN. The NCLEX test plans meet all of the industry standards. Nursing educators can use the test plans to map their courses and curriculum to help identify the essential knowledge, skills, and abilities their students will need upon entry into practice. By mapping courses and curriculum to the test plans, nursing educators may be able to identify gaps or redundancies in the curriculum. Furthermore, nursing educators can help students prepare for the NCLEX by familiarizing them with the test plan early in their studies, so the preparation for the NCLEX examinations is not so onerous. The 2004 NCLEX-RN Frequently Asked Questions (Appendix 13.3) can be quite useful to educators as they explain the test plan to students.

With the rapid changes in health care, it is important for nursing educators to keep abreast of changes related to the NCLEX examinations. For updated information about the NCLEX, visit the National Council of State Boards of Nursing website at www.ncsbn.org. For easy access to this site, insert the CD-ROM that accompanies this book into the drive. Go to Chapter 13 on the CD and click on the URL.

Learning Activities

1. Write several test items using the alternate item type format. Ask students to answer these questions. Discuss with students their feelings about these item types.

2. Consider a test you created for a course you are teaching. Or, write a sample test. Identify which category each item fits into on the NCLEX test plan.
3. Compare and contrast the test plans for the NCLEX-RN and NCLEX-PN.

End Notes

[1] The *Standards for Educational and Psychological Testing* defines validity as the appropriateness, meaningfulness, and usefulness of the specific inferences made from test scores. Validity refers to the degree to which evidence and theory support the interpretation of test scores entailed by proposed uses of tests. Validity is not all or nothing. Rather, the test developer collects evidence that helps establish the validity of the examination and rule out competing hypotheses.

[2] In April 2004, the NCSBN Board of Directors raised the passing standard for the NCLEX-RN examination from –0.35 logits to –0.28 logits on the NCLEX-RN examination scale. The NCSBN Board of Directors used multiple sources of information, including a criterion-referenced recommendation, to guide its evaluation and discussion regarding the change.

[3] To pass the NCLEX examination, the candidate's performance on the examination must **exceed** the passing standard. (A criterion-referenced method is used to help make a decision regarding the passing standard.) Ideally, NCSBN wants to be at least 95 percent certain of pass-fail decisions. Therefore, after the minimum number of items has been answered, when NCSBN is 95 percent certain that the candidate's ability is above or below the passing standard, no more questions are administered. Candidates pass if their scores are above the standard; they fail if their scores are below the standard. Candidates with very high or very low abilities tend to receive minimum-length tests. However, some candidates will have a true ability that is so close to the passing standard that even 1,000 items would not be enough to arrive at a decision with 95 percent confidence. Because it would be impractical to administer 1,000 items, a maximum number of items has been established for each type of examination. When these candidates answer the maximum of items, their ability estimates are rather precise, but not enough to make a decision with 95 percent certainty. Because the precision is quite good in these cases, the 95 percent certainty requirement is waived. If candidates' ability estimate is above the passing standard, they pass; if it is at or below the passing standard, they fail. If the examination ends because time runs out, it means that the candidate has not

demonstrated with 95 percent certainty that he or she is clearly above or below the passing standard, nor has the candidate answered the maximum number of items. Because the primary mission of boards of nursing is to protect the public, it can be argued that candidates should not pass when they have not demonstrated that they are competent. However, the response patterns for some of these people have indicated that there are candidates who appeared to have a **true ability** that is above passing and who have been performing consistently above the passing standard—the key word here is **consistently**. A mechanism is provided for these candidates to pass. If a candidate's performance has been consistently above the passing standard, then he or she will pass, despite running out of time.

References

American Educational Research Association, American Psychological Association, National Council on Measurement in Education. (1992). *Standards for educational and psychological testing.* Washington, DC: American Psychological Association.

Anderson, L. W., & Krathwohl, D. R. (Eds). (2001). *A taxonomy for learning, teaching, and assessing. A revision of Bloom's taxonomy of educational objectives.* New York: Addison Wesley Longman.

Bloom, B. S., Engelhart, M. D., Furst, E. J., Hill, W. H., & Krathwohl, D. R. (1956). *Taxonomy of educational objectives: The classification of educational goals, Handbook 1.* New York: David McKay.

Browning, A., & Bugbee, A. (1996). *Certification: A NOCA handbook.* Washington DC: National Organization of Competency Assurance.

Kane, M. (2002, Spring). Validating high-stakes testing programs. *Educational measurement: Issues and practices*, 31-42.

National Council of State Boards of Nursing (2003). *Test plan for the National Council Licensure Examination for Registered Nurses (NCLEX-RN).* Chicago: Author.

Rasch, G. (1980). *Probabilistic models for some intelligence and attainment tests.* Copenhagen: Danmarks Paedogogiske Institute. Reprint, Chicago: University of Chicago Press.

Schmitt, K. (1995). What is licensure? In J. Impara (Ed.), *Licensure testing: Purposes, procedures, and practices.* Lincoln, NE: Buros Institute.

Smith, J., & Crawford, L. (2003). *Report of findings from the 2002 RN practice analysis: Linking the NCLEX-RN examination to practice.* Chicago: National Council of State Boards of Nursing.

Wang, N. (2003, Fall). Use of the Rasch IRT model in standard setting. *Journal of Educational Measurement, 40*(3), 231-253.

Wright, B., & Mok, M. (2000). Rasch models overview. *Journal of Applied Measurement, 1*(1), 3-10.

Wright, B., & Stone, M. H. (1979). *Best test design.* Chicago: MESA Press.

Teaching Nursing: The Art and Science

Appendix 13.1
NCLEX-RN Test Plan
Test Plan for the National Council Licensure Examination for Registered
Nurses
(NCLEX-RN Examination)

Reproduced from the NCSBN Web site (www.ncsbn.org) and used with
permission from the National Council of State Boards of Nursing (NCSBN),
Chicago, Illinois.

Introduction

Entry into the practice of nursing in the United States and its territories is
regulated by the licensing authorities within each jurisdiction. To ensure public
protection, each jurisdiction requires candidates for licensure to pass an exam
that measures the competencies needed to perform safely and effectively as a
newly licensed, entry-level registered nurse. The National Council of State Boards
of Nursing, Inc. (NCSBN) develops a licensure exam, the National Council
Licensure Examination for Registered Nurses (NCLEX-RN), which is used by
state and territorial boards of nursing to assist in making licensure decisions.
Several steps occur in the development of the NCLEX-RN Test Plan. The
first step is conducting a practice analysis that is used to collect data on the
current practice of the entry-level nurse (Report of Findings from the 2002 RN
Practice Analysis: Linking the NCLEX-RN Examination to Practice, Smith &
Crawford, 2003). More than 4,000 newly licensed registered nurses are asked
about the frequency and priority of performing more than 130 nursing care
activities. These activity statements are then analyzed in relation to the frequency
of performance, impact on maintaining client safety and the client care settings
where the activities are performed. This analysis guides the development of a
framework for entry-level nursing practice that incorporates specific client needs
as well as processes fundamental to the practice of nursing. The second step is
the development of the NCLEX-RN Test Plan which guides the selection of
content and behaviors to be tested.
The *NCLEX-RN Test Plan* provides a concise summary of the content and
scope of the licensing exam. It serves as a guide for exam development as well
as candidate preparation. Each NCLEX-RN candidate exam is based on the test

plan. Each exam assesses the knowledge, skills, and abilities that are essential for the nurse to meet the needs of clients requiring the promotion, maintenance, or restoration of health. The following sections describe beliefs about people and nursing that are integral to the exam, cognitive complexities that will be tested in the exam and specific parts of the NCLEX-RN Test Plan.

Beliefs

Beliefs about people and nursing underlie the NCLEX-RN Test Plan. People are finite beings with varying capacities to function in society. They are unique individuals who have defined systems of daily living reflecting their values, motives and lifestyles. Additionally, people have the right to make decisions regarding their health care needs and to participate in meeting those needs.

Nursing is both an art and a science, founded on a professional body of knowledge that integrates concepts from the liberal arts and the biological, physical, psychological, and social sciences. It is a learned profession based on an understanding of the human condition across the life span and the relationships of an individual with others and within the environment. Nursing is a dynamic, continually evolving discipline that employs critical thinking to integrate increasingly complex knowledge, skills, technologies, and client care activities into nursing practice. The goal for nursing care in any setting is preventing illness; alleviating suffering; and protecting, promoting, and restoring health.

The registered nurse provides a unique, comprehensive assessment of the health status of the client (individual, family, or group), and then develops and implements an explicit plan of care. The nurse assists clients in the promotion of health, in coping with health problems, in adapting to and/or recovering from the effects of disease or injury, and in supporting the right to a dignified death. The registered nurse is accountable for abiding by all applicable federal, state, and territorial statues related to nursing practice.

Classification of Cognitive Levels

The exam consists of items that use Bloom's taxonomy for the cognitive domain as a basis for writing and coding items (Bloom, et al, 1956; Anderson & Krathwohl, 2001). Since the practice of nursing requires application of knowledge, skills and abilities, the majority of items are written at the application or higher levels of cognitive ability, which requires more complex thought processing.

Test Plan Structure

The framework of Client Needs was selected for the NCLEX-RN exam because it provides a universal structure for defining nursing actions and competencies across all settings for all clients.

Client Needs

Four major categories of Client Needs organize the content of the NCLEX-RN Test Plan. Two of the four categories are further divided into a total of six subcategories. The Client Needs categories and subcategories that define the content of the NCLEX-RN Test Plan are:

- Safe Effective Care Environment
  - Management of Care
  - Safety and Infection Control
- Health Promotion and Maintenance
- Psychosocial Integrity
- Physiological Integrity
  - Basic Care and Comfort
  - Pharmacological and Parenteral Therapies
  - Reduction of Risk Potential
  - Physiological Adaptation

Health Promotion and Maintenance and Psychosocial Integrity categories do not have subcategories.

Integrated Processes

The following processes are fundamental to the practice of nursing and are integrated throughout the four major Client Needs categories:

- **Nursing Process.** A scientific problem-solving approach to client care that includes assessment, analysis, planning, implementation, and evaluation.
- **Caring.** Interaction of the nurse and client in an atmosphere of mutual respect and trust. In this collaborative environment, the nurse provides hope, support, and compassion to help achieve desired outcomes.
- **Communication and Documentation.** Verbal and nonverbal interactions between the nurse and the client, the client's significant other, and the other members of the health care team. Events and activities associated with client care are validated in written or electronic records that reflect quality and accountability in the provision of care.
- **Teaching/Learning.** Facilitation of the acquisition of knowledge, skills, and attitudes promoting a change in behavior.

Distribution of Content

The percentage of test questions assigned to each Client Needs category and subcategory of the NCLEX-RN Test Plan is based on the results of *the Report of Findings from the 2002 RN Practice Analysis: Linking the NCLEX-RN Examination to Practice* (Smith & Crawford, 2003), and expert judgment provided by members of the NCSBN Examination Committee.

Client Needs	Percentage of Items From Each Category/ Subcategory
Safe, Effective Care Environment	
Management of Care	13%-19%
Safety and Infection Control	8%- 14%
Health Promotion and Maintenance	6%- 12%
Psychosocial Integrity	6%- 12%
Physiological Integrity	
Basic Care and Comfort	6%- 12%
Pharmacological and Parenteral Therapies	13%-19%
Reduction of Risk Potential	13%-19%
Physiological Adaptation	11%-17%

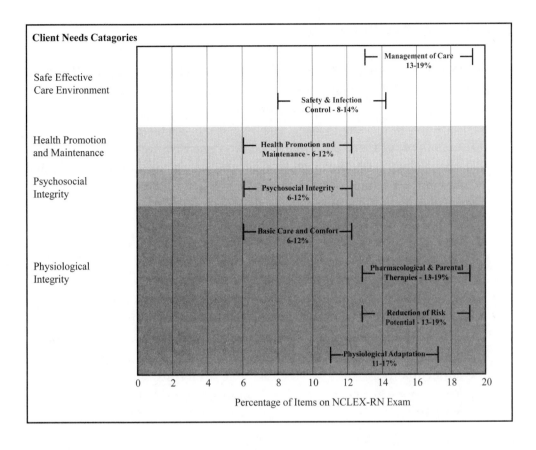

Client Needs Catagories

Safe Effective Care Environment
- Management of Care 13-19%
- Safety & Infection Control - 8-14%

Health Promotion and Maintenance
- Health Promotion and Maintenance - 6-12%

Psychosocial Integrity
- Psychosocial Integrity 6-12%

Physiological Integrity
- Basic Care and Comfort 6-12%
- Pharmacological & Parental Therapies - 13-19%
- Reduction of Risk Potential - 13-19%
- Physiological Adaptation 11-17%

Percentage of Items on NCLEX-RN Exam

The following processes are integrated into all Client Needs categories of the Test Plan: Nursing Process, Caring, Communication and Documentation, and Teaching and Learning.

Again, note that the Health Promotion and Maintenance and Psychosocial Integrity categories do not have subcategories.

Overview of Content

All content categories reflect client needs across the life span in a variety of settings.

Safe, Effective Care Environment

The nurse promotes achievement of client outcomes by providing and directing nursing care that enhances the care delivery setting in order to protect clients, family/significant others and other health care personnel.

- **Management of Care**. Providing and directing nursing care that enhances the care delivery setting to protect clients, family/significant others, and health care personnel.

Related content includes but is not limited to:

- Advance Directives,
- Advocacy,
- Case Management,
- Client Rights,
- Collaboration with Multidisciplinary Team,
- Concepts of Management,
- Confidentiality,
- Consultation,
- Continuity of Care,
- Delegation,
- Establishing Priorities
- Ethical Practice
- Informed Consent
- Legal Rights and Responsibilities
- Performance Improvement (Quality Assurance)
- Referrals
- Resource Management
- Staff Education
- Supervision

- **Safety and Infection Control**. Protecting clients, family/significant others, and health care personnel from health and environmental hazards.

Related content includes but is not limited to:

- Accident Prevention
- Disaster Planning
- Emergency Response Plan
- Error Prevention
- Handling Hazardous and Infectious Materials
- Home Safety
- Injury Prevention
- Medical and Surgical Asepsis
- Reporting of Incident/Event/ Irregular Occurrence/Variance
- Safe Use of Equipment
- Security Plan
- Standard/Transmission-Based/ Other Precautions
- Use of Restraints/ Safety Devices

Health Promotion and Maintenance

The nurse provides and directs nursing care of the client and family/significant others that incorporates the knowledge of expected growth and development principles; prevention and/or early detection of health problems, and strategies to achieve optimal health.

Related content includes but is not limited to:

- Aging Process
- Ante/Intra/Postpartum and Newborn
- Developmental Stages and Transitions
- Disease Prevention
- Expected Body Image Changes
- Family Planning
- Family Systems
- Growth and Development
- Health and Wellness
- Health Promotion Programs
- Health Screening
- High Risk Behaviors
- Human Sexuality
- Immunizations
- Lifestyle Choices
- Principles of Teaching/ Learning
- Self-Care
- Techniques of Physical Assessment

Psychosocial Integrity

The nurse provides and directs nursing care that promotes and supports the emotional, mental, and social well-being of the client and family/significant others experiencing stressful events, as well as clients with acute or chronic mental illness.

Related content includes but is not limited to:

- Abuse/Neglect
- Behavioral Interventions
- Chemical Dependency
- Coping Mechanisms
- Crisis Intervention
- Cultural Diversity
- End of Life
- Family Dynamics
- Grief and Loss
- Mental Health Concepts
- Psychopathology
- Religious and Spiritual Influences on Health
- Sensory/Perceptual Alterations
- Situational Role Changes
- Stress Management
- Support Systems

- Therapeutic Communications
- Therapeutic Environment
- Unexpected Body Image Changes

Physiological Integrity

The nurse promotes physical health and wellness by providing care and comfort, reducing client risk potential, and managing health alterations.
- **Basic Care and Comfort**. Providing comfort and assistance in the performance of activities of daily living.

Related content includes but is not limited to:

- Alternative and Complementary Therapies
- Assistive Devices
- Elimination
- Mobility/Immobility
- Nonpharmacological Comfort Interventions
- Nutrition and Oral Hydration
- Palliative/Comfort Care
- Personal Hygiene
- Rest and Sleep

- **Pharmacological and Parenteral Therapies**. Providing care related to the administration of medications and parenteral therapies.

Related content includes but is not limited to:

- Adverse Effects/Contraindications and Side Effects
- Blood and Blood Products
- Central Venous Access Devices
- Dosage Calculation
- Expected Outcomes/Effects
- Intravenous Therapy
- Medication Administration
- Parenteral Fluids
- Pharmacological Agents/ Actions
- Pharmacological Interactions
- Pharmacological Pain Management
- Total Parenteral Nutrition

- **Reduction of Risk Potential**. Reducing the likelihood that clients will develop complications or health problems related to existing conditions, treatments, or procedures.

Related content includes but is not limited to:

- Diagnostic Tests
- Laboratory Values
- Monitoring Conscious Sedation
- Potential for Alterations in Body Systems
- Potential for Complications from Surgical Procedures and Health Alterations

- Potential for Complications of Diagnostic Tests/ Treatments/Procedures
- System Specific Assessments
- Therapeutic Procedures
- Vital Signs

- **Physiological Adaptation**. Managing and providing care for clients with acute, chronic, or life threatening physical health conditions.

Related content includes but is not limited to:

- Alterations in Body Systems
- Fluid and Electrolyte Imbalances
- Hemodynamics
- Illness Management
- Infectious Diseases

- Medical Emergencies
- Pathophysiology
- Radiation Therapy
- Unexpected Response to Therapies

Administration of the NCLEX-RN Examination

The NCLEX-RN exam is administered to the candidate by Computerized Adaptive Testing (CAT). CAT is a method of delivering exams that uses computer technology and measurement theory. Items go through an extensive review process before they can be used as items on the exam. Items on a candidate's exam are primarily four-option, multiple-choice items. Other types of item formats may include multiple-choice items that require a candidate to select one or more responses, fill-in-the-blank items, or items asking a candidate to identify an area on a picture or graphic. Any of the item formats, including standard multiple-choice items, may include charts, tables, or graphic images.

With CAT, each candidate's exam is unique because it is assembled interactively as the exam proceeds. Computer technology selects items to administer that match the candidate's ability level. The items, which are stored in a large item pool, have been classified by test plan area and level of difficulty. After the candidate answers an item, the computer calculates an ability estimate based on all of the previous answers the candidate selected. An item determined to measure the candidate's ability most precisely in the appropriate test plan area is selected and presented on the computer screen. This process is repeated for each item, creating an exam tailored to the candidate's knowledge and skills while fulfilling all *NCLEX-RN Test Plan* requirements. The exam continues with items selected and administered in this way until a pass or fail decision is made.

All registered nurse candidates must answer a minimum of 75 items. The maximum number of items that the candidate may answer during the exam period is 265. Exam instructions (tutorial interface), sample items, and all rest breaks are included in the measurement of the time allowed for a candidate to complete the exam.

More information about the NCLEX exam, including CAT methodology, is listed on the NCSBN website, www.ncsbn.org.

References for Appendix 13.1

American Nurses Association. (2003, February). *Nursing's social policy statement 2003.* Draft posted for public comment. Retrieved April 7, 2003, from http://www.nursingworld.org/practice. review of core documents/draft open standards

American Nurses Association. (2003, January). *Nursing: Scope and standards of practice.* Draft posted for public comment. Retrieved April 7, 2003, from http://www.nursingworld.org/practice. review of core documents/draft open standards

American Nurses Association. (2001). *Code of ethics for nurses with interpretive statements.* Washington DC: Author.

Anderson, L. W., & Krathwohl, D. R. (Eds). (2001). *A taxonomy for learning, teaching, and assessing. A revision of Bloom's taxonomy of educational objectives.* New York: Addison Wesley Longman.

Bloom, B. S., Engelhart, M. D., Furst, E. J., Hill, W. H., & Krathwohl, D. R. (1956). *Taxonomy of educational objectives: The classification of educational goals.* (Handbook I.) New York: David McKay.

National Council of State Boards of Nursing. (2002). *Model nursing administrative rules.* Chicago: Author.

Smith, J., & Crawford, L. (2003). *Report of findings from the 2002 RN practice analysis: Linking the NCLEX-RN examination to practice.* Chicago: National Council of State Boards of Nursing.

Appendix 13.2
NCLEX-PN Test Plan
Test Plan For The
National Council Licensure Examination
For Practical/Vocational Nurses
(NCLEX-PN Examination)

Reproduced from the NCSBN Web site (www.ncsbn.org) and used with permission from the National Council of State Boards of Nursing (NCSBN), Chicago, Illinois.

Introduction

Entry into the practice of nursing in the United States and its territories is regulated by the licensing authorities within each jurisdiction. To ensure public protection, each jurisdiction requires a candidate for licensure to pass an examination that measures the competencies needed to practice safely and effectively as a newly licensed, entry-level practical/vocational nurse. The National Council of State Boards of Nursing, Inc., develops a licensure examination, the *National Council Licensure Examination for Practical/ Vocational Nurses (NCLEX-PN Examination)*, which is used by state and territorial boards of nursing to assist in making licensure decisions.

The initial step in developing the NCLEX-PN Examination is the preparation of a test plan to guide the selection of content and behaviors to be tested. In this plan, provision is made for an examination reflecting entry-level practical/ vocational nursing as identified in the study entitled *Linking the NCLEX-PN National Licensure Examination to Practice: 2000 Job Analysis of Newly Licensed Practical/Vocational Nurses in the U.S.* (Smith, Crawford & Gawel, 2000). The activities identified in this study were analyzed in relation to: (1) the frequency of their performance, (2) their impact on maintaining client safety, and (3) the settings in which they were performed. This analysis guided the development of a framework that delineates specific client needs and integrated concepts and processes for entry-level practice. The variations in each jurisdiction's laws and regulations guide the development of the test plan.

The test plan derived from this framework provides a concise summary of the content and scope of the examination. The plan also serves as a guide for both examination development and candidate preparation as well as a guide for feedback for the unsuccessful candidate. Based on the test plan, each unique NCLEX-PN examination reflects the knowledge, skills, and abilities essential for the practical/vocational nurse to master in order to meet the needs of clients requiring the promotion, maintenance, and restoration of health. The following sections describe beliefs about nursing and clients that are integral to the examination, the cognitive abilities that will be tested in the examination, and the specific components of the NCLEX-PN Test Plan.

Beliefs

Beliefs about people and nursing underlie the NCLEX-PN Test Plan. People are viewed as having varying capacities to function in society. They are unique individuals defining their own systems of daily living which reflect values, cultures, motives, and lifestyles. Additionally, they are viewed as having the right to make decisions regarding their health care needs and participate in meeting those needs. The profession of nursing makes a unique contribution in helping clients (individuals or families/significant others) to achieve an optimal level of health in a variety of settings.

Nursing is an art and a science that integrates concepts from the liberal arts and the biological, behavioral, and social sciences. The nature of nursing is dynamic and evolving. The goal of nursing in any setting is to promote health and assist individuals throughout the life span to attain an optimal level of functioning by responding to the needs, conditions, or events that result from actual or potential health problems (American Nurses Association, 1995). The domain of nursing and the relevant knowledge, skills, and abilities exist along a continuum and are organized and defined by professional and legal parameters.

The practical/vocational nurse utilizes "specialized knowledge and skills which meet the health needs of people in a variety of settings under the direction of qualified health professionals" (NFLPN, 1996). The practical/vocational nurse uses a clinical problem solving process (the nursing process) to collect and organize relevant healthcare data and help identify the health needs and problems of clients throughout the clients' life span and in a variety of settings. The entry-level practical/vocational nurse, under appropriate supervision, provides competent care for clients with commonly occurring health problems having predictable outcomes. "Competency implies knowledge, understanding, and skills that transcend specific tasks and is guided by a commitment to ethical/legal principles" (NAPNES, 1999).

Levels of Cognitive Ability

The NCLEX-PN examination consists of multiple-choice items (questions) written at the cognitive levels of knowledge, comprehension, application, and analysis (Bloom et al, 1956).

Test Plan Structure

The framework of client needs was selected because it provides a universal structure for defining nursing actions and competencies for a variety of clients across a variety of settings and is congruent with state laws and statutes.

Client Needs

Four major categories of client needs organize the content of the test plan. These client needs are further divided into subcategories that define the content each category contains. These categories and subcategories are:

- Safe, Effective Care Environment
  - Coordinated Care
  - Safety and Infection Control
- Health Promotion and Maintenance
  - Growth and Development Through the Life Span
  - Prevention and Early Detection of Disease
- Psychosocial Integrity
  - Coping and Adaptation
  - Psychosocial Adaptation
- Physiological Integrity
  - Basic Care and Comfort
  - Pharmacological Therapies
  - Reduction of Risk Potential

- Physiological Adaptation

Integrated Concepts and Processes

The following concepts and processes fundamental to the practice of nursing are integrated throughout the four categories of Client Needs.

- Clinical Problem Solving Process (Nursing Process), a scientific approach to client care that includes data collection, planning, implementation and evaluation.
- Caring, the interaction of the nurse and client in an atmosphere of mutual respect and trust. In this collaborative environment, the nurse provides support and compassion to help achieve desired outcomes.
- Communication and Documentation, the verbal and/or nonverbal interactions between the nurse and client, significant others and members of the health care team; events and activities associated with client care as validated through a written or electronic record that reflects standards of practice and accountability into the provision of care.
- Cultural Awareness, the knowledge of and sensitivity to the beliefs and values of the client and nurse, and the integration of such awareness in the provision of nursing care.
- Self-Care, the practice of assisting clients of various abilities to meet their own health care needs, including maintenance of health and/or restoration of function.
- Teaching/Learning, the facilitation of the acquisition of knowledge, skills and attitudes that leads to a change in behavior.

Distribution of Content

The percentage of test questions assigned to each Client Needs subcategory in the NCLEX-PN Test Plan is based on the results of the study entitled *Linking the NCLEX-PN National Licensure Examination to Practice: 2000 Practice Analysis of Newly Licensed Practical/Vocational Nurses in the U.S.* (Smith, Crawford, & Gawel, 2000). Expert judgment was provided by members of the National Council's Examination Committee and by the 2000 Practice Analysis Panel of Experts.

Categories	Percentage of Test Questions
Safe, Effective Care Environment	
Coordinated Care	6%- 12%
Safety and Infection Control	7%- 13%
Health Promotion and Maintenance	
Growth and Development Through the Life Span	4%- 10%
Prevention and Early Detection of Disease	4%- 10%
Psychosocial Integrity	
Coping and Adaptation	6%- 12%
Psychosocial Adaptation	4%- 10%
Physiological Integrity	
Basic Care and Comfort	10%-16%
Pharmacological Therapies	5%- 11%
Reduction of Risk Potential	11%-17%
Physiological Adaptation	13%-19%

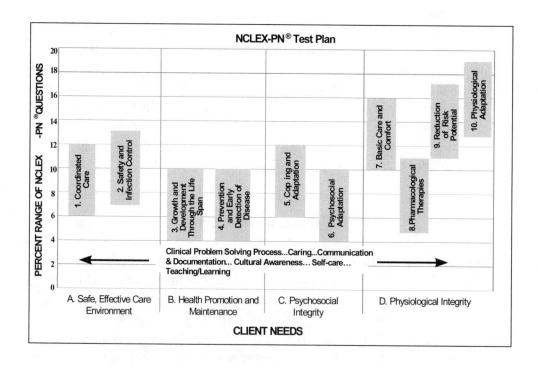

Overview of Content

All content categories reflect client needs across the life span in a variety of settings.

Safe, Effective Care Environment

The practical/vocational nurse provides nursing care and collaborates with others to enhance the care delivery setting and to protect clients, significant others and other health care personnel through:

- **Coordinated Care**. The practical/vocational nurse collaborates with other health care team members to facilitate effective client care.
  Related content includes, but is not limited to:

- Advance Directives
- Advocacy
- Client Care Assignments
- Client Rights
- Concepts of Management and Supervision
- Confidentiality
- Consultation with Members of the Health Care Team
- Continuity of Care
- Continuous Quality Improvement
- Establishing Priorities
- Ethical Practice
- Incident/Irregular Occurrence/ Variance Reports
- Informed Consent
- Legal Responsibilities
- Referral Processes
- Resource Management

- **Safety and Infection Control**. The practical/vocational nurse protects clients and health care personnel from environmental hazards.
  Related content includes, but is not limited to:

- Accident/Error Prevention
- Disaster Planning
- Handling Hazardous and Infectious Materials
- Medical and Surgical Asepsis
- Standard (Universal) and Other Precautions
- Use of Restraints

Health Promotion and Maintenance

The practical/vocational nurse provides and assists in directing nursing care, and promotes and maintains health through incorporating knowledge of the following areas:

- **Growth and Development Through the Life Span.** The practical/vocational nurse assists the client and significant others during the normal expected stages of growth and development from conception through advanced old age.

Related content includes, but is not limited to:

- Aging Process
- Ante/Intra/Postpartum and Newborn
- Developmental Stages and Transitions
- Expected Body Image Changes
- Family Interaction Patterns
- Family Planning
- Human Sexuality

- **Prevention and Early Detection of Disease.** The practical/vocational nurse provides client care related to prevention and early detection of health problems.

Related content includes, but is not limited to:

- Data Collection Techniques
- Disease Prevention
- Health Promotion Programs
- Health Screening
- Immunizations
- Lifestyle Choices

Psychosocial Integrity

The practical/vocational nurse provides nursing care that promotes and supports the emotional, mental and social well-being of the client and significant others in the following areas:

- **Coping and Adaptation.** The practical/vocational nurse promotes the ability of the client and/or significant others to cope, adapt and/or problem-solve situations related to illnesses, disabilities, and stressful events.

Related content includes, but is not limited to:

- Behavior Management
- Coping Mechanisms
- End of Life Issues
- Grief and Loss
- Mental Health Concepts
- Religious and Spiritual Influences on Health
- Sensory/Perceptual Alterations

- Situational Role Changes
- Stress Management
- Support Systems
- Therapeutic Communication
- Unexpected Body Image Changes

- **Psychosocial Adaptation.** The practical/vocational nurse participates in recognizing and providing care for clients with maladaptive behavior and assists with behavior management of the client with acute and/or chronic mental illness and cognitive psychosocial disturbances.

Related content includes, but is not limited to:

- Abuse and Neglect
- Behavioral Interventions
- Chemical Dependency
- Crisis Intervention

- Mental Illness Concepts
- Suicide
- Therapeutic Environment

Physiological Integrity

The practical/vocational nurse promotes physical health and well-being by providing care and comfort, reducing client risk potential and assisting to manage the client's health alterations.

- **Basic Care and Comfort.** The practical/vocational nurse provides comfort and assistance in the performance of activities of daily living.

Related content includes, but is not limited to:

- Assistive Devices
- Elimination
- Mobility/Immobility
- Non-pharmacological Pain Interventions

- Nutrition and Oral Hydration
- Palliative Care
- Personal Hygiene
- Rest and Sleep

- **Pharmacological Therapies.** The practical/vocational nurse provides care related to the administration of medications and monitors clients receiving parenteral therapies.

Related content includes, but is not limited to:

- Adverse Effects
- Expected Effects
- Medication Administration

- Pharmacological Actions
- Pharmacological Agents
- Side Effects

- **Reduction of Risk Potential.** The practical/vocational nurse reduces the client's potential for developing complications or health problems related to treatments, procedures or existing conditions.

Related content includes, but is not limited to:

- Diagnostic Tests
- Laboratory Values
- Potential Complications of Diagnostic Tests, Procedures, Surgery and Health Alterations

- Potential for Alterations in Body Systems
- Therapeutic Procedures

- **Physiological Adaptation.** The practical/vocational nurse participates in providing care to clients with acute, chronic or life-threatening physical health conditions.

Related content includes, but is not limited to:

- Alterations in Body Systems
- Basic Pathophysiology
- Fluid and Electrolyte Imbalances
- Medical Emergencies

- Radiation Therapy
- Respiratory Care
- Unexpected Response to Therapies

Administration of the NCLEX-PN Examination

The *NCLEX-PN Examination* is administered via computer using computerized adaptive testing (CAT). CAT is a method for administering tests that uses current computer technology and measurement theory. Movement through the examination, including the selection of answers, was accomplished via a computer mouse for the first time in the April, 2001, administration of the examinations. A drop-down calculator was also available to candidates for the first time during that testing.

With CAT, each candidate's test is unique: It is assembled interactively as the individual is tested. Each examination item (question) is subjected to an extensive review and pre-testing process. Those items that have met pre-established criteria may be used in the examination. The test items, which are stored in a large item pool, are classified by test plan area and level of difficulty. As the candidate answers each item, the computer calculates a competence estimate based on all earlier answers. An item determined to measure the candidate's ability most precisely in the appropriate test plan area is selected and presented on the computer screen. The process is repeated for each item, creating an examination tailored to the individual's knowledge and skills while fulfilling all NCLEX test plan requirements. The examination continues in this way until a pass or fail decision is made.

Candidates answer a minimum of 85 and a maximum of 205 items during the testing period. The maximum five-hour time limit to complete the examination includes the tutorial, sample questions, and all breaks.

A copy of this document may be downloaded from the National Council's website, www.ncsbn.org.

References for Appendix 13.2

Bloom, B. S., Engelhart, M. D., Furst, E. J., Hill, W. H., & Krathwohl, D. R. (1956). *Taxonomy of educational objectives: The classification of educational goals.* (Handbook I.) New York: David McKay.

National Association for Practical Nurse Educators and Service. (1999). *Standards of practice for LPN/VNs.* Silver Spring, MD: Author.

National Federation of Licensed Practical Nurses. (1996). *Nursing practice standards for the licensed practical/vocational nurse.* Raleigh, NC: Author.

Smith, J. E., Crawford, L. H., & Gawel, S. H. (2000). *Linking the NCLEX-PN National Licensure Examination to practice: 2000 practice analysis of newly licensed Practical/Vocational Nurses in the U.S.* Chicago: National Council of State Boards of Nursing.

Appendix 13.3
NCLEX-RN Frequently Asked Questions

NCSBN

Leading in Nursing Regulation

National Council of State Boards of Nursing, Inc.
111 E. Wacker Drive, Suite 2900
Chicago, IL 60601-4277
312-525-3600 NCSBN
866-293-9600 Toll Free
312-279-1036 Testing Services fax

Frequently Asked Questions about the *2004 NCLEX-RN Test Plan*

What was the basis for making changes to the 2004 *NCLEX-RN Test Plan*?

NCSBN reviews both the NCLEX-RN and NCLEX-PN test plans once every three years. The recommended changes to the *2004 NCLEX-RN Test Plan* are based upon empirical data collected from newly licensed nurses, which can be found in the study published by NCSBN entitled *Report of Findings from the 2002 Practice Analysis: Linking the NCLEX-RN Examination to Practice.*

The practice analysis provides evidence regarding those activities that entry-level nurses are performing and the importance of those activities. In this study, more than 4,000 newly licensed nurses were surveyed regarding the frequency and priority of performing 138 nursing care activities. The data were analyzed and used to determine whether changes were needed in the test plan. Based upon the most recent survey results, as well as expert opinion and feedback from stakeholders, the NCSBN Delegate Assembly unanimously adopted the *2004 NCLEX-RN Test Plan* in August 2003.

What were the specific changes and rationale for the changes to the test plan?

Based upon empirical data from the practice analysis, expert judgment, and feedback from stakeholders, *client needs* was retained as the framework for the

274

2004 NCLEX-RN Test Plan.

Rationale: The practice analysis data and expert opinion supported retaining this structure. In addition, the client needs structure provides a common framework that is easily understood by candidates and other stakeholders. This structure also allows content to be updated without changing the test plan and facilitates reliable item coding. The four Client Needs categories have been retained, and the titles of the subcategories safe, effective care environment and physiological integrity have been retained as well. Also, the health promotion and maintenance and psychosocial integrity categories have been retained. However, there are no subcategories under health Promotion and maintenance and psychosocial integrity.

The 10 subcategories of the 2001 NCLEX-RN Test Plan were condensed into eight categories and subcategories for the 2004 NCLEX-RN Test Plan. The content from growth and development through the life span and the content from prevention and early detection of disease subcategories were combined and placed in the health promotion and maintenance category. The content from the coping and adaptation and psychosocial adaptation subcategories were combined and placed in the proposed psychosocial integrity category.

Rationale: The practice analysis data and expert opinion supported this framework in order to have conceptually coherent categories with sufficient content to allow for meaningful measurement of competencies.

The integrated concepts and processes section is now known as integrated processes because the two concepts, cultural awareness and self care, are distributed to specific content categories. In the proposed test plan, cultural awareness is part of psychosocial integrity and self care is part of health promotion and maintenance.

Rationale: Changing the title to **integrated processes** was necessary because this part of the test plan included only processes that apply to all categories and subcategories of the proposed test plan. For the purpose of maintaining conceptually consistent subcategories, the concept of cultural awareness was placed in the psychosocial integrity category and the self-care concept was placed in the health promotion and maintenance category.

The percentage of test items allocated to each client needs category and subcategory was revised. As illustrated in the chart below, there was a reduction in the percentage of test items in psychosocial integrity and health promotion and maintenance. There was a concomitant increase in the percentage of test items allocated to management of care, safety and infection control and pharmacological and parenteral therapies.

Rationale: The percentage of test items is based upon empirical data from the practice analysis study as well as psychometric considerations regarding the minimum number of examination items that are necessary to reliably sample a content category.

Some of the content listings (bulleted concepts) within each of the test plan categories/subcategories were revised, and new content listings were added.

Rationale: These changes were necessary based upon a review and assignment of each of the 2002 practice analysis task statements to a category/subcategory of the client needs structure. Other revisions are necessary for reasons of conceptual clarity, currency, and correction of redundancy.

2004 RN TEST PLAN

Client Needs Categories/Subcategories	Percentage of Items
Safe Effective Care Environment	
• Management of Care	13%-19%
• Safety and Infection Control	8%-14%
Health Promotion and Maintenance	6%-12%
Psychosocial Integrity	6%-12%
Physiological Integrity	
• Basic Care and Comfort	6%-12%
• Pharmacological and Parenteral Therapies	13%-19%
• Reduction of Risk Potential	13%-19%
• Physiological Adaptation	115-17%

2001 RN TEST PLAN

Categories	Percentage of Items
Safe, Effective Care Environment	
• Management of Care	7%-13%
• Safety and Infection Control	5%-11%
Health Promotion And Maintenance	
• Growth and Development Through the Life Span	7%-13%
• Prevention and Early Detection of Disease	5%-11%
Psychosocial Integrity	
• Coping and Adaptation	5%-11%
• Psychosocial Adaptation	5%-11%
Physiological Integrity	
• Basic Care and Comfort	7%-13%
• Pharmacological and Parenteral Therapies	5%-11%
• Reduction of Risk Potential	12%-18%
• Physiological Adaptation	12%-18%

What are the cognitive levels of the test items on the *2004 NCLEX-RN Test Plan*?

Since the practice of nursing requires the application of knowledge, skills and abilities, the majority of items on the NCLEX-RN examination are written at the application or higher levels of cognitive ability using Bloom's taxonomy and revised taxonomy (Bloom, 1956; Anderson and Krathwohl, 2001). These higher-level items require more complex thought processing and problem solving. Just as in nursing practice, many of the items in the NCLEX-RN examination address complex client problems and situations. For example, a pediatric client undergoing a medical procedure may have a concomitant mental illness and all factors must be considered in order to prepare the client for the procedure and to correctly answer the item.

What percentage of test items are allocated for nursing practice specialty areas such as psychiatric and mental health nursing?

The framework for the test plan is based on clients needs; therefore, it is not possible to specify the percentage of test items that address a particular nursing specialties such as psychiatric and mental health nursing. Content related to this nursing practice specialty can be found in many areas of the test plan. For example, the ANA/APNA *Standards for Psychiatric and Mental Health Nursing* mention promotion of self-care activities, health teaching, and health promotion and maintenance as global interventions used by the psychiatric nurse. Many of these activities, and thus examination items assessing these competencies, are categorized in the health promotion and maintenance category of the 2004 NCLEX-RN Test Plan. The psychobiological interventions and thus examination items assessing these competencies may be categorized in the pharmacological and parenteral therapies test plan subcategory.

Case management activities and examination items assessing these competencies may be categorized in the management of care subcategory of the test plan. At first glance, it may seem that the only test plan category that assesses the psychiatric and mental health nursing competencies of the entry-level nurse is the psychosocial integrity category, a more detailed analysis reveals that many test plan areas address the core competencies needed for psychiatric and mental health nursing. Thus, there are many opportunities within the structure of the 2004 NCLEX-RN Test Plan to assess the core competencies that are mentioned in the *Standards for Psychiatric and Mental Health Nursing*. There are analogous circumstances for other nursing practice specialties and subspecialties such as pediatric nursing and geriatric nursing.

What impact will these test plan changes have on nursing curricula?

It is difficult to determine if there will be any impact on nursing curricula because of the test plan changes. There is a significant variation in the nursing education programs' missions and philosophies, and this variety is reflected in their curricula. Since nursing practice is a continually evolving discipline, and practice analyses are conducted every three years, it may not be practical to revise a curriculum based on the minor changes in the 2004 NCLEX-RN Test Plan. However, the test plan may be a useful document for nursing programs to consider when reviewing a curriculum because the test plan is based upon the knowledge, skills, and abilities that are needed to practice nursing safely and effectively at the entry level.

Who are the stakeholders that provided feedback on the test plans?

Recommendations regarding the 2004 NCLEX-RN Test Plan were sent to boards of nursing, the NCSBN board of directors, the subcommittee of NCSBN's examination committee, the item review subcommittee, the practice analysis panel of experts, and NCSBN legal counsel. All of these stakeholders were asked to provide feedback to the examination committee regarding the test plan recommendations. The feedback was reviewed and changes were made to the test plan as appropriate. The examination committee then recommended the test plan changes to NCSBN's governing body, the delegate assembly. This process helped ensure a comprehensive review of the test plan and involvement of groups with a variety of viewpoints.

What was the timeline for implementing the test plan?

- January 2003: Examination committee received results of 2002 RN practice analysis and recommended revisions to the 2004 NCLEX-RN Test Plan.
- February 2003: Proposed test plan circulated to stakeholders, requesting feedback by March 31.
- April 2003: Examination committee reviewed feedback and approved the proposed 2004 NCLEX-RN Test Plan.
- May 2003: Examination committee submitted 2004 NCLEX-RN Test Plan to the delegate assembly for approval.
- August 2003: Delegate assembly approved test plan and implementation timeline.
- April 2004: 2004 NCLEX-RN Test Plan implemented.

This timeline was needed to ensure adequate time is available to analyze the data and the stakeholders to provide feedback. Additionally, NCSBN needs time to communicate about changes to the test plan. So, while there is pressure to implement the test plan as soon as possible because there has been a change in practice, there is counterpressure to communicate the change so everyone is informed.

When will the NCLEX-RN test plan be reviewed again ?

Since practice analyses are conducted every three years, the current timeline represents almost a continuous process of evaluating the test plan for necessary changes. Data collection for the 2005 registered nurse practice analysis is anticipated to begin in the spring of 2005. Consequently, the NCSBN delegate assembly would be expected to vote on a new test plan in 2006, with implementation occurring in 2007.

What background references may be helpful for individuals interested in the test plans?

American Educational Research Association, American Psychological Association, National Council on Measurement in Education. (2000). *Standards for educational and psychological testing.* Washington, DC: American Educational Research Association.

Anderson, L. W., & Krathwohl, D. R. (Eds). (2001). *A taxonomy for learning, teaching, and assessing. A revision of Bloom's taxonomy of educational objectives.* New York: Addison Wesley Longman.

Bloom, B. S., Engelhart, M. D., Furst, E. J., Hill, W. H., & Krathwohl, D. R. (1956). *Taxonomy of educational objectives: The classification of educational goals.* (Handbook I.) New York: David McKay.

Smith, J., & Crawford, L. (2003). *Report of findings from the 2002 RN practice analysis: Linking the NCLEX-RN examination to practice.* Chicago: Author.

Focus on Curriculum

Unit 4

Chapter 14: Engaging Students for Affective Learning
            Throughout the Curriculum
        Arlene Morris, BSN, MSN, RN,
        and Lynn Norman, BSN, MSN, RN

Chapter 15: Using Educational Theory as a Basis for Leveling
            Nursing Laboratory Simulation Experiences
        Arlene Morris, BSN, MSN, RN

Chapter 16: Benchmarking for Progression: Implications for
            Students, Faculty, and Administrators
        Ainslie Taylor Nibert, MSN, PhD, RN, CCRN

Chapter 17: Academic Program Review
        Jeffrey Papp, MS, PhD, RT(R)(QM)

Chapter 14: Engaging Students for Affective Learning Throughout the Curriculum

Arlene Morris, BSN, MSN, RN,
and Lynn Norman, BSN, MSN, RN

Attitude, professionalism, and caring—these are all important in the making of a nurse. Most people can learn to perform nursing psychomotor skills, but performing those skills in a caring, respectful manner is the hallmark of a true nurse. This chapter reminds us of the importance of developing a professional attitude and give us guidance for integrating this lesson throughout the curriculum. – Linda Caputi

Educational Philosophy

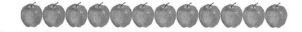

My teaching philosophy includes two core values that are also inherent in my nursing philosophy: the dignity of the individual and an emphasis on quality. I believe the individual student brings personal attributes and experiences to the learning environment. Nurse educators are challenged to build on these to assist the student in developing both a commitment to learning and a self-expectation of providing the highest quality nursing care. Transformation in both student and faculty occurs through collaboration as students are actively engaged in seeking their highest level of knowledge and professional nursing performance. – Arlene Morris

Students enter classroom settings with a variety of backgrounds and personal experiences that make each individual unique. The teacher or learning facilitator should utilize this uniqueness as a building block to help learners explore steps toward achieving their learning goals. The facilitator can employ cognitive, psychomotor, and affective teaching strategies in a climate conducive to making learning practical and fun. – Lynn Norman

Introduction

Nursing is a rapidly expanding body of knowledge that continues to evolve. This evolution demands that faculty constantly reevaluate what must be included in nursing curricula. One of the main dilemmas in nursing education is selecting the content for courses, and placing these courses within the curriculum. Krathwohl, Bloom, and Masia (1964) developed a comprehensive list of instructional objectives, divided into three major domains: cognitive, psychomotor, and affective. Curriculum design must account for student achievement in the cognitive domain of learning, such as that tested in traditional examinations, and in the psychomotor domain, such as performance of nursing skills in clinical settings. In developing curriculum concepts, the tendency may be to overlook the affective domain of learning (Martin and Briggs, 1986). The neglect of affective learning outcomes may be more evident in the current era of ever-changing, evidence-based nursing practice.

Reasons to Incorporate Affective Learning

There are valid reasons to include the affective domain of learning throughout the nursing curriculum. Affective learning helps form the character of the professional nurse. Nursing literature addresses this need. The American Association of Colleges of Nursing (AACN) (1998) includes "development of professional values and value-based behaviors" (p. 8) as foundations for practice. The central concept for nursing education is caring and consists of the following suggested professional values:
- Altruism;
- Respect for client autonomy;
- Respect for human dignity;
- Integrity; and
- Respect for social justice (AACN, 1998, pp. 8-9).

Certain disciplines, such as nursing, involve interpersonal interactions that must be based on a set of values that are vital to the caring perspective (Zimmerman & Phillips, 2000).

Affective learning may also be overlooked because of the ethical questions, "Should teachers teach values?" and "Should indoctrination be part of the instructor's role?" (Martin, 1989, p. 16). However, Brookfield (1989) supposed that emotions are **essential** in the process to stimulate critical thinking. Nursing is a discipline in which situations arise that require critical thinking. Students must be prepared to critically think about their own values for client interactions in varying situations.

Enhancing Cognitive Retention

Belanger and Jordan (2000) wrote that using the affective domain enhances cognitive retention. In their work evaluating and implementing distance learning, they asserted that affective strategies raise the student's level of interest and engagement in the instructional content, and that affective learning engages the learner when the instructional material engages multiple senses. In addition to cognitive learning, learners feel, see, and touch, enabling them to use more senses than they would by sitting passively in lecture-based course environments.

One method of appealing to multiple senses is through audiovisual presentations. A brief display of graphics coupled with a song related to the pictures can have a powerful affect on the emotional response of students. This response can set the tone for a subsequent lecture. On the CD-ROM accompanying this book is a video called *Safe Home*, which was produced by College of DuPage as an introduction to a lecture on domestic violence. Readers are invited to view this video and use it with their students.

Valuing

Valuing also increases motivation to change behavior. Martin and Briggs (1989) have researched the integration of the affective and cognitive domains. They claim that in order for a change in behavior to occur, the student must develop an attitude of valuing the behavior. It is important that the instructional design be planned to enable the student to develop the desired value.

The socialization of nursing students progresses along levels of attaining professional nursing values and attitudes. Krathwohl, et al (1964), differentiate levels of affective learning that progress from receiving, responding, and valuing, to the organization of values into a system with the ultimate development of a characteristic lifestyle. Included in their definition of affective learning is the principle of internalization, "… the process by which the phenomenon or value successfully and pervasively becomes a part of the individual" (p. 28).

Levels of Affective Learning

The beginning point of teaching in the affective domain is gaining the attention of the individual nursing student to some concept. An awareness begins as the nursing student pays attention to that concept. Thus, the lowest level of affective learning is **receiving**, in which an emotional connection gradually is formed with the concept. The next level is **responding**, in which the nursing student's reactions to similar stimuli become more consistent. Professional nursing **valuing**, the next level, continues to form in an internalization process as the student develops a preference for, or commitment to, the concept. The next step involves the nursing values being organized into a personal value system. Successful **internalization** of the values taught in the beginning nursing courses enables the student to use these values in situations throughout the curriculum and to continue the valuing process until their individual value system for the nursing profession becomes organized. Finally, the values are interrelated, or **organized**, in a structure or worldview that the student brings to new problems, and the student responds consistently to value-laden situations as a professional nurse (Krathwohl, Bloom & Masia, 1964, pp. 33-35).

Faculty may encounter difficulty in planning to include affective teaching strategies and methods to evaluate the learning attained from those strategies. Measurable outcomes for student learning should be specified for each level of affective learning attained. The receiving level involves the student attending to a stimulus and can be evaluated by observation of the student's engagement in the content. The responding level entails the student showing a behavior such as answering questions. The valuing level includes the student showing involvement or commitment, and may be evaluated by how the student is beginning to use the newly learned concept. The organization level occurs as the student incorporates the behavior into nursing practice, and may be evaluated by observation in classroom or clinical settings. The characteristic lifestyle level of affective learning has associated behavior changes in which the concept is more consistently demonstrated (Krathwohl, et al, 1964). Emphasis on the responding and valuing levels allows more immediate evaluation, whereas the organization and development of a characteristic lifestyle level may occur post-graduation or later in the graduate's nursing practice. The goals of faculty are to recognize the need for affective learning in nursing curriculum design, identify strategies to engage students in affective learning, and offer methods for effective evaluation.

The Climate for Affective Learning

Consideration of the climate for affective learning is essential. Nursing faculty must take into account the learners' attitudes, values, and experiences. Instruction in the affective domain may be disorienting if the student's attitudes, values, or experiences conflict with those of the nursing profession, or if the student has not reflected on personal values before beginning the course (Mezirow, 2000). The following suggestions may help when planning a climate for affective learning:

- Provide a climate of acceptance of student differences in attitudes and values, and of encouragement to ponder the values presented, to promote student reflection and integration.
- Allow time for student reflection or pondering of issues. Hall discussion, peer group discussion, pre- or postclinical conference, or appointments with faculty may be helpful especially if strong feelings have been aroused.
- Consider what is happening during the learning activity. Is there so much activity that the situation will be distracting and cloud the value being taught? Simple to complex educational strategies are more effective when teaching in the affective domain.
- Identify the value to be gained prior to structuring the assignment. Structure the assignment to achieve the goal of value development. Design lessons to simultaneously influence achievement of both affective and cognitive behaviors (Martin, 1989).

Timing in the curriculum is also highly important for students to relate the intended value to actual life experiences. First-semester nursing students need stories, role playing, or interactive activities because they may lack a background of experiences with clients. More advanced students may recall experiences with clients from previous courses, and may be able to associate new learning with their experience. For example, the value of human dignity may be introduced as a role play for first-semester students in which there is an obvious lack of respect for an individual in a healthcare setting. Students may then brainstorm methods to improve the interaction to include respect for human dignity. Thus, an early example can provide a basis for interaction with clients in later semesters or clinical settings.

Planning activities to engage students throughout the curriculum provides teachers an opportunity to encourage development of the values close to the time the student will experience similar situations in clinical settings, and allows the stu- dent to reflect on how the values can be applied in various situations. Dignity of client and empathy are recurring themes in all nursing content. Reinforcement of affective content in courses throughout the curriculum promotes revisiting "valued" concepts in later semesters. Also, revisiting issues helps faculty determine if students' behavior has changed.

Structured learning activities allow students to experience the dilemmas of potential value conflict in the traditional classroom, nursing laboratory, or web-based distance learning environment. Faculty should encourage alternative feelings and provide feedback (Mezirow, 2000). The internalization of the value—when it becomes a characteristic of the student's lifestyle or as part of nursing practice—may actually occur later in the curriculum following several experiences (Martin & Briggs, 1986).

Evaluation Strategies to Determine Outcome

Evaluation is actually twofold: Did the learner achieve the outcome? Was the teaching strategy effective? To assess affective learning, the faculty should first write affective objectives or outcomes.

An example of a short-term outcome is: Did the students feel the content?

An example of a long-term outcome is: Do the students use the outcome in actual nursing practice?

Several tools may be used to assess the effectiveness of affective learning (Martin & Briggs, 1986):

- Questionnaires;
- Interviews;
- Self-reporting; and
- Behavioral observations.

Additionally, attitudinal questions can be included in written examinations or case studies.

Often, the development of a value takes longer than classroom time allows. That is why assessment of attainment of the objectives may occur several months or years after the value has been introduced. Behavioral changes are the best indicators that a change in affective learning has taken place. For the nursing student, the outcomes are heightened awareness of potential client needs and the development of attitudes for providing higher quality nursing care—changes in behavior. A postgraduation survey may be needed to evaluate long-term changes in behavior.

Suggested Affective Learning Strategies Throughout the Curriculum

A variety of affective teaching strategies can be incorporated throughout the curriculum.

Nursing Fundamentals

An activity during students' first semester should involve a type of values clarification exercise. One method of incorporating personal values is to have the students identify values that are most important to them and incorporate those values into a personal nursing philosophy. Students are encouraged to review their personal nursing philosophy throughout the curriculum and make revisions based on new learning or experiences. A final nursing philosophy is submitted during the capstone course.

Students can be exposed to the broad concept of caring through many teaching strategies. Probably the most important teaching method is encouraging students to take note of the caring attitudes and behaviors of teachers, peers, and staff nurses. The curriculum can provide early opportunities for students to record observations of caring activities in clinical settings with the observed responses of clients, family, and interdisciplinary healthcare team members. However, other learning activities can be included in the presentation of course content. Triads of students can be asked to brainstorm synonyms for **caring**, and to write brief narratives of a time when they experienced caring. The narratives can then be reviewed to determine what aspect of caring was effectively demonstrated. Students can be assigned to write a response to an article such as Benner's "The Wisdom of Our Practice" (2000), in which a professional nurse leader discusses caring concepts. Photos and brief summaries of nurses' experiences, such as those included in Smeltzer and Vlasses' (2003) *Ordinary People, Extraordinary Lives: The Stories of Nurses*, can be used as introductions to various topics.

During the first-semester nursing concepts course, a role play may be used in which some students act as clients being admitted for a routine surgery and others pose as the healthcare providers they encounter (Alderman and Brien,

1987). In the script, calling the client by terms referring to the service to be provided— for example, the broccoli dietary tray, the gall bladder x-ray, the broken call bell, the red pill—provides opportunity for students to identify a need for dignity, respect, and courteous interaction with all clients. The scripted interaction of interdisciplinary healthcare providers rapidly entering the client's hospital room focusing on tasks instead of the client provides an opportunity for beginning nursing students to respond to the need to address the client holistically. This activity should be held prior to the initial clinical experience. The intended learning outcome is the valuing of human dignity through awareness of healthcare team members' verbal and nonverbal communication and transmission of attitudes to a client in the vulnerable situation of hospital admission.

A faculty-created role play may be used during the semester in which acute care or end-of-life issues are taught. Several members of the nursing faculty act as clients near death, while intergenerational family members are in conflict regarding end-of-life decisions. Exaggerated costumes and dramatic acting can be used to quickly engage the students' attention in the learning activity. End-of-life issues can be emotionally charged for students and faculty, and a role play promotes a safe environment in which students can explore personal feelings before encountering the situation in an actual clinical setting. Portrayal of diverse family members' conflicting desires related to end-of-life issues presents the value of respect for the client's autonomy and informed consent. This role play is performed once with faculty making blatant errors in dealing with the client, family, and healthcare team members, as well as with the actual nursing care and environment. Students individually identify and list errors, compare the list with a peer, and then engage in a class discussion to determine more effective methods of dealing with the difficult and emotionally charged end-of-life situation. The role play and discussion allow recall of personal experiences and exploration of effective methods of interacting with clients and family members. Immediately following the class discussion, a second role play should be performed with several student volunteers to act as the healthcare providers and the same faculty playing the client and family members. Prompts from students who are not participating in the role play are welcomed. End-of-life issues that students once regarded as depressing become real, and an opportunity to provide the ideal nursing care for client and family is realized. The classroom is a safer environment for reflection on the emotionally charged concepts than an unexpected clinical situation with an actual client. The outcomes of valuing client autonomy can be evaluated immediately by student discussion, and then later evaluated in the clinical setting when similar situations occur.

Cultural awareness can be promoted by many teaching strategies. Online discussion can provide valuable insight about student perceptions and learning. The faculty can present findings from interviews with people from cultural backgrounds different from that of the student. International nursing classes can link via the Internet to discuss cultural and healthcare issues. Teachers can arrange games of BaFá BaFá (Shirts, 1977), an interactive activity developed to promote sensitivity to cultural customs. Following presentation of content that may be culturally sensitive, students may wish to express their feelings, especially if a dilemma has occurred (Mezirow, 2000). Planned opportunities for continued discussion may be needed.

Fundamental Skills

The basic skill of handwashing can be taught with an emphasis on the affective domain. The affective learning objective for handwashing is to impact the student's attitude regarding the importance and relevance of proper handwashing technique. A teaching strategy to demonstrate the importance of the thoroughness of handwashing involves the use of a product called Glo Germ. Students are instructed in handwashing, rinsing, and drying techniques. Glo Germ, an oil-based liquid that glows under ultraviolet light, is then placed on their hands. Students wash their hands, then view them under fluorescent lighting. An orange glow indicates where bacteria would have remained on their hands. Initially, students are startled by how much "bacteria" remains after they washed their hands so thoroughly. At the end of the semester, a follow-up questionnaire assesses any change in student behavior regarding handwashing in clinical and personal settings. Students state increased awareness of the importance of thorough handwashing, and report changes in behaviors such as washing hands more diligently and more often.

Changing soiled gloves is another important skill for aseptic technique in nursing fundamentals. Teaching a student to remove gloves requires little innovation unless affective learning is a goal. Using chocolate pudding to demonstrate soiled gloves is an effective strategy (G. Langham, personal communication, September 12, 2003). Students don clean gloves and are asked to close their eyes and place their hands in front of them. The instructor places a dollop of pudding in the palm of each student's hands and tells the students to gently rub their hands together. With the student's eyes still shut, the instructor describes a scenario in which the nurse must empty a bed pan or attempt to dislodge a fecal impaction. The students are instructed to look at the gloves and then remove them using proper technique. The chocolate pudding reminds students to be cognizant of the correct way to remove gloves. Evaluation is evidenced by student comments and behavior changes in the clinical setting.

Beginning nursing students often have had limited experience touching and caring for strangers. Morning care, which includes bathing, oral care, and hair care, is a common routine that students perform on themselves every day. To incorporate affective learning, students are required to brush each other's teeth in the laboratory setting prior to attending clinical. Each student chooses a partner, brings a toothbrush and toothpaste, and performs oral care on his or her partner. In classes led by the authors, students have commented that it is easier to perform the skill on themselves than on each other. Performing the skill on each other enhances the students' awareness of how it feels to have someone provide supportive care for them, before they face an actual situation in which they must provide supportive care to a client. Learning outcomes of empathy can be evaluated by student comments and actual behaviors in the clinical setting.

Maternal/Newborn Nursing Course

A canvas apron, a partially inflated beach ball, and scuba diving weights can be used as props to teach students about the changes of late pregnancy for an affective learning in a maternal/newborn course. To simulate the last few weeks of pregnancy, attach eight pounds of scuba weights to the apron so that when a student wears the apron, the weights put pressure on the student's bladder. The ball is inflated to the extent needed to represent the effect of a term uterus pushing up on the diaphragm. Each student wears the apron for one or two hours during the semester. They experience the challenge of getting in and out of their desks or picking up a pencil from the floor.

Six months later the students are surveyed for their reaction and to ascertain if their behavior changed when caring for late-term pregnant clients. Student responses to this exercise have been positive, with several students, including men, stating that this strategy gave them a better appreciation for pregnant clients' challenges and influenced their provision of care. The students reported that they allowed more time for maternal clients to change positions, ambulate, and perform simple activities.

Pediatric Nursing Course

Parents speaking to students about the intense feelings they experienced when their child required care for serious health problems can help students become more aware of family needs. The affective learning outcome at the **receiving** level is achieved as students listen to the parents, then question them about their experiences with nursing care for their infant children who had major anomalies and subsequently died. Evaluation of the affective learning level of **responding** is also evident by the students' emotional reactions, including attempts to comfort the parent as students and speaker share tears. The level of **valuing** may be evaluated in the clinical setting as the needs of family members are addressed.

Care of Older Adult/Chronicity Nursing Course

Several teaching strategies can promote the nursing value of human dignity when providing nursing care to older adults. Having students play the role of the client is very effective for giving students the opportunity to experience how older clients perceive the environment and/or deal with physical changes (Tsushima & Gecas, 2001). Sensory alterations of aging can be simulated with:
- Construction paper glasses with distorted lenses to create the effect of multiple eye disorders;
- Cotton in the ears;
- Audiotapes in which consonants are less audible than vowels; and
- Masking tape around the fingers to limit flexibility.

With these alterations, each student is asked to retrieve a dime from a small plastic bag. The affective learning goal of **valuing** the challenges of functionality when dealing with effects of aging or chronic illness is realized.

Another strategy is having students sit in a wheelchair with vest and wrist restraints for the duration of a class. Students generally comment at the end of an hour they need to change positions. Students also comment about the feelings they experience while watching other students leave the room for a break.

A third role play taps into student creativity. Students are asked to attend class dressed to represent a chronic illness, with body image or psychosocial implications demonstrated in the design. During class, each student briefly describes the disease process, psychosocial implications, functional limitations, and methods the student believes might be helpful in dealing with the issues identified.

Videos also can help convey respect for the dignity of older adults. Short clips may provide a model of caring behaviors of caregivers toward older adults. For example, the portion of the motion picture *Driving Miss Daisy* (Zanuck, Zanuck & Beresford, 1989) in which a gentleman feeds pie to an older nursing home resident can promote discussion regarding meaningful interaction with older adults and methods of providing feeding. The video *Tucked in Tight* (Gauldin & Caputi, 2001) uses music and images to depict caring interactions of a caregiver with an elderly lady in an extended care facility. Portions of this video and a discussion about the instructional design used to develop this piece are included in Chapter 14 of the CD-ROM accompanying this book.

Mental Health Nursing Course

Reflective journaling can be utilized throughout the nursing curriculum and is especially useful in mental health nursing. Stories by students and clients about coping with stressful events encourage contemplation and promote student attainment of the affective level of **valuing** of effective interventions. Reflective journaling also can be used throughout the curriculum for students to identify areas in which they have demonstrated professional growth, thereby providing a method to evaluate the **organization** level of attainment of professional nursing behaviors and values.

The online environment can be used to provide more time to reflect on, and respond to, value-laden assessments. The online environment also affords privacy with responses that is not possible in the classroom.

Community Health Nursing Course

Student involvement in community assessments promotes awareness of the needs of individuals and groups in various communities. Communication with individuals and community leaders fosters interaction and gives students the opportunity to care for people whose backgrounds might be different than their own. The empathy developed can enhance the socialization of nursing students and make them more aware of the professional nursing value of social justice. Planning effective community interventions enables students to achieve the affective learning level of **valuing** the residents' needs.

Summary

Goleman (1994) wrote that increased empathy can be linked to increased motivation to intervene. Those engaged in nursing as a discipline must develop motivation to intervene and provide quality care for their clients. Planning educational strategies to promote affective learning is a necessary component of nursing education. Strategies that incorporate the affective domain can be integrated with content for the cognitive or psychomotor domain.

The effectiveness of affective teaching must be evaluated using different criteria than is used to evaluate cognitive or psychomotor teaching. Learner participation, engagement, enjoyment, or motivation are outcomes that can be measured for the **receiving** and **responding** levels of affective learning. Did the teaching strategy achieve the intended outcome of student **valuing** and **internalizing** the concept? Are professional nursing **behavioral patterns** being formed that can be observed in student interactions with clients?

The educational strategies presented in this chapter are intended to provide suggestions for incorporating the affective domain in nursing education, with the hope that they will spark ideas for many more effective affective strategies among creative nursing educators.

Learning Activities

1. Write two or three affective learning objectives.
2. Associate the above learning objectives to Krathwohl's levels of attainment in the affective domain—receiving, responding, valuing, organization, or characterization.
3. Plan teaching strategies to promote attainment of the learning objectives in Learning Activity 1.
4. Develop a survey tool that can be used to evaluate affective learning, focusing on both immediate and long-term behavior changes. The following table may be helpful for completing this learning activity

Student Learning Objective	Level of Affective Attainment	Teaching Strategy	Method of Evaluation

5. Identify affective teaching strategies that can best be used for distance learning.

References

Alderman, S., & Brien, A. (1987). *I am the broccoli.* Customer Communication Systems.

American Association of Colleges of Nurses. (1998). *Essentials of baccalaureate nursing education.* Washington, DC: Author.

Belanger, F. & Jordan, D. (2000). *Evaluation and implementation of distance learning: Technologies, tools, and techniques.* Hershey, PA: Idea Group.

Benner, P. (2001). The wisdom of our practice. *American Journal of Nursing, 100*(10), 99-105.

Brookfield, S. D. (1990). *The skillful teacher.* San Francisco: Jossey-Bass.

Gauldin, D., & Caputi, L. (2001), *Tucked in tight.* [videotape]. Glen Ellyn, IL: College of DuPage.

Goleman, D. (1994). *Emotional intelligence.* New York: Bantam.

Glo Germ Co. (2004). Retrieved Febraury, 2004, from http://www.glogerm.com.

Krathwohl, D. R., Bloom, B. S., & Masia, B. B. (1964). *Taxonomy of educational objectives: The classification of educational goals. Handbook II: Affective domain.* New York: Longman.

Martin, B. L. (1989). A checklist for designing instruction in the affective domain. Retrieved April 5, 2004 from http:// plaza.v-wave.com/kegj/mar.html.

Martin, B. L., & Briggs, L. J. (1986). *The affective and cognitive domains: Integration for instruction and research.* Englewood Cliffs, NJ: Educational Technology Publications.

Mezirow, J., & Associates. (2000). *Learning as transformation: Critical perspectives on a theory in progress.* San Francisco: Jossey-Bass.

Shirts, R. G. (1977). *BaFá BaFá A cross culture simulation.* Del Mar, CA: Simulation Training System.

Smeltzer, C. H., & Vlasses, F. R. (2003). *Ordinary people, extraordinary lives: The stories of nurses.* Indianapolis, IN: Sigma Theta Tau International.

Steins, G. (2000). Motivation in person perception: Role of the other's perspective. *Journal of Social Psychology, 140*, 692-707

Tsushima, T., & Gegas, V. (2001). Role taking and socialization in single-parent families. *Journal of Family Issues, 22*, 267-288.

Zanuck, R. D., & Zanuck, L. F. (Producers) & Beresford, B. (Director). (1989). *Driving Miss Daisy* [Motion picture]. United States: Warner Bros.

Zimmerman, B. J., & Phillips, C. Y. (2000). Affective learning: Stimulus to critical thinking and caring practice. *Journal of Nursing Education, 39*, 422-428.

Chapter 15: Using Educational Theory as a Basis for Leveling Nursing Laboratory Simulation Experiences

Arlene Morris, BSN, MSN, RN

Nursing practice is becoming more and more complex. Critical thinking and problem solving are on-demand skills used throughout all of nursing care. It is not enough to merely perform a nursing skill; nurses must be prepared to think on their feet. Simulated laboratory experiences across the curriculum help provide experience in practicing this on-demand thinking. – Linda Caputi

Introduction

Nursing students represent a diverse population in terms of age and experience (Billings & Halstead, 1998). Traditional college-age students (18 to 22 years old) and adult learners may be enrolled in the same class. Traditional students may have limited prior experience with the healthcare delivery system, and may be working part-time or full-time in areas not related to health care. However, these traditional students bring varied life experiences to the nursing education environment. Students older than traditional college-age students, some of whom may be returning for a second or third degree, also bring varied life experiences.

Educational Philosophy

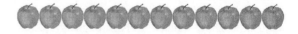

My teaching philosophy includes two core values that are also inherent in my nursing philosophy: the dignity of the individual and an emphasis on quality. I believe the individual student brings personal attributes and experiences to the learning environment. Nurse educators are challenged to build on these to assist the student in developing both a commitment to learning and a self-expectation of providing the highest quality nursing care. Transformation in both student and faculty occurs through collaboration as students are actively engaged in seeking their highest level of knowledge and professional nursing performance. – Arlene Morris

296

Prior experiences with health care provide a foundation on which to build nursing knowledge in the formal educational setting.

This wide range of prior student experiences should impact curricular planning and delivery. The wise teacher, cognizant of instructional design (the educational process), builds on these identified characteristics of students (Caputi, 2004). The teacher can design teaching-learning strategies that account for these student characteristics while using educational theory to develop experiential laboratory situations in which students can form a foundation for new learning. This chapter addresses this approach to instructional development.

Adult Learners as Nursing Students

Adult education—andragogy—has been described as "an organized and sustained effort to assist adults to learn in such a way that enhances their capability to function as self-directed learners" (Mezirow, 1981, p. 21).

From interviews with nurse educators, Jinks (1997) compiled four basic tenets upon which andragogy can be applied to nursing education:

1. A change in self-concept from one of total dependence to increasing self-directedness;
2. Life experiences, which enable learners to become rich resources for teaching and provide a broad base from which to relate to new learning;
3. A readiness to learn, based upon need to prepare for developing professional roles; and
4. A problem-solving approach to learning, which utilizes the desire to apply learning to current situations (p. 9).

Long (2004) also addresses the diversity of adult learners. Nursing students enter their educational programs at different levels, with prior preparation as a patient care technician, vocational nurse, or associate degree/diploma-prepared registered nurse. Many learners entering nursing programs have prior associate, baccalaureate, master's, and doctoral degrees in other disciplines. These life, work, and educational experiences all affect the student's learning.

Long discusses **participation** as the key motive for learning for adult learners. Thus, to enhance the effectiveness of teaching-learning situations, nursing faculty should design situations in which experiences can be shared or devise learning environments in which simulated situations can be experienced by all learners.

Necessary Learner Characteristics and Skills for Effective Simulations

Motivation for Active Learning

One objective of the simulation experience is to help the student assume responsibility for individual learning. Many of the learner characteristics necessary for effective use of the simulation teaching-learning strategy involve characteristics of the adult learner, such as being self-directed or self-motivated and desiring relevance of information presented However, many nursing students have been socialized in education experiences with passive learning. Some of the students have not developed the self-direction and self-motivation to learn the material other than memorizing lecture notes. Presenting the psychomotor skill validation of a simulated experience facilitates awareness of similar situations in which knowledge, critical thinking, and problem solving will be necessary. Thus, motivation to actively participate—or engage—in the experience is increased as students become aware of potential applications of the knowledge.

Attaining Necessary Knowledge

Another objective of the learner in a simulation experience is attaining knowledge necessary for completing the critical thinking and for the psychomotor skill performance. The knowledge necessary for the critical thinking component may be presented in theory courses, as rationale for nursing actions. This knowledge is then incorporated with the psychomotor skill performance, at increasingly higher levels, as adaptations and modifications in the performance of the psychomotor skill are indicated in the simulation scenario.

Honest Self Evaluation

An honest self evaluation by the student is a necessary step for simulations to be effective. The student should complete a self evaluation of the skill validation process prior to receiving evaluation from the faculty. Awareness of one's own strengths and areas for improvement can provide reinforcement for retention of the learned material and provide for a cumulative effect if it correlates with the faculty's evaluation. This is helpful because students often identify learning needs that were not determined by the faculty evaluator.

Learning Theory and Nursing Students

Brain research supports the constructivist learning theory that "new and higher-level neural structures have to connect or grow from structures (knowledge) already there" (Smilkstein, 2003, p. 71). A link is formed to connect prior knowledge or experience to new information.

Chaining is a term for the correct sequencing of appropriate responses or links. "Each chain is seen as a series of stimulus and response units that leads to appropriate further stimulus-responses. Each subtask or smaller chain must be taught" (Huckabay, 1980, p. 60).

When students' personal experiences with healthcare delivery relate to topics discussed in coursework, they should be encouraged to recount these experiences in small-group or classroom settings. This discussion of actual past experiences may provide a link for other students to connect the new knowledge. Faculty should be cautious, however, because some personal experiences with healthcare delivery may be less than ideal and may not provide the desired foundation for nursing students to build upon. Nursing faculty can help students make these cognitive links by contriving simulations that proceed from simple to complex.

Other aspects of learning theory in nursing education include (Jinks, 1997; Van Hoozer, et al, 1987):

- The learning objectives commonly used in nursing education are essentially behavioristic in theory, in that the nursing process and its associated problem-solving approach is a behavioral approach.
- The theory of nursing practice primarily relates to the cognitive domain.
- Practical application of motor skills involves the psychomotor domain.
- Attitudes, beliefs, and values are predisposing factors to actions, and involve the affective domain of learning.

Contriving scenarios that are similar to actual life experiences can establish effective teaching-learning situations to combine all of the learning theories and domains. Learners use cognitive recall and application of the theoretical principles of pathophysiology and effective nursing interventions, in combination with choosing or valuing from the affective domain, to determine the most important nursing action for the simulated scenario. The psychomotor skill demonstration can then be accomplished with evaluation of appropriate step-by-step procedures.

Required Skills for Expert Use of Simulations

The nursing faculty evaluating skills performance must be proficient in the actual psychomotor skill procedure and be familiar with the anticipated healthcare practice settings. Awareness of adult learning theory is important to promote the student's progression to active, self-directed learner, and to allow for the student's self evaluation. Teacher skill in providing verbal and written feedback is important for observing the student's performance in the least-threatening environment possible, and providing positive feedback and constructive criticism.

Planning for Leveled Laboratory Simulations

To plan a simulation, the teacher must analyze the steps performed in the psychomotor skill and identify equipment and props needed for the simulation. It is important to plan the appropriate timing for simulations in the curriculum, to ensure adequate background information has been presented. The case scenario should reflect what is anticipated in actual clinical experiences in that semester. Faculty who are knowledgeable and experienced in the practice area used in the simulation should develop the simulation and, if possible, teach the skill.

When developing skill performance scenarios, consider a task analysis that addresses all domains: cognitive, affective, and psychomotor. Each category's subtasks—including application of nursing process, communication, psychomotor skill performance, and self-evaluation of learning and performance—also should be factored into the process. Each subtask can be further broken down into step-by-step procedures.

The teacher must have adequate personnel and time to evaluate the demonstration (Gilley, 2004). Much time is needed to analyze the tasks involved in the demonstration, set up the simulation environment with appropriate props, and evaluate the return demonstration using the simulated environment cues. Institutional support to allow time for planning these activities also is necessary.

Selecting the Environment in Which to Teach Psychomotor Skills

Interviews revealed that the majority of nursing educators view teaching certain nursing skills prior to clinical experiences to be of prime importance. Jinks reported comments such as (1997):

- "Unless we address it (skills acquisition) in a safe environment, then some schools run the risk of being exposed to malpractice in some form."
- "The students were feeling very insecure about if they were seeing enough in the clinical areas." (pp. 114-115).

Jinks summarized findings from research with nursing educators:

Generally an impression is gained that skills teaching in clinical areas is the ideal but for a variety of reasons this is not occurring and therefore a number of institutions are undertaking this type of teaching now, or planning to do so in the future, in the form of skills workshops. However, it can be seen that skills needed for nursing practice are not solely defined in terms of psycho-motor skills. A number [of those interviewed] mentioned developing skills needed for effective communication and interpersonal relationship attributes. (p. 115)

Often nursing students enter the program of study with minimal or no experience in providing health care. Navigating the healthcare delivery system can be a dilemma in itself. An awareness of services provided on different levels of delivery can be gained by using scenarios in the nursing simulation laboratory. Simulations are an effective method of instruction in many areas of learning— in military simulated weekend warrior training, in business, and in education. Nursing education especially profits from the use of scenarios in which students are exposed to situations in a structured and safe environment that promotes critical thinking skills (Purtee, Ulloth & Caputi, 2004; Ulloth & Purtee, 2004).

Learning nursing requires the student to acquire both knowledge and skill. Demonstration and simulation techniques are effective methods for assessing students' progress in acquiring both knowledge and skill. Psychomotor skills may be differentiated as **closed**, in which the environment and stimuli remain constant across settings (such as handwashing), or as **open**, in which the stimuli and environment change (DeYoung, 1990). Using scenarios that replicate real-life—or open—situations provides an opportunity for adult nursing students to progress in psychomotor skill performance in a simulated environment with varying stimuli. Patient simulators have been used in nursing education (Luppien & George-Gay, 2001) to replicate physiological changes that could occur in nursing care of actual clients. However, adding environmental stimuli, such as a client's family, equipment, and other personnel, affects prioritization of client needs. The resulting choice of appropriate nursing actions can provide challenging situations in a less costly fashion.

Laboratory Conditions for Effective Simulations

Nursing simulation laboratories traditionally have included mannequins, on which various nursing intervention skills can be practiced, and other healthcare equipment to replicate a typical hospital room. The addition of areas to simulate a neonatal nursery, intensive care unit, or community setting increases the versatility of the nursing laboratory and allows the student to conceptualize the nurse's role as a client advocate in a variety of settings. One area could be arranged with equipment from an intensive care unit: oxygen, suctioning, and monitors. If no actual monitors are available, equipment can be simulated. For example, a cardboard box can be covered with a drawing or computer printout of reading from an electrocardiogram or aortic balloon pump. Another possibility is using a portion of a large simulation laboratory to replicate an assisted living environment, including a kitchenette, laundry area, sitting area, bedroom, and bathroom. The choice of the simulation setting should reflect the area of clinical practice being studied during that semester.

Developing and Teaching Leveled Simulations
in the Nursing Laboratory

Nursing educators must plan instruction to be relevant to the current healthcare delivery system, yet take into consideration the varying experiences of diverse learners. "The primary task in education is to develop learning experiences that take into account individual differences to promote the fullest development of the individual" (Huckabay, 1980, p. 474). Active learning involves students using cognitive processes, senses, and activity, any of which may meet the needs of students with different learning styles.

Teaching strategies and learning activities are purposely selected throughout the nursing curriculum to foster students' development for various nursing roles. Learning activities and experiences must be designed to offer students the opportunities to achieve curriculum outcomes by providing practice in applying specific areas of content and processes to client care. Learning experiences that require some student participation may actually make it easier to assess students' learning (Norton, 1998). However, students may feel it is stressful to have their active participation observed by a faculty evaluator. Reminding students that the simulation laboratory is a safe place to refine thinking and skills before they enter settings in which clients, families, and healthcare team members will be observing their actions may lessen their anxiety.

Demonstration First then Return Demonstration

Psychomotor skills may be demonstrated using video performances of nursing skills, computer-assisted instruction (CAI) modules, or interaction with a teacher, another student, or a group of students. It may be most helpful for students to first view videos or CAI skill performances to obtain an overview of the procedures, read a clinical skills or nursing fundamentals text for the theory, and then observe a teacher's demonstration. The teacher should take care to ensure all students have an unobstructed view of the demonstration and provide an opportunity for students to ask questions about the procedure. After viewing the demonstration, students should be given opportunities to practice individually, in dyads, or in triads in the nursing simulation laboratory and encouraged to practice at home with their own equipment. (Students should have purchased their own equipment at the beginning of the curriculum.) It is suggested that one student perform the skill while the rest of the class critiques issues related to the student's performance—for example whether he or she maintained a sterile field. Repeating the procedure can help students retain knowledge, so students should then switch roles. In the nursing simulation laboratory, a teacher may be available for questions while several pairs of students practice simultaneously. Each student can progress at a self-determined pace until accurate imitation of the skill is attained (Morris, 2004). Faculty should meet with each student individually to validate that the student can properly perform the skill. Requiring this appointment—and successful demonstration of the skill—before the student is allowed to participate in a clinical experience each semester can ensure that students follow through.

Progressive Leveling of Skill Performance

During the initial semester in which a psychomotor skill is learned, a simple case scenario can be devised that requires the student to accurately repeat the steps of the skill performance and complete a self-evaluation. During successive semesters, **progressive** levels of psychomotor skill performance should be expected. A critical-thinking component may be added to the skill validation by incorporating a contrived scenario that requires problem solving, prioritization, and creativity. The scenarios for each semester should simulate situations the students are expected to encounter during that semester's clinical experience. For example, during the geriatric course, simulations related to experiences with older adults are presented; for the pediatric course, simulations are developed using scenarios with children and families as clients.

An Approach to Leveling a Psychomotor Skill Simulation

A simulation early in the nursing curriculum can be used to evaluate the skill of measuring vital signs. This is a nursing assessment that is familiar to all students, and therefore less intimidating than a more complex skill. However, the evaluation of the simple vital sign assessment can be enhanced to include an awareness of variations in the healthcare delivery system. Using a scenario of a blood pressure screening at a health fair in a shopping mall, students can be asked to play the roles of nurse, client, and family members. The level at which the student will be intervening with the client and the family should be designed into the scenario to relate to the concepts presented in the curriculum to date. For example, a client scenario can include a request for a vital sign check of a healthy adult with all results within normal limits. However, the scenario can be made slightly more complex, by giving the student a situation in which the client has difficulty communicating. The student must explore methods to deal with this scenario; the situation can also be made more complex by including higher-level decision making.

Learning Outcomes

Nursing students are expected to demonstrate behaviors characteristic of the role of the professional nurse. These characteristics can be included in learning outcomes identified in the laboratory simulations. The following learning outcomes proceed from simple to complex, and can be incorporated at appropriate levels throughout the nursing curriculum:

- Professionalism may be established in demeanor, dress, and preparation for caring for the client.
- Professional communication may be demonstrated by a student interacting therapeutically with the simulated client, family, significant other, and other healthcare providers.
- The role of client advocate may be practiced as students determine client needs and make appropriate referrals.
- Critical thinking can be demonstrated by the student comparing client data to standards to determine areas of possible concern or actual problems.
- Reviewing simulated situations for safety hazards, such as electrical wires across clients in emergency scenarios, encourages critical thinking.
- Reviewing care for comparison with standards and evidence-based practice enables students to determine whether interventions are effective or ineffective.
- Prioritizing client needs provides an opportunity for students to determine from the scenario which needs, if unmet, have most potential for harm. For example, students determine which client need is potentially life-threatening and selects that as the priority for intervention.
- Prioritizing interventions requires student awareness of desired outcomes of each intervention. For example, providing intravenous fluids not only hydrates the client, but also provides a way to administer medications or infuse dextrose in a client with low blood sugar.

Learning outcomes related specifically to the steps of the nursing process include the following:

- Assessing the client as indicated in the scenario and assessing the environment;
- Identifying potential and actual problems with related nursing diagnoses;
- Planning for priority interventions and gathering needed equipment;
- Implementing interventions, including the validation of psychomotor skill performance and appropriate client/family teaching; and
- Evaluating the client, including documenting the assessment findings that indicate the need for the appropriate nursing intervention, documenting the actual skills performed, and documenting post-intervention assessment findings to evaluate if outcomes are met.

Sample Scenarios

Following are several scenarios for simulation experiences (Figures 15.1 - 15.5). These are basic and may be made more complex to require higher levels of critical thinking, communication, nursing process, and delegation. To better simulate an actual clinical setting, faculty can write the physician's orders on a chart, with abbreviations, to simulate actual orders. This helps prepare students for reading actual charts in clinical settings. Including questionable orders in the scenario provides opportunity for students to critically think and problem solve. Additionally, creating a medication administration record in the format that students will use during the following semester's clinical experience provides practice in accurate medication tracking and documentation.

 To help faculty provide consistent evaluations, a faculty page is included with the simulation materials. These faculty pages provide information about what the teacher is looking for in the student's performance. These pages might include information about areas that students should identify as priority nursing interventions and potential threats to client safety (Morris, 2004). See the CD-ROM that accompanies this book for sample faculty pages.

Figure 15.1 - Pediatric-Mental Health Scenario

Pediatric-Mental Health Scenario

S. K., a 7-year-old with spina bifida, is admitted with depression, weight loss, and severe dehydration. He has a stage III green and black pressure ulcer to the right buttocks, which his mother has been treating at home. He is crying and upset at this time. He weighs 25 kg.

Medical orders
Admit with Dx: depression, wt loss, & dehydration
Diet: soft as tolerated
Activity: up to W/C TID
VS: q 4 hrs
Allergies: iodine
IVF: D5 ½ NS @ 100 cc/hr
Medications
Haldol 0.5 mg IM PRN agitation
300 mg Depakene per NG bid
Ceftin 1 gram IVPB q 12 hrs
Give #2 MMR sq today
Insert NG tube for feeding
One can Ensure every 4 hr; hold if residual >50 cc. Follow with 50 cc H_2O.
Continue wound care from home
Surgery consult re: debridement
Straight cath QID per home protocol

Continued
S. K. is now one day post-op from surgical debridement of his pressure ulcer. A trachesotomy was performed after respiratory complications during surgery. VS: T-99, 96, 20, 100/60. Respirations are even and unlabored. His dressing is saturated with serosanguinous drainage.

Medical orders
Resume pre-op orders
Trach care and suction q 4 hrs PRN
Wound care: Sterile wet to dry dressing with NS to wound BID

Figure 15.2 - Adolescent Scenario

Adolescent Scenario

E. P., a 15-year-old female, is admitted with a diagnosis of weight loss and possible anorexia nervosa. Ht. 5'7", wt. 92 lbs. She had a severe allergic reaction to a medication and after an episode of respiratory distress, a tracheostomy was performed. Respirations are even and unlabored. Urine output was 80 cc last shift, and her bladder is slightly distended. VS: 97, 64, 24, 88/58.

Medical orders
Admit Dx: wt loss, dehydration, possible anorexia
Activity: BR
VS: routine
NKDA
IV D5 ½ NS @ 125 cc/hr
NG tube for feeding; consult dietary for cont. feeding
100 cc H$_2$O per NG q 4 hr
Diet: soft
Medications
Milk of Magnesia 30 cc per NG QID
20 mg Pepcid IVPB q 12 hr
Fragmin 2500 IU sq q am
Update immunizations—Td today
Trach care q shift; suction q shift and q 2 hr prn
Straight cath q 12 hr if UOP < 200 cc/ shift

Figure 15.3 - Maternal Scenario

Maternal Scenario

O. B., a 25-year-old para 2 gravida 2, is admitted to the OB unit with gestational diabetes and gonorrhea. She is 27 weeks gestation.

Medical orders
Admit Dx: Gestational diabetes, gonorrhea; 27 weeks gestation
Diet: 2000 cal ADA
Activity: Up as tolerated
VS: q 4 hr
Straight cath U/A, C&S
Clean wound to labia with NS, apply antibiotic oint. BID
Medications
Rocephin 125 mg IM x 1 dose
Tylenol 650 mg p.o. q 6 hr PRN discomfort
Insulin 6 units Humulin R/14 units Humulin N sq q am before breakfast
Glucoscan QID
TB Mantoux test today ID

Figure 15.4 - Adult Medical-Surgical Scenario

Adult Medical-Surgical Scenario

J. S., a 52-year-old man, is admitted with bowel obstruction and N/V. He reports a history of IDDM x 6 years, and CA of the larynx 4 years ago with trach placement which the pt maintains at home independently. Exploratory lap scheduled for 7 am in the morning.

Medical orders
Admit Dx: N/V, bowel obstruction
Diet: NPO
Activity: BR with BRP
VS q 2 hr x 4 then q 4 hr
Allergies: PCN
IVF: ½ NS @ 150 cc/hr
Insert NG to low intermittent suction
FSBS q 4 hr, FBS @ 6 am, pre-op lab work
S/S insulin: BS <150 = no coverage
        BS 150-250 10 units Humalog insulin sq
        BS 251-350 20 units Humalog insulin sq
        BS >350 call MD
Reglan 50 mg in 50 cc ½ NS q 8 hrs
Vistaril 25 mg IM q 6 hr PRN nausea
Trach care and suction PRN
TB mantaux ID today
OR permit for exploratory laparotomy

Figure 15.5 - Older Adult Scenario

Older Adult Scenario

C. K., a 90-year-old man, is admitted to the unit with urinary retention. His bladder is slightly distended and he states he last voided approximately 12 hours ago. He has a history of stomach cancer and heart disease.

Medical orders
Admit Dx: urinary retention
Diet: regular as tolerated
Activity: up with assistance
VS: q 4 hr x 4 then q shift
IVF: D5 ½ NS @ 50 cc/ hr
Insert foley cath to BSD
Call if UOP < 30 cc/hr
Lanoxin 0.25 mg p.o. q day

Summary

The discipline of nursing is rapidly changing with new research-based evidence providing new directions for best practice. It can be daunting for educators to disseminate this information. Creating scenarios that allow students to peruse new techniques, decide the appropriateness of application of the new information, and state the rationale for the decision making is one new way to teach nursing students. The motive for these types of experiences continues to be that the experience in a nursing simulation environment provides the stage for developing critical thinking, problem solving, and interventions when in actual client care settings.

Learning Activities

1. Visit a facility in which students will have clinical experiences. Identify frequent admitting diagnoses and discuss them with the nursing staff. Develop a simple scenario based on client experiences in that clinical area, including at least three psychomotor nursing interventions.
2. Using the scenario in Learning Activity 1, determine the priority nursing interventions and write brief rationale for these choices on a faculty page. These are used as a reference to promote consistency among faculty evaluators.
3. Analyze the scenario and nursing interventions from Learning Activity 1 to create an appropriate simulated environment in the nursing simulation laboratory. Gather the necessary props and equipment. Select the appropriate student skills evaluation tool for the number of interventions that the students will be expected to validate.
4. Review your institution's curriculum. Determine at which level students would be expected to demonstrate non-psychomotor skills such as therapeutic communication; delegation, referral, and management; and awareness of diversity, family, community, and environmental issues. Identify specific times in the curriculum at which simulations can be made more complex to include these roles of the nurse.
5. Discuss the scenario in Learning Activity 1 with faculty colleagues or staff nurses. Consider how the scenario might be made more complex with the

addition of safety hazards, coexisting disease processes, need for interdisciplinary healthcare team delegation or referral, errors in medication (eg, expiration date, safe dosage, incomplete order, incorrect route), or by changing the client's age, ethnicity, or environment. Determine which student behaviors would be required to meet the additional needs.

6. Brainstorm with other faculty colleagues or staff nurses about memorable client situations. These situations can provide a template for creating scenarios. Assure clients' confidentiality by changing pertinent data. Often it is easiest to create a student scenario by beginning with a complex situation from actual experience, then changing certain aspects of the simulation to create a simpler situation. Encounters in the healthcare arena that require problem solving are perfect for scenario creation, and will enable students to practice critical thinking in the safe environment of the simulation laboratory.

References

Billings, D. M., & Halstead, J. A. (1998). *Teaching in Nursing: A guide for faculty.* Philadelphia: Saunders.

Brookfield, S. D. (2004). Critical thinking techniques. In M. W. Galbraith (Ed.), *Adult learning methods: A guide for effective instruction* (3rd ed.). Malabar, FL: Kreiger.

Caputi, L. (2004). An overview of the educational process. In L. Caputi & L. Engelmann, (Eds.) *Teaching nursing: The art and science*, Vol. 1 & 2. Glen Ellyn, IL: College of DuPage Press.

DeYoung, S. (1990). *Teaching nursing.* Redwood City, CA: Addison-Wesley Nursing.

Gilley, J. W. (2004). Demonstration and simulation. In M. W. Galbraith (Ed.), *Adult learning methods: A guide for effective instruction* (3rd ed.). Malabar, FL: Kreiger.

Gredler, M. E. (2001). *Learning and instruction: Theory into practice* (4th ed.). Upper Saddle River, NJ: Merrill Prentice Hall.

Huckabay, L.M. (1980). *Conditions of learning and instruction in nursing: Modularized.* St. Louis: Mosby.

Jinks, A. M. (1997). *Caring for patients, caring for student nurses: Developments in nursing and health care.* Brookfield, VT: Ashgate.

Long, H. B. (2004). Understanding adult learners. In M. W. Galbraith (Ed.), *Adult learning methods: A guide for effective instruction* (3rd ed.). Malabar, FL: Kreiger.

Lowenstein, A. J. (2001). Strategies for innovation. In A. J. Lowenstein & M. J. Bradshaw (Eds.), *Fuszard's innovative teaching strategies in nursing* (3rd ed.). Gaithersburg, MD: Aspen.

Chapter 16: Benchmarking for Progression: Implications for Students, Faculty, and Administrators

Ainslie Taylor Nibert, MSN, PhD, RN, CCRN

"And our pass rate is..."   These words strike at the heart of every nursing faculty. Why? Because faculty diligently work to educate caring, compassionate, and knowledgeable nurses but often feel they have failed if students' pass rates on the NCLEX® are lower than expected. One of the many facets of helping students succeed on NCLEX is identifying those at risk for failure so we can help them before they take the exam. In this chapter, Dr. Nibert offers us help with that very important task. – Linda Caputi

Educational Philosophy

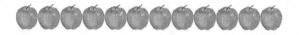

The nurse educator must have the ability to impart to the student sound clinical practices rooted in expert knowledge and skill. Recent advances in educational technology, including computer-assisted instructional packages and web-based programming, have virtually eliminated the need for a teacher-as-expert-lecturer; however, nothing can replace the value of the expert nurse educator directing student learning in the clinical environment. The educator's use of reliable and valid evaluation methods is as important as effective teaching. Without sound measures to determine individual students' remediation needs and a curriculum evaluation plan to assess total program outcomes, educators cannot adequately determine if educational goals have been accomplished. The end product of good teaching and evaluation in nursing is always the development of outstanding nursing students who are destined to become outstanding professional nurses. – Ainslie Taylor Nibert

Introduction

In recent years, nursing has received significant attention in the media. With news about medication errors made by nurses, aggravated by increasing workloads and the current nursing shortage, the public has been bombarded with information about the problems facing the nursing profession (American Nurses Association, 2003). Because the U.S. population is aging and the need for nursing care is increasing, these problems are of greater concern now than at any other time in history. The public is demanding accountability—not only of the financial accountability of healthcare delivery systems, but also from the higher education institutions that are preparing individuals to practice nursing. In these days of extreme nursing faculty shortages, nursing schools are grappling more than ever with the issue of accountability and asking, "How can we measure students' readiness for progression through the curriculum and for the National Council Licensure Examination for Registered Nurses (NCLEX-RN)?"

Through their actions, key stakeholders already have responded to this question. Increasingly, nursing faculties have adopted the use of reliable and valid evaluation criteria to monitor student progress throughout their nursing curricula. The purpose of this chapter is to describe the use of computerized nursing exams to measure student achievement through the nursing curriculum and readiness for graduation, defined in part by their preparedness for the NCLEX-RN. In addition, this chapter describes related benchmarking-for-progression practices that incorporate NCLEX-RN scores which serve as indicators of achievement of curricular competencies. The author has chosen Health Education Systems, Inc. (HESI) exams to serve as examples of reliable and valid tests administered throughout the nursing curriculum to benchmark for progression.

Review of the Literature

A review of the literature reveals two main areas relevant to the topic of benchmarking for progression. These two areas are:
- Public demand for accountability; and
- Achieving NCLEX-RN success.

Public Demand for Accountability

The public's increased demand for accountability among nursing professionals is in no small way related to the recent accounting scandals that have occurred throughout the United States and throughout the world. The images of corporate chief executive officers being led away in handcuffs, charged with bankrupting their publicly held companies while personally profiting at the expense of their stockholders, are responsible for a heightened public distrust of corporate America and increased regulatory controls enacted through legislation. Likewise, academic institutions are undergoing scrutiny by accrediting agencies and the federal government, the watchdog entities typically charged with enforcing professional standards and identifying corporate malfeasance. In this climate of intense scrutiny, it is no surprise that public outrage has resulted from the exposure of waste and mismanagement in academic and healthcare institutions. Legislatures are no longer willing to fund academic programs without clear evidence of the need for these programs and the application of outcome measures that provide objective data regarding curricular effectiveness in achieving program goals (Arone, 2003; Burd, 2003; Schmidt, 2002).

The demand for accountability in higher education also has affected nursing programs (Langston, Cowling & McCain, 1999; Minnick & Halstead, 2001). The well-publicized nursing shortage not only has adversely affected healthcare delivery systems, but also has negatively impacted academic settings. The American Association of Colleges of Nursing (AACN) (2004) reported a faculty vacancy rate in 2003 of 8.6 percent, an increase from 7.4 percent in 2002. The faculty vacancy rate is expected to skyrocket in the next five to 10 years, as the doctorally prepared nurses who hold faculty positions reach retirement age at a rate of 200 to 300 per year between 2004 and 2012 (American Association of Colleges of Nursing, 2003b). Compounding the problem is the dearth of younger faculty to replace the massive number of retirees expected to leave schools of nursing within the next decade (American Association of Colleges of Nursing, 2003c). Today, fewer advanced practice nurses are selecting teaching as their career path. Often this choice is financially motivated: Average salaries for master's-prepared nursing faculty positions across all ranks are as much as $10,000 lower than average salaries for master's-prepared nurse practitioners working in clinical settings (American Association of Colleges of Nursing, 2004; Olsen, 2003).

Nurses who persevere in academic settings and retain faculty appointments describe the mounting challenges they face to provide effective teaching. These challenges are described at length in the nursing literature:

- Increasing numbers of part-time faculty (Adams, 1995);
- Increasing numbers of academically at-risk students enrolling in nursing programs (Fearing, 1997; Jalili-Grenier & Chase, 1997; Jeffreys, 1998; Yoder, 2001); and
- Increasing pressure on nursing faculties to maintain ever-higher levels of achievement on key program outcome indicators, such as the NCLEX-RN (Arathuzik & Aber, 1998; Ashley & O'Neil, 1994; Barkley, Rhodes, & Dufour, 1998; Frierson, Malone & Shelton, 1993; Lyons, Young, Haas, Hojat & Bross, 1997; Patton & Goldenberg, 1999; Smith & Crawford, 2002).

Despite these challenges, the public has stepped up its demands for financial accountability within institutions of higher learning and student achievement at the end of educational programs. To meet the demands for financial accountability, positions are being eliminated when faculty and staff leave through retirement or attrition. Furthermore, adjunct faculty are increasingly being hired to replace college and university faculty as clinical instructors for nursing courses. Although these part-time faculty primarily cover clinical teaching assignments left unfilled due to the high vacancy rate among full-time positions, they typically have limited teaching experience. They also frequently lack direct involvement in development of, and evaluation activities for, the courses they are assigned to teach. There is little doubt that administrators and faculties alike are feeling the pressure to do more with less, as funding for faculty and staff has succumbed to federal, state, and institutional cutbacks (Bowler, 2003).

To demonstrate accountability for student learning, nursing faculties must clearly define the educational outcomes for their nursing programs and must objectively measure attainment of these outcomes. High-stakes testing is increasingly being used by faculties as an objective measure of curricular effectiveness (Bowler, 2003; Hacsi, 2004; MacGillis, 2003). These standardized exams are given throughout the curriculum as gatekeepers, with student progression contingent upon satisfactory performance. Students who fail to meet the designated educational outcome may not graduate until they have demonstrated the required end-of-program competencies (Nibert, Young & Britt, 2003).

Achieving NCLEX-RN Success

NCLEX-RN failures create numerous problems for graduates, faculties, and employers, and they significantly contribute to the nursing shortage by delaying new nurses' access to employment in registered nurse positions.

Candidates who fail the licensure exam lose out on the higher-paying salaried positions they would have received if licensed, and they are often forced to take lower-paying technical positions while they await the opportunity to re-test. Vance and Davidhizar (1997) reported that NCLEX-RN failure results in personal losses, including feelings of shame and low self-esteem, that are even more distressing to candidates than the loss of higher salaries.

Consistently low pass rates on the NCLEX-RN by a school's graduates can damage the school's reputation within the nursing community and within the community at large. The loss of the public's trust can lead to fewer applicants, which ultimately can affect the school's very existence. Most state boards of nursing, as well as the Commission on Collegiate Nursing Education (CCNE) and the National League for Nursing Accrediting Commission (NLNAC), which grant program approval and accreditation, view NCLEX-RN pass rates as an important indicator of a program's effectiveness (American Association of Colleges of Nursing, 2003a; National League for Nursing Accrediting Commission, 1999a, 1999b).

NCLEX-RN failures also have significant consequences for graduates' prospective employers. The time required to orient newly graduated nurses represents a sizable investment of resources. Candidates who fail the licensing exam can become a financial liability for the institution.

To avoid the potentially devastating consequences of a program's low annual pass rate on the NCLEX-RN, nursing educators have attempted to determine the best predictors of NCLEX-RN success. Campbell and Dickson (1996) reported that while predictors of licensure success had been investigated for over four decades, no consistently reliable method had been adequately described in the nursing literature. However, a series of articles published beginning in 1999 offers evidence of one consistently accurate predictor, the HESI Exit Exam (E^2) (Lauchner, Newman & Britt, 1999; Newman, Britt & Lauchner, 2000; Nibert & Young, 2001; Nibert, Young & Adamson, 2002).

Purposes of Standardized Testing

For years, schools of nursing have employed standardized testing to accrue data for external curriculum evaluation. Morrison (in press) defined external curriculum evaluation as the "evaluation of students' abilities in comparison with the general population of nursing students in the U.S." Standardized testing is the method most often used to create this type of balanced, objective comparison. Another current use for standardized testing is formative evaluation as specified within internal curriculum evaluation plans. Morrison defined internal curriculum evaluation as the "evaluation of outcomes identified by the school of nursing; specifically, the evaluation of course objectives" (in press). Nursing faculties increasingly are using the results of standardized tests to establish benchmarks for student progression through the nursing curriculum (Morrison, Free & Newman, 2002; Nibert & Young, 2001; Nibert et al., 2003).

Incorporating standardized testing throughout a nursing program is particularly important when a new curriculum is implemented. Administering standardized tests at strategic intervals within the program allows nursing faculties to establish benchmarks, so that objective data are available for an initial curriculum evaluation. Scores on standardized tests are useful not only as indicators of the curriculum's effectiveness in covering important content areas, but also for identifying gaps in content. These gaps should be addressed when the curriculum is revised for the next implementation cycle.

Standardized testing is also useful for evaluating outcomes within established nursing programs. Faculties can use aggregate test results to identify content areas that are not being appropriately addressed within the curriculum. Trending of aggregate standardized test scores can serve as a measure not only of student performance, but also of faculty performance, and longitudinal data can be an objective measure of curricular effectiveness.

Benchmarking in Nursing Education

Benchmarking is a process for establishing an expected level of quality. The practice originated with surveyors who marked objects in the landscape to indicate a reference point for determining altitudes (Rudy, Lucke, Whitman & Davidson, 2001). It first gained recognition in business as a technique for quality improvement wherein companies identified best practices by comparing performances on specific variables. Benchmarking within the healthcare industry is used to identify and judge the quality of care through the interpretation of client outcome data. This led to the periodic publishing of hospital report cards to designate an institution's track record in meeting recognized standards for quality client care. Such reports also address the cost effectiveness of services provided (Rudy et al, 2001). The American Nurses Association (ANA) identified nursing-sensitive client outcome indicators to demonstrate the role that the nursing profession played in the delivery of quality client care and it began publishing an annual report card for nursing in 1995 (American Nurses Association, 1995, 1996).

Although benchmarking is an accepted practice in most industries, it has been adopted less frequently in higher education, and it is usually limited to setting admission criteria or determining scholastic awards (Billings, Connors & Skiba, 2001). For example, many schools set a minimum SAT score as a criterion for admission, and a benchmark PSAT score is established each year to select finalists for National Merit Scholarships (Hewitt, 2002). The nursing education literature focuses primarily on benchmarking for its use in conducting external curriculum evaluation, such as reaccreditation by NLNAC and CCNE (Wilson, 1999). Recently, the use of benchmarking has been expanded to include continuous quality improvement programs designed to measure achievement of educational standards (Yearwood, Singleton, Feldman & Colombraro, 2001).

Even though NCLEX-RN success is a top priority for stakeholders in nursing education, few authors have described specific benchmarks to identify students at risk of failing the exam. Professional judgment rather than empirical evidence historically has been used to identify students at risk of NCLEX-RN failure. However, a new and growing trend among nursing faculties is to develop progression polices based on benchmarks that provide objective evidence of nursing competence (Morrison et al, 2002; Nibert et al, 2003). These policies are designed to identify students in need of remediation prior to graduation and NCLEX-RN candidacy, so that success on the licensing exam can be achieved.

Morrison et al (2002) first described the use of the E^2 as a benchmark for progression. Administrators of seven nursing programs that had implemented policies that used E^2 scores as a benchmark for progression were interviewed regarding NCLEX-RN outcomes before and after implementing those policies. They reported that pass rates improved between 9 percent and 41 percent within two years of implementing the progression policy. However, criteria contained within these policies, including a specific benchmark indicating readiness for graduation, were not described. Nibert et al (2002) expanded on this study by surveying administrators at 158 nursing schools to assess trends in benchmarking-for-progression policies and found that 149 schools (94.3 percent) had used E^2 scores as a benchmark for remediation, and 45 (30.2 percent) of those schools had implemented policies that tied progression to a minimally acceptable E^2 score in order for students to graduate or to take the NCLEX-RN. A follow-up study indicates that the percentage of schools that have adopted benchmarking-for-progression policies increased again in 2001-2002, the most recent academic year for which survey data were available, and that more schools of nursing are addressing accountability issues by establishing such policies (Lewis & Young, 2004).

Establishing a Progression Policy

Although nursing faculties increasingly are adopting benchmarking-for-progression policies, the process of planning, developing, and implementing such a policy can seem intimidating. However, when a systematic method is employed and certain guidelines followed, faculties often find the process less difficult than they originally imagined. There are six basic steps for developing a progression policy:

1. Obtain faculty consensus regarding implementation of the policy.
2. Communicate the policy to all stakeholders.
3. Choose the measure that will be used as a benchmark for progression.
4. Identify the benchmark score that will be used in the progression policy.
5. Determine the consequences associated with the progression policy.
6. Evaluate outcomes following implementation of the progression policy.

Step 1: Obtain Faculty Consensus Regarding Implementation of the Policy

Often a faculty's decision to establish a progression policy based on standardized exam scores is motivated by less-than-desirable NCLEX-RN pass rates. However, some schools take a proactive stance and implement such policies to protect their current NCLEX-RN pass rates. Progression policies that are based on standardized exams can serve as validation for faculty evaluations because student performance on HESI exams usually parallels performance on teacher-made exams and clinical evaluations. Therefore, implementing a progression policy based on external curriculum evaluation measures can be supportive of faculty interventions with those students who need to remediate.

If the nursing faculty makes the decision to implement a progression policy, it is critical for program administrators to support the faculty in enforcing the policy. Otherwise, students will quickly determine that remediation following a poor performance on the standardized exams is not really required after all. Progression and remediation policies that are enforced inconsistently are of little value and may even be less effective than not having a policy at all.

Faculties should anticipate some student resistance initially when a progression policy is implemented. Students may feel threatened by the concept of having their standardized exam scores tied to progression, graduation, and/or NCLEX-RN candidacy. However, when pass rates increase because more students succeed on the NCLEX-RN, schools can better assess the value of these policies. In fact, faculties often report that although students are initially unhappy with the policy, they are far more positive after graduation when they realize that benchmark testing helped them to succeed on their first attempt at the NCLEX-RN.

Change is always difficult, and a change as important as implementing a progression policy requires consensus of the entire faculty. Nothing will cause more havoc among students and faculty than a dissenting faculty member sabotaging the policy by consorting with students regarding how "unfair" the policy is. It is absolutely essential that faculty members are united when implementing a progression policy. While a healthy dialogue among faculty that encourages arguments for and against the policy helps promote a productive teaching and learning environment, those on the dissenting side of the argument should not subvert the policy once the decision has been made to move forward. A lack of professionalism among faculty who openly disregard the benchmarking-for-progression policy can carry over into other areas of policy enforcement and permanently damage student-faculty relationships in the nursing program. Ultimately, it is the responsibility of the program director or dean to uphold the program's standards and to convey the behavioral and professional expectations to both students and faculty. Therefore, adoption of a progression policy should not be taken lightly. To achieve maximum effectiveness, the policy should be approved by the entire faculty and should receive a clear commitment of support from the school's administration prior to implementation.

Step 2: Communicate the Policy to All Stakeholders

Morrison et al (2002) advised that students should be notified of the school's progression policy in accordance with the university's administrative requirements. Some schools designate the catalog that was in force when a student entered the program as a binding contract between the student and the academic institution. In these situations, schools usually recognize that any policy changes implemented during the student's tenure that were not specified in the catalog when the student was admitted to the program do not apply to that student. In such situations, the contract is in force even if the student's graduation date extends beyond the inclusive dates of the catalog of record at the time of admission. Some schools even extend the original contract to students who re-enroll following an absence of more than one semester for either personal or academic reasons. Such students can pose concerns for the faculty since they may take months or even years to complete the program. It is wise for administrators and faculty committees to consider such circumstances when writing school policy.

Other schools acknowledge that policy changes occurring during a student's tenure in the program alter the contractual agreement implied under the specific published edition of the catalog that was in effect when the student entered the program. Therefore, before publishing or notifying students of the adoption of a progression policy, faculties should investigate the college's or university's official procedure for changing policy statements in the catalog. In particular, faculties should be aware of all steps in the procedure for changing graduation requirements and any related policies that dictate when such requirements take effect. This information is necessary to determine if students are exempt from existing policy statements or policy changes not included in the catalog of record at the time of their admission.

Morrison et al (2002) advised faculties to publish a paragraph that describes the progression policy in the school's catalog. They presented a sample of such a paragraph:

Students will be required to take nationally-normed tests throughout the curriculum and to make a satisfactory score on such tests. In the last semester/quarter of the curriculum, students will be required to take a comprehensive exam and to make a satisfactory score on such an exam prior to graduation/taking the licensing exam. (p. 96)

Note that the suggested paragraph does not mention the specific benchmark scores or exams that will be used. It merely gives faculty the power to implement the type of external curriculum evaluation it deems necessary to achieve program goals and to delineate and change as needed the benchmark scores required for progression throughout the curriculum. The policy statement, however, should be worded with enough specificity to indicate the institution's seriousness about achievement of the benchmark score.

Before any nursing faculty establishes a progression policy, key decision makers affiliated with the institution should consider the issue carefully, including the legal implications of this type of policy. Administrative approval should be sought prior to implementation of the progression policy. Risk managers within the college or university also should be consulted so that litigation stemming from policy enforcement can be avoided. If the risk manager believes that the school could face legal action based on policy enforcement, the nursing faculty needs to be advised about the best ways to word the policy, communicate the policy to stakeholders, and implement the policy, so that, if necessary, the school could successfully defend the use of the policy in a court of law.

One such case was filed in Florida (Brownfield, 2003). The outcome demonstrated that nursing faculty were justified in establishing benchmarks for progression within their program. Students are not likely to be successful in legal actions taken against a school if the school can demonstrate that all students who agreed to the policy were treated fairly and equally and that the enforcement of the policy was not done in a capricious or arbitrary manner. Of course, no administrator wants to devote resources to the defense of a lawsuit. Often legal action can be avoided by communicating to the students the need for the policy and the benefits of implementing accountability measures within the nursing curriculum.

Step 3: Choose the Measure That Will Be Used as a Benchmark for Progression

Once a nursing faculty determines the need for setting benchmarks throughout the curriculum, it then must identify standardized exams that provide accurate predictions of NCLEX-RN success. Reliable and valid exams that produce trustworthy scores should be chosen to benchmark students' readiness for nursing school and their competence at various stages throughout their undergraduate curriculum, as well as their preparedness for the licensure exam and clinical practice. HESI produces several exams that can be useful for establishing benchmarks.

HESI exams currently are used as components of internal and external evaluation at more than 500 schools of nursing throughout the United States. Research provides evidence of the effectiveness of HESI exams in producing reliable and valid measures of students' nursing knowledge and their ability to apply nursing concepts to clinically oriented problems. Published research findings regarding the accuracy of the HESI E^2 in predicting NCLEX-RN outcomes are likely the catalysts for the increased use of specific E^2 scores as benchmarks for progression (Heupel, 1994; Lauchner et al, 1999; Newman et al, 2000; Nibert & Young, 2001; Nibert et al, 2002; Nibert et al, 2003). These studies provided the data faculty needed to make decisions regarding curriculum evaluation and policy development, particularly as these decisions relate to progression-to-graduation and approval for NCLEX-RN candidacy.

Step 4: Identify the Benchmark Score That Will Be Used in the Progression Policy

HESI exams used to assess student achievement throughout the nursing curriculum provide two scores: a HESI score, which is a three-digit number that is calculated using the HESI Predictability Model (HPM), and a conversion score, which is a weighted percentage score. The HPM is a proprietary mathematical model, and four studies that reviewed the NCLEX-RN outcomes of 17,342 RN students found that the E^2 was between 96.36 percent and 98.30 percent accurate in predicting NCLEX-RN success (Lauchner et al, 1999; Newman et al, 2000; Nibert & Young, 2001; Nibert et al, 2002). The authors of these studies concluded that the HPM was highly accurate in determining NCLEX-RN success. Therefore, HESI scores can be used as benchmarks for progression-to-graduation and as predictors of NCLEX-RN outcomes.

In contrast to the HESI score, which is calculated using the HPM and considers the difficulty level of each **individual** test item, the conversion score is a weighted percentage score that does not use the HPM in its calculation and considers the **average** weight of the test items the student answered correctly and the **average** difficulty of all test items contained on the exam. The HESI conversion score can be used in the calculation of the student's final course grade if the faculty wishes, but it should not be used as a predictor of NCLEX-RN success (Morrison, Adamson, Nibert & Hsia, in press).

Educators directly engaged in classroom and clinical teaching are the most qualified to establish curricular benchmarks because they are responsible for articulating the mission, goals, and objectives of the program. However, published findings often help faculty make decisions regarding the benchmark score that is best for their particular population. Nibert et al (2002) assessed the degree of risk for NCLEX-RN failure that was associated with various HESI scoring intervals. Directors of 158 nursing programs, including associate degree, baccalaureate degree, and diploma programs, with a total of 5,903 RN students who took the E^2 in the 1999-2000 academic year, were asked to provide the number of students in each scoring interval who failed the NCLEX-RN. Based on the data from this survey, the authors concluded that the number of students who failed the NCLEX-RN was significantly higher in each successively lower

Figure 16.1 - NCLEX-RN Pass/Fail Rates by E^2 Scoring Intervals

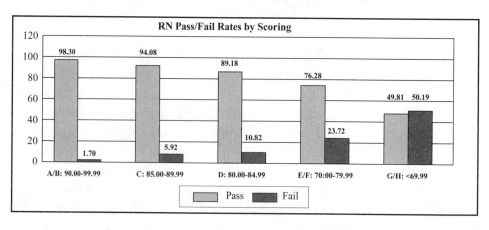

Used with permission – Nibert, A., Young, A., & Adamson, C. (2002). Predicting NCLEX success with the HESI Exit Exam: Fourth annual validity study. *CIN: Computers, Informatics, Nursing, 20*(6), 261-267.

E^2 scoring interval, creating a stepwise pattern of increasing frequency of NCLEX-RN failure. The authors further described the consistent pattern that was observed (see Figure 16.1).

Of the 2,059 RN students who scored in the A/B [highest-scoring] category, 35 (1.70 percent) failed the licensing examination; of the 1,014 students who scored in the C category, 60 (5.92 percent) failed; of the 980 students who scored in the D category, 106 (10.82 percent) failed, of the 1,324 students scoring in the E/F category, 314 (23.72 percent) failed, and of the 526 students scoring in the G/H [lowest-scoring] category, 264 (50.19 percent) failed. (p. 264)

Although this information is helpful in determining benchmark scores, faculties must also consider individual school and student characteristics when establishing the benchmark score that is best for their particular population. For example, programs that graduate small numbers of students are particularly vulnerable to scrutiny by state nursing boards and other accrediting organizations. In schools with few graduates, even one NCLEX-RN failure each quarter can severely lower the school's annual pass rate. For that reason, schools with small graduating classes often set their benchmark scores at higher levels so that their graduating students will have a lower risk for NCLEX-RN failure. Additionally, faculties who teach in schools with a large percentage of minority students or a large number of students for whom English is a second language often set their benchmark scores at higher levels. Published findings indicate that these students experience higher attrition rates and are at greater risk for NCLEX-RN failure than non-minority, English-speaking students (Arathuzik & Aber, 1998; Endres, 1997; Fearing, 1997; Frierson et al, 1993). Some faculties have decided that they do not wish to create stress for their students with an expectation that may be regarded as too high, so they have elected to set their benchmark E^2 HESI scores lower than 850 (designated by HESI as a minimally acceptable score), sometimes even as low as 800. Extrapolating the findings of Nibert et al (2002), schools that set their benchmark at 800 can be expected to maintain an annual NCLEX-RN pass rate of approximately 82 percent, while schools that set a benchmark of 850 can expect an annual pass rate of approximately 92 percent.

Some schools administer customized exams to evaluate students at the end of the first half of the curriculum. HESI refers to these 100-item exams as mid-curricular (MC) exams. MCs are essentially exit exams for the first half of the curriculum. Faculties usually set the same HESI score as a benchmark for the MC as the one they adopt for the E^2.

HESI specialty exams administered throughout the curriculum prior to the E^2 are often substituted for teacher-made exams. These 50-item exams, referred to by HESI as "generics," are designed to evaluate specific subject areas, such as fundamentals, medical-surgical, maternity, pediatrics, psychiatric-mental health, pharmacology, community, and leadership/management. Specialty exams also can be customized to evaluate the specific content of a particular course.

When HESI specialty exams are substituted for teacher-made final exams in nursing courses, the HESI **conversion** score should serve as the final exam grade. This provides an evaluation method in which the outcome (the student's final course grade) is not totally dependent on a HESI exam. The substitution of HESI specialty exam conversion scores for final exams ensures that students are taking professionally developed exams that contain critical-thinking test items that have met HESI's stringent criteria for test construction (Morrison et al, 2004). Furthermore, substituting HESI exams for final exams relieves the faculty of the arduous tasks of developing, scoring, and analyzing the final exams, and updating test items based on the item analysis.

Step 5: Determine the Consequences Associated with the Progression Policy

The consequences for students' failure to achieve benchmark scores should be those that are most effective in motivating students to perform their best on these exams. Nibert et al (2002, 2003) surveyed administrators at 149 schools of nursing to determine benchmarking and remediation policies of these schools during the 1999-2000 academic year. Of the 45 schools that used HESI scores as a benchmark for progression, 35 (77.78 percent) submitted either complete or partial progression policy statements (Nibert et al, 2003). Among the submitted policies, the consequences most often cited for students who did not achieve the benchmark E^2 score designated by the school's faculty were:

- Denial of eligibility for graduation (18 schools [51.43 percent]);
- Assignment of an incomplete or failing grade in the capstone course (12 schools [34.29 percent]); and
- Withholding approval for NCLEX-RN candidacy (5 schools [14.29 percent]).

These findings are summarized in Figure 16.2.

For students who do not meet the benchmark score, a minimum of four weeks—but preferably six weeks—of remediation should occur before they are re-tested using a different version of the exam. Students should be required to complete the assigned remediation, and faculties should hold students accountable for such completion by tying remediation requirements to the program's benchmarks.

Figure 16.2 - Progression Policies: Consequences of Benchmark Failure (*N*=35)

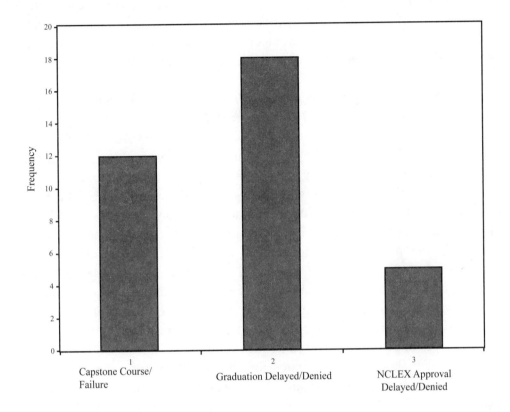

Without consequences attached to the remediation program, students are unlikely to follow through with the plan. In addition, faculties should evaluate the effectiveness of their remediation programs by re-testing students with a different version of the exam that follows the same blueprint as the original exam but does not contain test items that were included in the original. HESI offers three different versions of the E^2. For schools that elect to administer MCs, HESI suggests that two versions of the MC be designed and that the these exams be rotated for re-testing.

Much has been written about remediation strategies, and although some strategies have been found to be more effective than others, students do not readily avail themselves of remediation resources recommended by faculty (Ross, Nice, May & Billings, 1996). Today's students have many responsibilities outside of nursing school, including children, spouses, and jobs (often, full-time jobs), which place extreme constraints on their time and act as barriers to the additional school-work required to remediate. They must have remediation resources that are readily available, even if the student's only time to focus on nursing study is the middle of the night. Remediation therefore needs to be easily accessible, convenient, user-friendly, nonthreatening, and available virtually anywhere and at any time.

Step 6: Evaluate Outcomes Following Implementation of the Progression Policy

Faculty should evaluate the progression policy after the first semester of implementation—and annually thereafter—to determine if the program's goals are being met. This evaluation should be based on several criteria. First and foremost, faculties should determine whether the school's annual NCLEX-RN pass rate has improved since the progression policy was implemented. If the annual pass rate has increased, the faculty should determine if the magnitude of improvement is significant in comparison to the annual pass rate before the progression policy was implemented. If the faculty concludes that the pass rate did not significantly improve, they should investigate other factors that might have rendered the policy ineffective, such as a lack of adherence to stipulated consequences or resistance created by faculty dissenters.

Faculty also should review scores for all other standardized examinations that were administered throughout the curriculum. Students' mean scores on these exams should be reviewed to determine if they have improved from one class to the next. Other questions for the curriculum committee to consider for institutional research projects might include:

- Did students who took the specialty exams do better on the E^2 than those who did not take the specialty exams?
- Was there any difference between the NCLEX-RN outcomes of those students who took HESI specialty exams in place of teacher-made final exams and the results of those who took teacher-made final exams?

Faculty and student satisfaction with the policy should be determined through quantitative and qualitative analysis of responses by both groups. If satisfaction is low despite objective evidence of the policy's effectiveness, the program administrator may need to schedule face-to-face meetings with the unhappy constituents to re-explain the rationale behind adoption of the policy, and the faculty may consider making reasonable modifications to the policy that would diminish opposition. Many of these issues may be avoided by establishing good communication with all parties prior to implementing the policy, so all individuals feel that they were fully informed about the rationale for the policy. Additionally, follow-up studies with the program's graduates should include questions about the effectiveness of progression policies, as well as the graduates' feelings about such policies following their transition to professional nursing practice.

The faculty's choice of a specific benchmark score also should be re-evaluated periodically. Factors that might precipitate changing a benchmark include:

- Persistence of low annual NCLEX-RN pass rates;
- Incongruence of scores on teacher-made tests and HESI exams; and
- New research that demonstrates changing trends in benchmarking among nursing schools that use the same standardized exams to predict NCLEX-RN success.

Summary

There is an increasing need for accountability in nursing education, and this chapter describes the process for incorporating HESI scores as benchmarks for progression throughout a nursing program to provide such accountability. Nursing faculties should be aware of the potential pitfalls surrounding adoption of a progression policy. However, if a policy is adopted, the faculty should maintain their commitment to the policy and they should remain focused on the desired curricular outcomes, even in the face of the challenges it may present. Requiring students to demonstrate nursing competence using reliable and valid standardized exams through an objective, evidence-based approach empowers the faculty to establish accountability in nursing education.

It is of utmost importance that faculties carefully consider the ramifications before implementing a progression policy. Faculties would be wise to review the six steps presented in this chapter when developing or revising a progression policy. Attention should be paid to current research findings regarding benchmarking practices in nursing education, as well as new research findings as they become available.

Faculty must closely monitor students' outcomes—particularly for academically at-risk students—to determine whether their NCLEX-RN performance improves as a result of the benchmarking-for-progression policy. Ongoing evaluation is essential to determine whether existing progression policies should be maintained and to justify the efforts and expense required to implement remediation and re-testing. Faculties need to review standardized testing data to obtain objective evidence of achievement of program outcomes. This evidence is useful in demonstrating curriculum outcomes during reaccreditation and can contribute positively to the school's reputation.

Increasingly, major stakeholders are calling upon academic institutions to provide greater accountability for achieving educational outcomes. Faculties that establish benchmarking-for-progression policies demonstrate a clear commitment to accountability for the quality of their programs and the products they produce: new graduate nurses. Such a proactive approach fosters excellence in nursing education.

Learning Activities

1. Consider the NCLEX pass rates at a school of nursing of your choice. Do these pass rates indicate a need for a progression policy? Why or why not?
2. Discuss the use of a progression policy with nursing faculty from three different schools of nursing. Compare and contrast their opinions of these policies.
3. Develop a progression policy based on the six steps discussed in this chapter. Ask a colleague to critique your policy. What opposition do you anticipate will be offered by other faculty?

References

Adams, D. (1995). Faculty workload and collegial support related to proportion of part-time faculty composition. *Journal of Nursing Education, 34*(7), 305-311.

American Association of Colleges of Nursing. (2003a). *CCNE accreditation standards*, Retrieved March 15, 2004, from http://www.aacn.nche.edu/accreditation/new_standards.htm.

American Association of Colleges of Nursing. (2003b). *Faculty shortages in baccalaureate and graduate nursing programs: Scope of the problem and strategies for expanding the* supply. Washington, DC: Author.

American Association of Colleges of Nursing. (2003c). *Thousands of students turned away from the nation's nursing schools despite sharp increase in enrollment.* Washington, DC: Author.

American Association of Colleges of Nursing. (2004). *AACN's nursing faculty shortage fact sheet*. Retrieved February 15, 2004, from http://www.aacn.nche.edu/media/backgrounders/facutlyshortage.htm.

American Nurses Association. (1995). *Nursing report card for acute care*. Washington, DC: American Nurses Publishing.

American Nurses Association. (1996). *Nursing quality indicators, definitions and implications*. Washington, DC: American Nurses Publishing.

American Nurses Association. (2003). *ANA commends IOM report outlining critical role of nursing work environment in patient safety*. Retrieved February 15, 2004, from http://nursingworld.org/pressrel/2003/pr1105.htm.

Arathuzik, D., & Aber, C. (1998). Factors associated with National Council Licensure Examination-Registered Nurse success. *Journal of Professional Nursing, 14*(2), 119-126.

Arone, M. (2003). Lawmakers seek to hold colleges more accountable. *The Chronicle of Higher Education, 50*(18), A19.

Ashley, J., & O'Neil, J. (1994). Study groups: Are they effective in preparing students for NCLEX-RN? *Journal of Nursing Education, 33*(8), 357-364.

Barkley, T., Rhodes, R., & Dufour, C. (1998). Predictors of success on the NCLEX-RN. *Nursing and Health Care Perspectives, 19*(3), 132-137.

Billings, D., Connors, H., & Skiba, D. (2001). Benchmarking best practices in web-based nursing courses. *Advances in Nursing Science, 23*(3), 41-52.

Bowler, M. (2003, July 2). Community colleges reaching limits. *The Baltimore Sun*. Retrieved January, 2004 from www.baltimoresun.com.

Brownfield, C. (2003, September 13). B-CC wins nursing lawsuit; Student not misled about exit exam. *The Daytona Beach News-Journal*, p. 01C.

Burd, S. (2003). Accountability or meddling? *The Chronicle of Higher Education, 49*(4), A23-A25.

Campbell, A., & Dickson, C. (1996). Predicting student success: A ten-year review using integrative review and meta-analysis. *Journal of Professional Nursing, 12*(1), 47-59.

Endres, D. (1997). A comparison of predictors of success on NCLEX-RN for African American, foreign-born, and white baccalaureate graduates. *Journal of Nursing Education, 36*(8), 365-371.

Fearing, A. (1997). *Literature update on academic performance of minority baccalaureate nursing students* (ED3999920). Illinois.

Frierson, H., Malone, B., & Shelton, P. (1993). Enhancing NCLEX-RN performance: Assessing a three-pronged intervention approach. *Journal of Nursing Education, 32*(5), 222-224.

Hacsi, T. (2004, January 4). Tales out of school. *The New York Times*. Retrieved February 15, 2004, from http://query.nytimes.com/gst/fullpage.html?res=9503E2DE1F3FF937A35752C0A9629C8B63.

Heupel, C. (1994). A model for intervention and predicting success on the National Council Licensure Examination for Registered Nurses. *Journal of Professional Nursing, 10*(1), 57-60.

Hewitt, P. (2002, October 30). Keeping score academically: National Merit semifinalists rate as cream of crop. *Houston Chronicle*, p. 22A.

Jalili-Grenier, F., & Chase, M. (1997). Retention of nursing students with English as a second language. *Journal of Advanced Nursing, 25*, 199-203.

Jeffreys, M. (1998). Predicting nontraditional student retention and academic achievement. *Nurse Educator, 23*(1), 42-48.

Langston, N., Cowling, W., & McCain, N. (1999). Transforming academic nursing: From balance through integration to coherence. *Journal of Professional Nursing, 15*(1), 28-32.

Lauchner, K., Newman, M., & Britt, R. (1999). Predicting licensure success with a computerized comprehensive nursing exam: The HESI Exit Exam. *Computers in Nursing, 17*(3), 120-125.

Lewis, C., & Young, A. (2004). *HESI exams: Benchmarking for progression and remediation.* Unpublished manuscript.

Lyons, K., Young, B., Haas, P., Hojat, M., & Bross, T. (1997). *A study of cognitive and noncognitive predictors of academic success in nursing, allied health and medical students.* Paper presented at the annual meeting of the Association for Institutional Research.

MacGillis, A. (2003, December 30). Regents criticize Towson policy. *The Baltimore Sun.* Retrieved February 15, 2004, from http://www.baltimoresun.com/news/education/bal-md.towson30dec30,0,1149942.story?coll=bal-education-utility.

Minnick, A., & Halstead, L. (2001). Use of a faculty investment model to attain the goals of a college of nursing. *Journal of Professional Nursing, 17*(2), 74-80.

Morrison, S. (in press). Improving NCLEX-RN pass rates through internal and external curriculum evaluation. In M. Oermann & K. Heinrich (Eds.), *Annual review of nursing education* (Vol. 3). New York: Springer.

Morrison, S., Adamson, C., Nibert, A., & Hsia, S. (in press). HESI exams: An overview of reliability and validity. *CIN: Computers, Informatics, Nursing.*

Morrison, S., Free, K., & Newman, M. (2002). Do progression and remediation policies improve NCLEX-RN pass rates? *Nurse Educator, 27*(2), 94-96.

National League for Nursing Accrediting Commission. (1999a). *Accreditation manual 1999 for post secondary and higher degree programs in nursing.* New York: Author.

National League for Nursing Accrediting Commission. (1999b). *Accrediting standards and criteria for academic quality of postsecondary and higher degree programs in nursing* Retrieved February, 2004, from http://www.accrediting-comm-nlnac.org/2am_stds&crit_fnl.htm#III.

Newman, M., Britt, R., & Lauchner, K. (2000). Predictive accuracy of the HESI Exit Exam: A follow-up study. *Computers in Nursing, 18*(3), 132-136.

Nibert, A., & Young, A. (2001). A third study on predicting NCLEX success with the HESI Exit Exam. *Computers in Nursing, 19*(4), 172-178.

Nibert, A., Young, A., & Adamson, C. (2002). Predicting NCLEX success with the HESI Exit Exam: Fourth annual validity study. *CIN: Computers, Informatics, Nursing, 20*(6), 261-267.

Nibert, A., Young, A., & Britt, R. (2003). The HESI Exit Exam: Progression benchmark and remediation guide. *Nurse Educator, 28*(3), 141-145.

Olsen, N. (2003). Shortage of nurse educators? It shouldn't come as a surprise! *Reflections on Nursing Leadership*, 31.

Patton, R., & Goldenberg, D. (1999). Hardiness and anxiety as predictors of academic success in first-year, full-time and part-time RN students. *Journal of Continuing Education in Nursing, 30*(4), 158-167.

Ross, B., Nice, A., May, F., & Billings, D. (1996). Assisting students at risk: Using computer NCLEX-RN review software. *Nurse Educator, 21*(2), 39-43.

Rudy, E., Lucke, J., Whitman, G., & Davidson, L. (2001). Benchmarking patient outcomes. *Journal of Nursing Scholarship, 33*(2), 185-189.

Schmidt, P. (2002). Most states tie aid to performance, despite little proof that it works. *The Chronicle of Higher Education, 48*(24), A20-A22.

Smith, P., & Crawford, L. (2002). The link between entry-level RN practice and the NCLEX-RN examination. *Nurse Educator, 27*(3), 109-112.

Vance, A., & Davidhizar, R. (1997). Strategies to assist students to be successful the next time around on the NCLEX-RN. *Journal of Nursing Education, 36*(4), 190-192.

Wilson, M. (1999). Using benchmarking practices for the learning resource center. *Nurse Educator, 24*(4), 16-20.

Yearwood, E., Singleton, J., Feldman, H., & Colombraro, G. (2001). A case study in implementing CQI in a nursing education program. *Journal of Professional Nursing, 17*(6), 297-304.

Yoder, M. (2001). The bridging approach: Effective strategies for teaching ethnically diverse nursing students. *Journal of Transcultural Nursing, 12*(4), 319-325.

Chapter 17: Academic Program Review

Jeffrey Papp, MS, PhD, RT(R)(QM)

Nursing faculty certainly are accustomed to outside scrutiny of their programs through NLNAC and CCNE accreditation and state approval. But increasingly, programs also are being reviewed from within. Institutions are adopting internal program review policies, a form of self-monitoring for quality improvement. Fortunate educators teach in programs where all program reviews are coordinated and are used to produce the best possible program. Dr. Papp explains how the internal monitoring process works and how it differs from external reviews.
– Linda Caputi

Introduction

Academic program review has become commonplace among institutions of higher education, as practically every college, regardless of its size or mission, engages in some form of program review. Initially, academic program review was practiced at just a few institutions and for departments such as vocational programs in community colleges and graduate programs in universities. Today, the academic program review process is conducted at most institutions and applied to all academic programs as well as many administrative programs.

This chapter provides an overview of academic program review, including an explanation of the phases of the review process and a guide for how to proceed with each phase. A sample review report for a nursing program is included on

Educational Philosophy

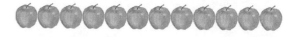

As a medical physicist, I teach many complicated concepts to students and then have them apply those concepts clinically. This requires explaining these concepts in ways that students can readily understand. To help accomplish this goal, I try to draw analogies between the technical concept they must understand and experiences in their everyday lives. I find that learning is much easier when you can relate a new concept to something that already exists in your memory. – Jeffrey Papp the CD-ROM accompanying this book. To access that report, launch the CD on your computer and go to Chapter 17.

Overview of Academic Program Review

Beginning in the late 1950s and early 1960s, various factors, primarily outside of higher education—such as dissatisfaction with public school education, increased federal funds for education, and the proliferation of vocational programs—resulted in pressure for greater effectiveness of educational programs (Popham, 1975). This pressure led to the development and refinement of evaluation processes, primarily at the elementary and secondary levels. This is often referred to as the **accountability movement**. By the late 1970s and early 1980s, similar pressure began to impact higher education. In response, many colleges, universities, systems, and state-level boards began to adopt a specialized form of evaluation known as **program review** (Conrad & Wilson, 2000; Barak, 1986). The term arose because the focus of this evaluation process was on academic programs, usually defined as a sequence of educational experiences leading to a degree or certificate (Conrad & Wilson, 2000). Today, program review is commonly used as an institutional evaluation process whereby reviews are conducted at various levels—program, department, institution, and statewide—and involve a variety of individuals—including faculty, administrators, students, staff, and alumni.

Program review differs from the traditional accreditation reviews, such as those conducted by the National League for Nursing Accrediting Commission (NLNAC) and the Commission on Collegiate Nursing Education (CCNE), because it seeks to evaluate all programs against a standard set of criteria. By using a standard set of criteria, faculty and administrators can make judgments concerning a program's effectiveness and develop processes to improve the program. Table 17.1 shows a comparison between institutional academic program review and accreditation review (Conrad & Wilson, 2000).

Program review typically is a three-stage process:

- In phase one, a plan is developed for the entire program review process. This includes a needs assessment, overall design considerations, and criteria for evaluation, assignment of responsibility, determining resource requirements, and scheduling.
- Phase two is the action stage, in which the review is conducted.
- In phase three, faculty and administrators summarize and follow up on

recommendations made in the program review report.

Table 17.1 - Comparison of Academic Program Review and Accreditation Review

Feature	Institutional Academic Program Review	Accreditation Review
Primary purpose	To develop program, analyze direction and content, and assess its quality	To assess whether program or institution meets minimum standards
Primary measures	Indicators of quality deemed appropriate by institutional or departmental personnel	Minimum approved standards of the discipline or profession
Primary evaluators	Departmental or institutional personnel	Peer reviewers
Secondary evaluators	Peer consultants, advisory groups representing profession, current students and graduates	Departmental or institutional personnel via self-study

Phase One: Planning for an Effective Review

For an academic program review to be successful, those affected by it (ie, nursing faculty), must be appropriately involved in the review process. In this respect, most nursing and allied health faculty have an advantage over educators in other disciplines in that they tend to be familiar with the concept of continuous quality improvement. In 1991, the Joint Commission on Accreditation of Healthcare Organizations began incorporating the tenets of continuous quality improvement (CQI) into its program for accreditation of healthcare organizations (Papp, 2001). CQI is based on the 14 Points for Management developed by W. Edwards Deming (1984; 2000). These points are presented in Figure 17.1.

338

Figure 17.1- Deming's 14 Points for Management

The following are summaries of Deming's 14 Points for Management:

1. Create constancy of purpose toward improvement of product and service, with the aim to become competitive and stay in business and provide jobs.
2. Adopt a new philosophy.
3. Cease dependence on mass inspection to achieve quality. Build quality into the product in the first place.
4. End the practice of awarding business on the basis of price alone. Instead, minimize total cost. Move toward a single supplier for any one item because of a long-term relationship built on loyalty and trust.
5. Improve constantly and forever the system of production and service to improve quality and productivity and thus reduce costs.
6. Institute training on the job.
7. Institute leadership to help people do their job better.
8. Drive out fear so that everyone can work effectively for the good of the organization.
9. Break down barriers between departments.
10. Eliminate slogans, exhortations, and targets for the work force.
11. Eliminate work quotas. Substitute leadership.
12. Eliminate merit-rating systems.
13. Institute a vigorous program of education and self-improvement.
14. Involve everyone in the organization in the transformation of total quality improvement.

Many of Deming's points are more applicable to healthcare services or workplace environments than to nursing education programs. However, the corporate-type quality improvement model is being applied to campus accreditation (Edler, 2004; Grant, Kelley, Northington & Barlow, 2002). The concept of involving everyone in the organization is especially applicable to academic program review.

Planning an effective program review is usually a five-step process that includes:

1. Conducting a needs assessment;

2. Designing the program review plan;
3. Assigning responsibility;
4. Determining resource requirements; and
5. Scheduling.

Step One: Conducting a Needs Assessment

Developing a successful program review begins with a needs assessment. The needs assessment is the basis for designing a viable and credible review plan that addresses the needs that have been identified. The needs assessment is used to define the purposes, objectives, and needs with respect to program review. The needs assessment can be conducted either formally or informally, but must ensure certain key factors are considered. Mims (1978) cited the following factors to consider in conducting a needs assessment:

- Key individuals and their appropriate levels of involvement;
- Problems to be addressed and likely solutions;
- Purposes to be addressed and likely solutions;
- Critical factors to be considered and appropriate strategies for their consideration;
- Constraints—such as deadlines, collective bargaining, personnel, and resources—and their likely impact; and
- Various alternative approaches to program review and their likely impact on the organization.

A task force or committee should be appointed by someone at the top of the institution's structure, such as the chancellor, president, or chief academic officer. The committee mix should incorporate people with knowledge of the organization's structure, its processes, resources, finances, academic affairs, political environment, and program reviews. Committees typically include key faculty—faculty senate members, important committee chairs, and respected faculty—institutional research staff, academic administrators and staff, and business office staff. The appointments should be accompanied by specific charges to the committee and a timetable for the review. The average review takes about one academic year.

The needs assessment should result in seven basic outcomes (Conrad & Wilson, 2000):

- A statement of purposes, expected results, and expected uses;

- Criteria for judging the design of specific reviews and the review results;
- Specification of administrative responsibilities and policies for conducting reviews, distributing results, monitoring implementation, and providing information;
- Design policies and guidelines;
- Procedures for identifying new information needs, updating review plans, and evaluating the review process itself;
- A budget for required staffing and dollars;
- A summary schedule for program reviews.

Step Two: Design the program review plan

Once the needs assessment is complete and a climate conducive for successfully conducting a review has been established, the next step involves conceptualizing the review process, defining tasks and roles, and establishing timetables for completing various tasks and the process itself. This phase results in a plan for the review. This is perhaps the most important aspect of program review because it determines who will be involved in the review, what their roles will be, when the review will take place, and how the review will be conducted.

The overall design of the program review process should be determined during this phase. There is no general consensus regarding the **best** process to follow. Descriptions of many different approaches—any of which can be modified to fit your program—can be found online. Your institution and state board of higher education also might have program review formats that your nursing program must utilize. Refer to the sample review process on the CD-ROM accompanying this book.

An important aspect of designing a program review process is determining the criteria by which the program will be judged. Common examples of these criteria are program need, program cost, and program quality. Depending on the size, nature, and composition of the group designing the review process, one or more of the following techniques can be used to define the criteria for program review:

- Small-group discussion;
- Large-group discussion;
- Surveys;
- Copying from others;

- Professional consultant expertise; and
- Administrative decision.

After the relevant criteria are selected, indicators for each of these criteria must be selected, which is often more difficult than selecting the criteria. Again, specific institutions or state boards of higher education might have specific indicators that must be included in these reports, which will make this task easier.Only indicators that are specific and distinct should be selected. Some indicators, such as cost per student credit hour and the number of graduates over a given period of time, are quantitative. Other indicators, such as adequacy of facilities and equipment, peer ratings, and assessment of leadership, can be qualitative. Clark, Harnett, and Baird (Conrad & Wilson, 2000) developed criteria for the selection of indicators, which include:

- Responsiveness to the needs and purposes of the review;
- Cost and cost-effectiveness of data collection and analysis;
- Simplicity, so indicators can be readily understood by those associated with the review;
- Validity, to ensure the indicators represent an accurate proxy for the criteria;
- Comprehensiveness, to ensure there are sufficient indicators to provide a well-rounded picture of a program;
- Reliability, to ensure the indicators actually reflect what they purport to represent;
- Credibility, to ensure the review itself is not brought into question;
- Objectivity, to avoid data bias;
- Uniformity, so data from all programs reviewed are reasonably consistent; and
- Relevance, to ensure a meaningful effort.

Step Three: Assigning Responsibility

It is important to assign duties and responsibility for the review to avoid confusion or a breakdown in the process. Typical responsibilities for most academic program reviews at a college or university are:

- Faculty in the program being reviewed: Undertake the self-study; assist in collecting and reviewing data;
- Faculty outside the program: Serve on the review committee; collect and

analyze data; survey students, alumni, and employers of graduates; oversee reviews; write the final report and make recommendations;

- Administrators: Respond to interviews or surveys; appoint the review committee; review recommendations and take steps for their implementation; and
- Students and alumni: Respond to interviews or surveys.

Step Four: Determining Resource Requirements

The resources required—both human and otherwise—for a program review depend on the nature and purpose of the review and the size of the institution. These resources should be estimated as part of the needs assessment to ensure they can be made available. They would include:

- Data collection and analysis;
- Faculty, staff, and administrative time;
- Travel and expenses;
- Printing and postage; and
- Computer hardware and software.

The direct cost of conducting a program review can easily exceed $50,000 per year at a large institution.

Step Five: Scheduling

Program reviews typically are conducted every five years. At the institutional, system, and state levels this means that one-fifth of the programs are being reviewed every year. The specific programs reviewed in a given year can be determined either by the institution—as it is with private colleges and universities—or the state board of higher education—as it is with state colleges and universities. For nursing programs, it would be ideal to have the program review one year before accreditation renewal by the NLNAC or CCNE, since much of the data in the review also is needed for the self-study. In addition, any recommendations identified in the program review report can be implemented prior to the accreditation visit.

Phase Two: Conducting the Review

Once the program review plan has been prepared, the next step is to conduct the review. This phase normally begins with the committee gathering data from various sources within the institution. This information must be assembled so the faculty review committee can make objective observations about the current state of the program and offer useful recommendations for improving the program. Because too much data can complicate the program review process and diminish its effectiveness, the data collected should address the basic criteria against which the program will be judged. Common data collected for assessing the program at this point include:

- Course enrollment information;
- Grade profiles of courses within the program;
- Demographic data, which may include the number of declared majors, status of former graduates, and degrees and certificates awarded; and
- Projected job market information for the program.

Normally, the institution's finance office compiles cost and revenue data for the specific program and the division and institution as a whole. Multiple sources are used to assess program quality, including student surveys, faculty surveys, administrative surveys, and graduates' success on the licensing examination.

Once the data are collected, they must be analyzed. People with expertise in data collection and knowledge of the program should have a role in analyzing the data. Certain departments may have special course requirements or teaching loads that may skew some data elements. For example, nursing programs may grade clinical courses on a pass-fail basis which may affect a teacher's grade point averages, which in turn can impact data used to evaluate that teacher. Someone familiar with the intricacies of the program can ensure the data is interpreted correctly. The analysis should relate the data to the review's questions, goals, and objectives. The analysis also should:

- Clearly identify the mission of the program under review;
- Provide sufficient detail about the program so the program's likely influences can be discovered;
- Identify and validate the sources of information used in the review;
- Use valid measurement in the data-gathering instruments and procedures;
- Use reliable instruments and procedures to ensure the information is dependable for the intended use;

- Use data control procedures to ensure accurate data collection, processing, and reporting; and
- Ensure the data used in the review are appropriately analyzed to produce supportable interpretations.

After data analysis is complete, a formal written program review report is created. The typical review report consists of the following sections, each tailored to the needs of the intended audience (Barak, 1986):
- A description of the program reviewed;
- A description of the review process (who, what, where, and when);
- An analysis of previous review findings and current review results and documents;
- A description of the program's strengths and weaknesses; and
- Recommendations and timetable for implementation.

Regardless of the format, the final report should be simple and clear and present actionable recommendations. Usually, the report is written by the chair of the program review committee or by a member of the committee with the chair serving as editor. Other members of the committee also should be given the opportunity to review the report and provide comments and suggestions. Faculty from the program should review a draft of the final report for factual errors and omissions. Statistical data such as enrollment information can be complex. To make the assimilation of this data easier, information analysis tools such as histograms can be utilized (Papp, 2001). It may be easier to present some data in a graphic format. A histogram, or bar graph, may be used to represent data such as enrollment trends.

The following checklist may help ensure the final report is clearly written and contains actionable recommendations (Conrad & Wilson, 2000):
- Could someone totally unfamiliar with the program understand it?
- Are parts of the report redundant?
- Is jargon kept to a minimum?
- Is statistical expertise necessary to understand the report?
- Are recommendations written in a clear and action-oriented manner?
- Are positive solutions listed?
- Are negative findings fairly stated? Are they stated in a problem-solving rather than a blame-setting context?
- Are the data upon which recommendations are made defensible?

Phase Three: Post Review

Once the report is finalized, it is up to the program's faculty and administration to utilize the findings to continuously improve the program. One of the most devastating results of a review is inaction (Conrad & Wilson, 2000). Faculty, administrators, and others soon lose faith in the review if it is not used in decision making.

If the review is not being integrated into the program, faculty should encourage administrators to do so. Smith (1988) proposed 15 ways to facilitate use of the review results:

1. Consider utilization at every decision point. By the end of the evaluation, the potential for using the results has been largely determined.
2. Answer the questions that are asked. Credibility involves more than methodological quality; it also involves responsiveness to specific policy questions. Focus data gathering on those factors that are amenable to manipulation and intervention with program efforts.
3. Frame findings in terms of the intended users. Findings set in a context of unfamiliar categories and concepts make it difficult for users to translate them into action.
4. Focus recommendations on incremental rather than comprehensive changes. Small-scale changes are less disruptive and less likely to meet with resistance.
5. State recommendations in prescriptive terms. Evaluators look back; decision makers look forward. Decision makers want to know what the findings signify for future programming actions.
6. State recommendations as goals rather than delineating specific courses of action. People may be more willing to do something if they can control how it is done.
7. Make sure there is an obvious link between the recommendations and the data. Otherwise, the recommendations may be conceived as ideologically or politically inspired—and therefore mistrusted.
8. Avoid calling into question the organization's beliefs and values.
9. Adhere to rigorous methodological standards of practice. A common strategy of those who oppose report findings is to discredit the methods.
10. Use a combination of approaches to secure information so the strengths of one can mitigate the weaknesses of another.
11. Time the presentation of findings to the decisions that will be affected.

12. Make findings clear, useful, and available to policymakers. This means ordering them in a policy context, and condensing and deleting what is not relevant.

13. Rediscover the anecdote. After learning the scope, range, frequency, direction, and characteristics of a problem, one of the most effective ways to present findings diplomatically is to illustrate the general findings via specific cases that focus attention on, or explain, the large points. Anecdotes should not be presented only as data; they are effective when used in conjunction with the facts and figures.

14. Reduce political barriers. Become thoroughly familiar with the political process, operate within it, recognize the political viability of possible solutions, and know what means are politically acceptable for getting the solutions implemented. Be flexible in dealing with key political players— compromise is the key to achievement. Demonstrate a willingness to consider others' views on matters of mutual interest.

15. Couch findings in the context of other work done in the area. Although a survey is important before a study is designed, it is often omitted in the interest of time or because evaluative information is mistakenly thought to be for decision makers only.

After a program review cycle has been completed, the program review process itself should be reviewed and evaluated for accuracy and effectiveness; and the program should regain or strengthen its commitment to the process and identify ways to improve the credibility of the process. In 1981 the Joint Committee on Standards for Educational Evaluation developed a set of standards for evaluating educational programs and it was subsequently revised as a result of extensive use in the field. A modified version of these standards applicable to the evaluation of program reviews in higher education is presented in Figure 17.2 - Standards for Evaluating Program Reviews in Higher Education.

Figure 17.2 - Standard for Evaluating Program Reviews in Higher Education

1.0 Utility Standards

The Utility Standards are intended to ensure that a review serves the practical information needs of those responsible for the reviews. These standards are:

1.1. *Audience Identification.* Persons involved in or affected by the review should be identified so that their needs can be adequately addressed. Depending on the nature and purpose of the reviews this could include program faculty, administrators, the public, and students.

1.2. *Evaluator Credibility.* The persons conducting the review should be trustworthy, objective, and competent to perform the review so that their findings achieve maximum credibility and acceptance both internally and externally.

1.3. *Information Scope and Selection.* Information collected should be of such breadth and depth and selected in such ways as to addresspertinent questions about the program being reviewed and be responsive to the needs and interests of those with an interest in the program.

1.4. *Valuational Interpretation.* The perspectives, procedures, and rationale used to interpret the findings should be carefully described so that the basis for value judgments is clear and this information is available to the various constituents.

1.5. *Report Clarity.* The program review report should describe clearly the program being reviewed and its context, as well as the purposes, procedures, and findings of the review, so that it will be readily understandable to all what was done, why it was done, what information was obtained, what conclusions were drawn, and what recommendations were made.

1.6. *Report Timeliness.* Release of reports should be timely so that recipients can best use the reported information. If the deadline cannot be met, there should be adequate notice of the new deadline. Reports that are delayed repeatedly tend to lose their credibility.

1.7. *Evaluation Impact.* Reviews should be planned and conducted in ways that encourage their use by the appropriate persons

2.0 Feasibility Standards

The Feasibility Standards are intended to ensure that a review will be realistic, prudent, diplomatic, and frugal. These standards are:

2.1. *Efficient Procedures.* The review procedures should be efficient so that the disruption is kept to a minimum and needed information can be obtained.

2.2. *Political Viability.* The review should be planned and conducted with anticipation of the different positions of various interest groups, so that their cooperation may be obtained and any attempt to curtail review operations or bias or misapply the results can be averted.

2.3. *Cost-Effectiveness*. The review should produce information of sufficient value to justify the resources expended.

3.0 Propriety Standards

The Propriety Standards are intended to ensure that a review will be conducted legally, ethically, and with due regard for the welfare of those involved, as well as those affected by its results. These standards are:

3.1. *Formal Obligation*. Obligations of the formal parties to a review (what is to be done, how, by whom, and when) should be agreed to in writing, so that these parties are obligated to adhere to all conditions of the agreement or formally to renegotiate it. This is especially true when the review is being conducted by outside contractors.

3.2. *Conflict of Interest*. Conflict of interest, frequently unavoidable, should be dealt with openly and honestly, so that it does not compromise the review process and results.

3.3. *Full and Frank Disclosure*. Oral and written reports on the review should be open, direct, and honest in their disclosure of pertinent findings, including the limitations of the review. They should also be available to anyone with a legitimate purpose.

3.4. *Public's Right to Know*. The formal parties to a review should respect and assure the public's right to know, within the limits of other related principles and statutes, such as those dealing with public safety and the right to privacy.

3.5. *Rights of Human Subjects*. Reviews should be designed and conducted so that the rights and welfare of the human subjects are respected and protected. This includes a concern about the privacy of individual student records.

3.6. *Human Interactions*. Reviewers should respect human dignity and worth in their interactions with other persons associated with a review.

3.7. *Balanced Reporting*. The review should be complete and fair in its presentation of strengths and weaknesses of the program, so that strengths can be built upon and weaknesses addressed.

3.8. *Fiscal Responsibility*. The reviewers' allocation and expenditure of resources should reflect sound accountability procedures and otherwise be prudent and ethically responsible.

4.0   Accuracy Standards

The Accuracy Standards are intended to ensure that a review will reveal and convey technically adequate information about the features of the program that determines its worth. The standards are:

4.1. *Object Identification.* The object of the program review should be sufficiently examined, so that the form of the program being considered in the review can be clearly identified.

4.2. *Context Analysis.* The context in which the program exists should be examined in sufficient detail that its likely influences can be determined.

4.3. *Described Purposes and Procedures.* The purposes and procedures of the review should be described in sufficient detail that the adequacy of the information can be assessed.

4.4. *Defensible Information Sources.* The sources of information for the review should be described in sufficient detail that the adequacy of the information can be assessed.

4.5. *Valid Measurement.* The information-gathering instruments and procedures used in the review should be chosen and then implemented in ways that will assure that the interpretation is valid for the given use.

4.6. *Reliable Measurement.* The information-gathering instruments and procedures used in the review should be chosen and then implemented in ways that will assure that the information is sufficiently reliable for the intended use.

4.7. *Systematic Data Control.* The data collected, processed, and reported in the review should be examined and corrected so that the results of the review will not be flawed.

4.8. *Analysis of Quantitative Information.* Quantitative information in the review should be appropriately and systematically analyzed to ensure supportable interpretations.

4.9. *Analysis of Qualitative Information.* Qualitative information in the review should be appropriately and systematically analyzed to ensure supportable interpretations.

4.10. *Justified Conclusions.* The conclusions reached in the review should be explicitly justified so that the audiences can assess them.

4.11. Objective Reporting. The review procedures should provide safeguards to protect the findings and reports against distortion by the personal feelings and biases of any party to the review.

While evaluating its own program review process, the University of California at Berkeley (2003) used several core values that would be of value to most academic institutions. They included:

- Maintain a review process that is faculty driven.
- Develop the potential of the program review process to promote key campus objectives within a decentralized organizational structure.
- Create a structure for the departmental self-study that is flexible and responsive to the individual needs of the department.
- Reaffirm the importance of statistical data in developing self-studies and providing better centralized support to departments in preparation and interpretation of such data.
- Assure that units address student learning outcomes in discipline-specific ways.
- Create better integration between external and internal reviews.
- Maintain a program review process that is distinct from professional or specialized accreditation.
- Make the dean's role in program review more prominent, especially as a means of promoting departmental follow-up and accountability.

Summary

Faculty and institutional staff agree that the most helpful part of the review process is what we learn about ourselves. Since the object of the review is to improve the program, knowing a program's strengths and weaknesses is critical in determining its strategic direction and future decision making.

Learning Activities

1. Interview two colleagues teaching in different nursing programs about their academic program review process. Compare and contrast the two systems.

2. Interview an administrator who oversees a nursing program. Discuss the pros and cons of the academic program review process. What are the top two concerns on both sides of the issue?
3. Talk with a faculty who teaches in a healthcare program other than nursing. Compare the academic program review process for that program with a nursing program's review process.
4. Compare and contrast the institutional academic review process with the NLNAC or CCNE accreditation process.

References

Conrad, C. F., & Wilson, R. F. (2000). *Academic program reviews: Institutional approaches, expectations, and controversies.* San Francisco: Jossey-Bass.

Deming, W. E. (2000). *The new economics for industry, government, education* (2nd ed). Cambridge, MA: MIT Press.

Deming, W. E. (1986). *Out of the crisis.* Center for Advanced Educational Services. Cambridge, MA.: MIT Press.

Edler, F. (2004, Winter). Campus accreditation: Here comes the corporate model. *The NEA Higher Education Journal: Thought & Action, 19*(2), 91-104.

Grant, L., Kelley, J., Northington, L., & Barlow, D. (2002). Using TQM/CQI processes to guide development of independent and collaborative learning in two levels of baccalaureate nursing students. *Journal of Nursing Education, 41*(12), 537-540.

Joint Committee on Standards for Educational Evaluation. (1981). *Standards for evaluations of educational programs, projects, and materials.* New York: McGraw-Hill.

Papp, J. (2002). *Quality management in the imaging sciences* (2nd ed.). St. Louis: Mosby.

Popham, W. J. (1975). *Educational evaluation.* Englewood Cliffs, NJ: Prentice-Hall.

Smith, M. F. (1988). Evaluation utilization revisited. In J. A. McLaughlin, et al. (Eds.). *Evaluation utilization. New Directions for Program Evaluation.* San Francisco: Jossey-Bass.

University of California at Berkeley. (2003). Educational effectiveness review. Retrieved June 1, 2004 from Campus Accreditation website: http://education.berkely.edu/accreditation.

Warmbrod, C. P., & Persavich, J. J. (1981). *Postsecondary program evaluation* Columbus: National Center for Research in Vocational Education.

Bibliography

Ingersoll, G., & Sauter, M. (1998). Integrating accreditation criteria into education program evaluation. *Nursing and Health Care Perspectives, 19*(5), 224-226.

Kyrkjebo, J., & Hanestad, B. (2003). Personal improvement project in nursing education: Learning methods and tools for continuous quality improvement in nursing practice. *Journal of Advanced Nursing, 41*(1), 1-15.

Yearwood, E., Singleton, J., Feldman, H., & Colombraro, G. (2001). A case study in implementing CQI in a nursing education program. *Journal of Professional Nursing, 17*(6), 297-304.

Focus on Critical Thinking

Unit 5

Chapter 18: Critical Thinking Online: Can It Be Conquered?
    Carol Boswell, MSN, EdD, RN,
    and Sharon Cannon, MSN, EdD, RN

Chapter 19: Ideas to Develop Critical Thinking
                in the Classroom and the Clinical Setting
    Lynn Engelmann, MSN, EdD, RN,
    and Linda Caputi, MSN, EdD, RN

Chapter 18: Critical Thinking Online: Can It Be Conquered?

Carol Boswell, MSN, Ed D, RN,
and Sharon Cannon, MSN, Ed D, RN

Nursing today requires dealing with complex client situations. This requires critical thinking. Volumes 1 and 2 of **Teaching Nursing: The Art and Science** *include several chapters on teaching critical thinking. This chapter focuses on teaching critical thinking online. If we are to teach our students critical thinking, then we must incorporate critical thinking opportunities into all delivery methods, including online instruction. This chapter offers ideas on how to do just that.*
— *Linda Caputi*

Educational Philosophy

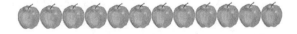

Lifelong learning is the hallmark of the educational experience. To help individuals understand the necessity of continuing to grow and learn is the ultimate reward for an educator. Helping learners develop the skills and confidence to persevere in the learning environment should be the aspiration for every teacher and facilitator. The teacher's role has evolved into that of a facilitator for the student's learning experience. By fostering the concept of lifelong learning, teachers can help students become self-motivated, passionate, and dedicated to advancing the practice of holistic nursing care for the clients they encounter. — Carol Boswell

Teaching is an interactive process that should be enjoyed by all. I believe that an emphasis on fun, or at least enjoyment, is essential to provide a positive environment for learning in nursing education. — Sharon Cannon

Introduction

Offering courses online is no longer an option but an expectation. Online courses can range from online-only to hybrid offerings, which combine face-to-face and online delivery of course material. In many cases faculty are being asked to assume the additional responsibility of developing online courses without being given the time to adequately prepare materials, or acquire skills, for this new educational delivery method. It is essential for teachers who write online courses to develop instructional approaches that not only teach content but also foster critical thinking.

This chapter addresses how to develop critical thinking activities in online nursing courses. It also discusses ways that many of the delivery methods used to teach critical thinking in a face-to-face setting can be modified for online education.

Thoughts For Online Instruction and Critical Thinking

Because faculty members often teach as they were taught, they frequently have no examples to emulate as they migrate to teaching online. Opportunities to formally prepare to teach using online methodologies seem to be few and far between. The challenge of learning to develop online instruction is increasingly problematic because of budget constraints that limit faculty development activities.

The National Council of State Boards of Nursing (NCSBN), accreditation agencies, and nursing educators emphasize the need for the development of critical thinking skills. Promotion of critical thinking in online courses must be carefully and thoroughly contemplated. Frequently, online courses are hurriedly developed by simply posting the notes from face-to-face lectures online for the Web-based student to print. A Web course should be more than just a printer for the teacher's lecture notes. Additional attention needs to be given to the development of content to be presented on a Web page and the integration of critical thinking activities.

When developing an online course, another important area to consider—one that can foster critical thinking—is the dialogue that takes place among students and between students and the teacher. According to Worrall and Kline (2002), a teacher needs to have continual presence during the online delivery but must be careful not to dominate the dialogue. The teacher's communication should help foster the student's professional development and encourage the learning process.

Critical Thinking in the Online Environment

Caputi studied the many existing definitions of critical thinking in nursing and developed a working definition for use in educational settings. This working definition is:

> Critical thinking "is a complex thinking process that is disciplined and self-directed, based on mastery of many thinking skills and abilities, best developed when applied to actual or simulated real world situations, involves thinking about the thinking process as it is occurring, and evaluates the decisions or problem solution against a standardized set of criteria" (Caputi, 2004, p. 698).

As a teacher contemplates how to enrich the critical thinking aspects of the online learning process, three aspects of this working definition of critical thinking emerge:
- Requires mastery of many thinking skills and abilities;
- Develops as a result of applying ideas to actual or simulated real-world venues; and
- Evaluates the decisions or solutions against a standardized set of criteria.

Each of these characteristics should be carefully considered as the teacher incorporates critical thinking ideas into online presentations. These three strategic facets are clearly applicable for online delivery. For the educational process conducted via the World Wide Web, the need to facilitate the students' thought processes and confirm decision-making abilities is fundamental for conveying the essential knowledge of the course.

Gathering Data

Caputi (2003) lists many skills and strategies used in critical thinking—the elements of critical thinking. One of these elements is gathering data. Four aspects of gathering data seem applicable for use in the advancement of critical thinking skills online. These four aspects are:

- Gathering complete and accurate data and then acting on that data;
- Determining the importance of information;
- Collaborating with coworkers; and
- Checking the accuracy and reliability of the data (Caputi, 2003).

Each of these four elements is of paramount importance for managing online offerings. The online teacher should consider ways to build these four elements into course assignments.

Asking Questions

It is essential for teachers developing an online instructional program (or module) to envision students' development of critical thinking skills. The process can be enhanced through the effective use of thought-provoking questions. Skillful questioning is a key part of the artistry of teaching in all educational environments. According to Nelson (2003), "well-crafted [questions] take thought and creativity and in turn require the same of students" (p. 115). Nelson (2003) writes that well-crafted questions have a mixture of believable solutions. Well-crafted questions should stimulate the students to dig deep for thoughtful responses. Given multiple believable solutions, the student is challenged to defend the selected answer, which encourages critical thinking about the problem.

Therefore, well-crafted questions can address the four aspects of gathering data. During the development of questions, careful consideration of the depth of data needed, the importance of the data, effective interaction with peers, and the accuracy and reliability of the data emerge as valuable components. While developing the instructional dialogue, the teacher should include thought-provoking, open-ended questions and limit the use of closed-ended questions.

Face-to-Face Strategies Modified for Online Delivery

Many of the strategies currently used in face-to-face sessions to invigorate student participation and critical thinking can be modified and used online. Activities such as debates, scavenger hunts, quizzes, one-minute papers, muddiest points, poster presentations, and case studies can be effectively adapted to online courses. In addition, activities like asynchronous bulletin boards (or discussion boards) and synchronous chat rooms—unique to the Internet—also can be used effectively.

Debate Session

A debate session is a face-to-face technique that can be modified for online delivery. Managing a debate requires critical thinking skills by the participants. The teacher establishes the ground rules for the activity, organizes the group, and posts questions for the debate online. Instead of being presented orally, the arguments are posted online for review. The arguments use the following critical thinking skills:

- Organizing data to support the process;
- Prioritizing the points for use in making the designated stance; and
- Confirming the dependability of the argument.

The debate format also allows the development of a collaborative process among the members of each group.

To manage of this type of online learning, individuals are assigned to summarize the affirmative and negative stances. The teacher establishes the number of interactions and the number of sentences the participants are allowed to use to defend their positions. Because it is important to carefully consider the quality of the information in a debate, at some point the debate is stopped and other members of the class are directed to discuss the strength of each argument.

Incorporating debate into the management of a course segment provides an introduction to the art of argument (Weston, 1987). Through the development of the skills needed to organize a strong argument, students become more adept at thinking critically and coordinating a defense that can be utilized in real-world healthcare settings. Students are expected to carefully consider the underlying conclusions and premises of the topic being debated. Within the process of establishing an effective argument, the students are asked to solidify their conclusions by presenting facts and evidences that provide the basis of the argument. The expected outcome of this process is a convincing answer to the "so what?" question. The entire process of organizing and presenting an argument for a debate combines the students' ability to critically think about decisions or solutions and the need to base these decisions and solutions on an established set of criteria.

Scavenger Hunts

Scavenger hunts allow students to search online for sources of information, which is one of the characteristics of critical thinking. During this learning strategy, students are expected to post their findings and comments on the value of the sources identified. This strategy is beneficial for facilitating critiques of online resources on a given topic. Students become familiar with accurate, reliable sources to better respond to clients who have used the Internet to find healthcare information.

This technique can be incorporated into a class by asking students to locate and critique websites related to any topic appropriate for the course. For example, students in a course on alternative medicine may be asked to search the Web for sites with information about stress management. The concept behind a scavenger hunt is to encourage the students to seek resources on the Internet that clarify or explain the topic under investigation. Students are encouraged to think critically about the websites by comparing and contrasting the sites against criteria established by the teacher and are required to post their findings and appraisals of the Web sites based on an established set of criteria. This process helps students appreciate the value of potential sources of information available within the healthcare arena.

Quizzes and Tests

Quizzes and tests are an integral part of the educational process. Relative to critical thinking, tests are viewed as a way to validate that students have acquired appropriate and accurate data. Developing online tests requires the same thought and consideration that goes into any examination. Although most online teaching software has a testing component within the program, teachers must carefully consider their expectations of the examination process.

As with any examination process, cheating is always possible online. If as much thought is given to the entire process prior to an online test as for face-to-face examinations, cheating can be minimized or prevented. One mechanism for controlling delivery of online examinations and possible cheating is establishing a time limit. With online delivery, the teacher can elect to have the test available to the students for a selected number of days. During that time, a student may enter the examination only once and must complete the test at that time. Imposing a time restriction makes it mandatory that students arrive at the testing session prepared for the assignment.

Identifying the purpose of the test is fundamental to administering any test. The teacher should examine the goal to be achieved when using a test as a learning strategy. When examining this goal, the teacher should consider allowing students to use textbooks during the examination. An open-book test is another mechanism for addressing concerns about cheating. If the goal is for students to know where and how to access information, then open-book testing is valuable.

The teacher may also arrange to have the examination proctored at a designated computer lab for the online student to ensure the integrity of the examination. The examination can be protected by a password to guard against inappropriate access. A password helps prevent cheating because the proctor provides the password to the students at the designated testing site.

Another consideration for online examinations is managing computer-related problems. If an examination is timed and the online platform becomes inaccessible, the teacher must address the student concerns that would result from not having access to the examination during the designated time period. Most platforms allow the course developer to reset the examination if students' access to the examination is restricted. The teacher needs to carefully consider the possibility of technology failure in advance to allow time to deal with the problem.

One-Minute Paper/Muddiest Point

Another interesting strategy used in face-to-face encounters is the one-minute paper/muddiest point. In both of these processes, the student is given the opportunity to acknowledge effective as well as ineffective classroom strategies. With the one-minute paper, students are asked to document—within one minute—the principal points learned during the face-to-face period. The muddiest point requires the student to document the points from the lesson that continue to be confusing.

These two strategies can easily be adapted for online presentation. With the asynchronous delivery method, a forum for one-minute papers/muddiest point assignments can be established. At intervals during the management of the course, the teacher can either incorporate this type of assignment into the class schedule or simply post an entry requesting the information. In a synchronous delivery method, such as during a chat, the teacher can ask the students to complete the one-minute paper or muddiest point just as the teacher would in a face-to-face delivery venue. Again, critical thinking skills are heightened when the students are asked to evaluate their understanding of information at a designated point in the learning process.

The authors are familiar with one online undergraduate research course that used the muddiest points concept to help students communicate difficult topics of discussion within the assigned modules. Four times during the semester, students were asked to post an asynchronous entry on any topic that they found confusing after they completed the other course assignments. The teacher then directly addressed these topics. The teacher realized that other students frequently had similar questions. By incorporating this assignment, the teacher was able to address the confusing issues to all students at one time.

Case Studies and Problem-Based Learning

Case studies and problem-based learning are becoming increasingly useful in face-to-face learning. These strategies can be readily converted to an online methodology. Teachers can use both asynchronous or synchronous methods. For the asynchronous delivery, the teacher posts a situation on an online discussion board with specific instructions for gathering and utilizing data to address the assigned situation. The teacher assigns the grouping of students, creating networking opportunities for the students. The teacher determines a time limit for working on the situation and each group's results are posted for comments by the rest of the class.

If synchronous delivery is used, the situation is posted on the discussion board before the chat-room time to allow students to gather complete and accurate data. During the chat room, the students are divided into small groups and sent to different chat rooms to discuss the problem. Following the small-group chat, the whole class reconvenes to discuss and evaluate the solutions to the problems selected in their individual group sessions.

A Closer Look at Online Discussions

Asynchronous discussion boards allow students and teachers to converse about topics of interest in order to promote thought and reflection, which are important components of critical thinking. Discussion board entries should indicate a growing understanding of the topic. To begin the process, a designated person—frequently the teacher—carefully constructs questions and posts them to the discussion board. These questions direct the participants to explore innovative areas of thought and thus promote critical thinking. Because the process is asynchronous, each and every individual becomes actively engaged in critical thinking.

One challenge inherent in online delivery is that the teacher is not able to look into the students faces' to ascertain if they understand the material. In face-to-face delivery, if a question results in blank looks, the teacher can re-word the question. Moallan (2002) discussed management of the student's confused look as the use of "scaffolding strategies" (p.180). The use of bridging techniques to reduce confusion and frustrations takes on a new meaning when used online.

This subjective feedback process is not possible in online presentation; the "blank look" is not in view. Therefore, the wording of the questions posted for discussion is of great importance. The facilitation of the thought process rests on the appropriateness and inspiration of the questions. The questions need to be broad enough to encourage diverse views and discussion, yet focused enough to ensure completion of the course objectives.

Faculty should also consider in advance their expectations of online discussions. It is important to build expectations around the goal of promoting critical thinking. Moallan (2002) relates that task structure and course organization profoundly affect the temperament and reputation of the entire course delivery.

Worrall and Kline (2002) recommended participation in the discussion board activity be a factor designated in the student evaluation. Does a student need to post six entries per topic to demonstrate understanding of the topic or will two entries suffice? Is the student evaluated by the number of entries or by the critical thinking demonstrated in the entries?

If an online class of 40 students, the teacher requires six entries per student per topic, and the course has six topics (modules), the teacher must address 1440 entries at a minimum on the course content alone. Faculty time is a major issue to be considered. An online course can very quickly overwhelm the teacher. Care must be given to the issue of how many and what level of asynchronous activities are necessary for satisfactory completion of the course. The teacher not only needs time to read and evaluate the postings, but also must have time to assess the level of critical thinking reflected in the students' posts to the discussion board.

Synchronous Chat Room

In many ways, the synchronous chat room experience has developed a bad reputation. Participants at workshops around the country have shared their comments concerning the difficulties of using synchronous chat rooms for academic assignments. Synchronous classes may be disruptive for students who have chosen online courses because of the flexible schedule they offer. Synchronous sessions are sometimes difficult when students live in different time zones or when the sheer numbers of posting from a large class makes it difficult to follow a discussion thread (Baumlein, 2004).

Synchronous discussions do have benefits. Synchronous activities allow students to interact with each other about real-world experiences or for group-paper discussions. According to Moallan (2002), "interaction is a vital element in the educational process and a collaborative interactive learning environment can lead to deeper understanding" (p. 175). A deeper understanding of an issue is fundamental to critical thinking.

Synchronous activities in online delivery platforms require specific, carefully developed outlines to aid the flow of the activity. The activity in chat rooms is usually rapid and somewhat detached. The teacher needs to take directed time prior to the chat room to determine appropriate expectations for the discussion. The flow within the chat room is much like a room full of people all trying to talk at the same time. Unless someone takes control of the discussion, the volume in that room can be formidable. The same is true in a chat room. The teacher must set clear discussion guidelines for the participants. When students depart from the guidelines during the discussion, they must be re-directed to the objective.

Since the process moves very rapidly, archiving the chat discussion following its completion allows students to examine more deeply the content and to think critically about the comments posted. The students can then contact the teacher to discuss concerns or misunderstandings they have about the discussion.

Another advantage of synchronous opportunities is their potential to help establish a community of scholars. Regular interactions allow students to become more directly involved with other individuals in the course. This promotes the critical thinking skill of collaborating with coworkers.

Synchronous chat rooms also can be used to simulate office hours for the faculty. Since the expectation in online courses is that students will be on campus rarely—if at all—designated office hours via chat rooms is one mechanism that allows faculty to be available to students. When the chat room is used for office hours, the faculty should clearly state the expectations. If the teacher sets online office hours for 3 PM until 4 PM, it is important for the faculty to be available online for the entire time.

Summary

Online teaching methods can promote critical thinking regardless of the content offered. Faculty can use and adapt teaching strategies typical of the more traditional face-to-face approach without extensive training for online teaching. The   strategies suggested in this chapter can provide a stimulating, thought-provoking educational experience.

Techniques specifically developed for online courses are also valuable resources for the development of critical thinking skills. The asynchronous methodology easily lends itself to the use of actual and simulated situations. Online teaching requires additional preparation and thought to maximize students' critical thinking. A teacher should not wait and let the course develop its own flow. Innovative and creative thought by the faculty before the beginning of the class will ensure greater success in developing students' critical thinking skills.

Learning Activities

1. You are the faculty assigned to convert a community health RN-BSN course to an online-only delivery format. One of the assignments used in the traditional face-to-face delivery has been a debate on the value of community-based health care versus hospital-based health care. Develop the instructions

you would post in the online syllabus to direct the students to complete this debate online.

2. Document the criteria needed to accomplish a treasure-hunt critique of Internet sites that provide information about alternative medicine.

3. Interview three to four students currently enrolled in an online course. Ask them what type of assignments they have been assigned for this course. Solicit their recommendations for improving the instructions that were provided for those assignments and ideas for making the instructions more understandable.

4. Develop four open-ended, critical thinking questions that could be used in an asynchronous discussion venue on the topic of client education issues for the professional nurse.

References

Baumlein, G. (2004). Internet-based education. In L. Caputi & L. Engelmann (Eds.), *Teaching nursing: The art and science, Vol. 1 & 2*. Glen Ellyn, IL: College of DuPage Press.

Caputi, L. (2003). *The critical thinking tutorial software program*. Glen Ellyn, IL: College of DuPage Press.

Caputi, L. (2004). Operationalizing critical thinking. In L. Caputi & L. Engelmann (Eds.), *Teaching nursing: The art and science, Vol. 1 & 2*. Glen Ellyn, IL: College of DuPage Press.

Moallan, M. (2002). Designing and implementing an interactive online learning environment. In P. Comeaux (Ed.), *Communication and collaboration in the online classroom: Examples and application*. Bolton, MA: Anker Publishing.

Nelson, L. B. (2003). *Teaching at its best*. (2nd ed.). Bolton, MA: Anker Publishing.

Weston, A. (1987) *A rule book for arguments*. Indianapolis: Hackett.

Worrall, P., & Kline, B. (2002). Building a communication learning community. In P. Comeaux (Ed.), *Communication and collaboration in the online classroom: Examples and application*. Bolton, MA: Anker Publishing.

Chapter 19: Ideas to Develop Critical Thinking in the Classroom and the Clinical Setting

Lynn Engelmann, MSN, EdD, RN,
and Linda Caputi, MSN, EdD, RN

Critical thinking—that recurring but elusive concept! This chapter offers more ideas for developing critical thinking in nursing students. The ideas are simple yet effective. – Linda Caputi

Educational Philosophy

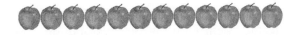

The teacher who artfully engages students in an atmosphere rich in trust, rapport, and resources is well on the way to developing a climate that is just right in which to learn. Students need to feel safe to explore and question, in order to gain meaning from their experiences. Students also need focus and perspective. In a collaborative atmosphere, both teacher and student are learners. It is equally important for teachers to be well ensconced in a positive working environment—one that fosters personal growth and enhancement. – Lynn Engelmann

My educational philosophy is succinct: Give the best educational experience possible. I feel faculty should continuously challenge themselves to provide creative, interesting, and sound education—students soon learn that education doesn't have to be boring; they become self-motivated, enthusiastic, and interested…learning then follows. – Linda Caputi

Introduction

Many factors impact how well students will succeed in their nursing programs. Everyone has high expectations, but sometimes students fall short of the expectations. Two major consideration are the nature of instructional design and the expertise with which it is delivered. Inherent in the instructional design is the modeling and teaching of critical-thinking skills.

Critical thinking is highly valued in all educational realms. Not to be confused with problem solving, critical thinking is "careful, deliberate, outcome-focused (results-oriented) thinking" (Alfaro-LeFevre, 2002, p. 23). It would be difficult to find current nursing literature that does not attest to the need for enhanced critical thinking skills in nursing students and graduates—the future artists and scientists in nursing. The mission of nurse educators is not simply to assign grades, but to educate students to think, learn, and make well-associated connections.

This chapter explores practical interventions faculty may use to enhance instruction for classroom and clinical experiences through the use of specially designed critical thinking tools. The tools are offered for faculty to use or modify as they see fit.

The first section of this chapter introduces the topic of critical thinking tools and the advantages of using them. The second section discusses the process faculty can use to develop their own critical thinking tools. The third section focuses on concept mapping as a critical thinking activity that may be used in the classroom, or with independent study, to enhance student study skills and knowledge of a particular topic. A concept map created by one student is used to illustrate how concept maps may be used to augment the study of nursing care for the client with thyroid dysfunction. The fourth and final section discusses the value and application of select critical-thinking tools to enhance student understanding of client care in the clinical setting.

Expertise in Teaching and Learning

Faculty, regardless of their teaching background, usually have one common characteristic: They have a perspective on the practice of nursing. It is this perspective, gained over years of experience, that enables faculty to provide insights for students and direct them in both the art and science of nursing. Students learning about the role of the nurse, and all it encompasses, lack such experience, and cannot possibly foresee how all the pieces fit. However, students do not lack the desire or the ability to put it all together. They simply need guidance to learn how to solve problems and think critically. Therefore, the expertise students develop is directly proportional to the guidance faculty provide. A major part of this guidance is the modeling of critical thinking. One way to model critical thinking is to provide a frame of reference for a given situation or client condition. Critical thinking tools provide this frame of reference.

Advantages of Using Critical Thinking Tools

There are several advantages for both faculty and students when critical thinking tools are developed and used.

Faculty Expertise

Developing critical-thinking tools not only facilitates students' learning, but also refines the faculty's knowledge and expertise, because faculty must be knowledgeable about the content they wish to address. Most importantly, students have a focus, and faculty have a way to structure and evaluate that focus. One of the most important things faculty can do to help students learn is to provide focus, or a direction for learning.

Comprehending the Task at Hand

When developing critical-thinking tools, faculty must think clearly and must clearly communicate the objectives of a given exercise, so that everyone involved knows exactly what the task is. By devising these tools in advance, faculty can design instruction that enables students to seek information in a well-organized, orchestrated fashion. Students who are given such tools understand the task at hand and find the information they need to provide competent, informed care.

Perspective

When critical-thinking tools are employed, students gain a clear perspective of what the task is and have a definite plan to follow. Such tools provide not only direction, but also a written means of communication giving students an opportunity to write about their understanding of a topic and for teachers to evaluate the students' level of knowledge about particular content. This allows a dialogue to take place between student and faculty. If the tools are used in group discussions, all students may benefit from one student's experience.

Direction

By organizing important concepts of an assignment into manageable segments, students can use these tools independently, or with a buddy, to enhance their knowledge of a particular content area. By developing the tools in advance, and planning when they might best be implemented, the faculty has greater control over experiences that are provided and can plan instruction in an organized fashion. For example, with eight to 10 students simultaneously asking questions in a clinical setting, it is often difficult to keep a class organized, or keep students on task. Having planned instructional approaches for the situations students are likely to encounter can help faculty avoid scrambling to assess or provide student goals for client care. As novices, students often do not know the most important focus when they are planning care. Critical-thinking tools can help students decide where their priorities rest. To that end, carefully selected tools, like the one developed for a client with congestive heart failure (see Figure 19.7), may be used. Tools may also be more general in nature depending on the level of learner.

Application for All Students

Ultimately, the information students learn from the critical thinking tools can be shared in group sessions. Students are able to bring important highlights of their experience to others, and this in turn builds self confidence and self esteem. Also, if there are any misperceptions, or misinterpretations of data, the teacher can redirect students' thinking. Thus, critical thinking tools may be used to evaluate a student's ability to relate theory to practice.

Critical thinking activities benefit not only those who complete them, but also classmates who hear the organized delivery of their fellow student's client history. Students and faculty often are tired at the end of a busy clinical day. During postconference, when client care is discussed, it can be challenging to summon the energy to put facts together. Using a critical-thinking tool to present information to fellow students is especially helpful because it provides a blueprint of the content and direction for the discussion. In some instances, this leads to fellow students asking even more probing questions and seeking information they otherwise might not explore.

The authors have found such critical-thinking activities to be effective teaching tools, and have used several different types of tools. All these tools were developed as remedies for deficits in student preparation, understanding, and application of concepts to client care situations. These tools range from chart exploration—for the novice student who needs to learn how to navigate charts and where to find information that relates to the overall client picture—to tools specific for clients that present with a particular diagnosis or condition. Each of these types of tools is discussed later in the chapter.

Creating Critical-Thinking Tools: A Guide for Nurse Educators

Before discussing actual tools that have been used with students, it may be helpful to explain a process designed to help educators develop their own tools (Caputi & Engelmann, 2003). The following steps are employed:

1. Identify the teaching challenge. Think of a situation your students have encountered that you would have liked the students to be better prepared to handle.
2. Formulate your purpose and approach. Consider the:
   a. General goal; and
   b. Specific criteria: objectives you hope to achieve.
3. Create the tool.
   a. What would the student need to know to handle this situation and what steps would the student need to work through? Write down those steps. This is perhaps the most difficult part to develop. As an expert, the teacher may have a difficult time identifying all the thinking that takes place in any particular nursing intervention. The answers to the following questions will help determine the steps that are included in the tool for the student:
      i. What thinking processes do I use when I approach this problem or intervention?
      ii. What questions do I ask myself?
      iii. What information do I need?
   b. Plan a tool that walks the student through each of those steps. When possible, relate it to a critical thinking skill or strategy. Following are several critical thinking skills and strategies (Caputi, 2004):

i.   Identifying signs and symptoms;

ii.   Assessing systematically and comprehensively;

iii.   Checking accuracy and reliability;

iv.   Clustering related information;

v.   Collaborating with coworkers;

vi.   Determining the importance of information;

vii.   Distinguishing relevant from irrelevant information;

viii.   Gathering complete and accurate data, and then acting on that data;

ix.   Judging how much ambiguity is acceptable;

x.   Recognizing inconsistencies;

xi.   Using diagnostic reasoning;

xii.   Applying the nursing process to develop a treatment plan;

xiii.   Communicating effectively;

xiv.   Predicting and managing potential complications;

xv.   Resolving conflicts;

xvi.   Resolving ethical dilemmas;

xvii.   Setting priorities;

xviii.   Teaching others;

xix.   Evaluating and correcting thinking;

xx.   Evaluating data; and

xxi.   Supporting conclusions with evidence.

Tool Development Considerations

When developing a critical thinking tool, faculty should consider:

- **Level of learner.** At what stage of critical-thinking development is the learner: basic, complex, or committed? (Ignatavicius, 2004)
- **Learning context.** Where will the tool be used? In a clinical or classroom setting, or in a nursing laboratory or nursing specialty area?
- **Student activation.** Put the student in the role of nurse, using the thinking skills the nurse would use. For example, if it is important for the student to prioritize, the tool should guide the student through the steps of prioritization.

The teacher must delineate all of the critical-thinking skills and strategies used by the nurse to meet the specific objectives (eg, integrate concepts, prioritize, delegate, or plan care). The teacher, as the expert, has to think through how that specific objective is achieved, and then guide the student through the same process. The tool provides a tangible framework and direction for a course of action for the student to take. It uses the expert nurse's critical thinking skills and strategies as models for the student. In this way, students actively learn as they go through the guided process you have developed.

Creating Critical Thinking Tools: A Process for Nurse Educators Example

1. Identify the teaching challenge.
   Think of a situation you have encountered with your students that you wish the students had been better prepared to handle.

> **Safe administration of medications taking into consideration all important information.**

2. Formulate your purpose and approach.
   a. General goal

> **The student will safely administer medications to clients after careful consideration of all important data.**

   b. Specific criteria (objectives you hope to achieve)

> **Student will collect and analyze data pertinent to:**
> 1. **Client's history;**
> 2. **Client's current condition;**
> 3. **All aspects about the medication relevant to this particular client; and**
> 4. **Proper administration of the medication.**

3. Plan the strategy that will best guide the process. Will it be role playing, a critical-thinking activity or exercise, or a case study? etc.

> **Critical-thinking exercise.**

4. Create the tool
   a. What would the student need to know to handle this situation and what steps would the student need to work through? Write down those steps.

---

1. **Gather information about the client.**
2. **Consider information about the medication and how it relates to the client.**
3. **Determine how to safely administer the medication.**

---

   b. Plan a tool that walks the student through each of the steps.

See Figure 19.1. A printable version of this tool is contained on the CD-ROM accompanying this book.

Critical Thinking Applied to Self

Students and faculty need to work together to foster a successful school experience. This means that students must have a clear understanding of the faculty's expectations and how they might meet these expectations. For this purpose, student success plans may offer a way for students to think critically to focus their energies on the goal: successfully completing the program.

Student Success Plan

Students may benefit from outlining their personal strategy for success each term. Some teachers include such plans in their syllabi. Reviewing students' success plans can augment the faculty's ability to support students in their approach to the term. A student success plan is presented in Figure 19.2, and a printable version is included on the CD-ROM accompanying this book.

Figure 19.1 - Sample Critical-Thinking Exercise

**Medication Administration
Critical Thinking Exercise**

1. Gather information about the client.
Medication to be administered _____ Classification _____
Client Diagnosis _____
Allergies _____
Surgical Procedure _____
Chronic Conditions _____

2. Consider information about the medication and how it relates to the client.
Reason the medication is prescribed for this client __
How does this medication relate to the client's H&P?
Other prescribed medications that relate to this medication and affect the administration of this medication _____
Expected therapeutic effects _____
Side effects to consider _____
When was the last time this medication was given? _____
What were the effects of the medication the last time it was given? _____

3. Determine how to safely administer the medication.
Any pertinent assessments to make? _____
Any parameters to consider? _____
Any contraindications to giving this medication? _____
Any reason to hold this medication? _____
What dosage will be given? _____
What route will be used? _____
IV? _____ Compatible with IV solution? ___ Compatible with other meds in the line? __
Flush needed? __ _____
Oral?____ Can it be crushed?_____ Given with food? _____
Can it be given with other medications? _____
Evaluation data to collect _____
Collect evaluation data how long after administering the med? _____
Pertinent information to document _____

Critical thinking skills and strategies used:
- Gathering complete and accurate data
- Identifying signs and symptoms
- Understanding and applying the physiology of body systems
- Analyzing data
- Distinguishing relevant from irrelevant data
- Determining the importance of information
- Clustering related information

Figure 19.2 - Student Success Plan

Student Success Plan

The goals of this exercise are to consider carefully all factors that impact your ability to succeed in this program and to design an individual success plan. Please identify obstacles with which you might need help, or any resources that you feel might help you meet your goals. Please consider the following as you think about how to succeed this term.

1. What is your overarching goal this term?
2. How do you anticipate meeting this goal? Please consider:
   a. When and how you will study:
      i. Independently
      ii. In a study group
      iii. With a tutor
      iv. Other
   b. Number of hours you will need to work per week
   c. Childcare needs
3. What are your resources to help with the following?
   a. Understanding theoretical concepts
   b. Time management
   c. Study skills
   d. Home maintenance
   e. Personal time

Critical Thinking in the Classroom: Using Concept Maps

Concept maps are very helpful tools for developing critical thinking (Couey, 2004). Knowing that the endocrine system is often confusing for students, the author, Dr. Engelmann, elected to use maps in conjunction with classroom lecture and case study to augment students' knowledge of this challenging topic.

Concept Maps Used During Lecture

A total of five hours of lectures on the care of clients with dysfunction of the thyroid, parathyroid, adrenal, and pituitary glands were presented to the class using PowerPoint presentations. Throughout the lectures, case studies were used to illustrate key concepts and aspects of nursing assessment, care, and evaluation. During the final 30 minutes of each class, students were asked to break into groups of six to develop a concept map on the topic of their choice. Before beginning this exercise, students were presented with a sample concept map on another topic and introduced to the design and purpose of the activity. There were some students who were quite familiar with the use of concept maps and others who had never heard of concept mapping.

As might be expected, there was some student resistance to developing a concept map. Some students were not sure how to begin, what to do, what topic they should select, or whether they would do it right. Simple suggestions were offered, such as:

- Place the client with a particular condition in the center of the page.
- Pick one of the topics you think you understand.
- Choose a topic you want to learn more about.
- Refer to your notes and texts.

Soon students began to write their ideas. When they began to draw lines and circles, linking information, such as lab values and certain disease states, it was apparent they had the correct information associated with the corresponding endocrine dysfunction.

Once the groups completed their concept maps, they shared them with other members of the class. Fellow students were able to see how classmates processed information and make note of ideas their own groups hadn't considered. Students made linkages in creative, interesting ways, and there was variety in both the style and presentation of the concept maps.

One way to further increase students' comprehension is for their concept maps to be copied and distributed to the class, so that each student has a concept map for all major endocrine dysfunctions. This provides students four or five pages of the necessary information about the disease or body system in a visual format, as opposed to several pages of notes. This serves to present a concise clinical picture of the particular disease or condition, which helps students focus their study. Using a concept map for this particular material is especially beneficial because students might not have the opportunity to care for clients diagnosed with some of the conditions presented during the lectures.

In our classroom one student reported that at first she did not want to do this exercise, but admitted she had learned from the experience. Another student stated she had a teacher in high school who used concept maps and she loved that class. She had earned a high grade in that class and thought she learned well with concept mapping.

Students learn in a variety of ways. Using concept maps in conjunction with lecture, discussion, and case studies engages students in learning and provides a visual representation of the material being presented. It also allows faculty to question cross links or associations that students make to determine if students comprehend the material.

Please refer to the CD-ROM that accompanies this book to view a concept map related to the care of clients with pathology of the thyroid.

Concept Maps as a Study Method

Several students who wanted to improve their test scores sought help from the one of the authors, Dr. Engelmann, prior to taking an exam on the endocrine system. That author examined lecture notes and talked with students about their study habits and the challenge of keeping the information straight. It was suggested that students create concept maps for major areas of study and divide the content by studying one concept map each day, with the last day reserved to review all the concept maps. This intervention served as a focused review of the material and helped students avoid feeling overwhelmed with the subject matter.

It was also suggested that if students worked in a study group, members of the group could create concept maps for certain segments of information, and then share their maps and explain the relationships they drew. Students could then consult with faculty to validate their associations. Using the concept maps for teacher-student consultation provides a focal point for discussion, and the visual aid allows the teacher to easily identify gaps in knowledge and point students in the right direction for further study.

Critical-Thinking Tools for the Clinical Setting

The following section discusses approaches that may be used to facilitate critical thinking in the clinical component of a nursing course and presents several critical thinking tools as they apply to care of clients. Readers are free to implement these tools for use with their students.

Critical-thinking tools that organize and facilitate student experiences in the clinical setting serve to direct students in their clinical duties, provide structure, and frame their practice. In addition, such tools provide a springboard for students to gain momentum in their nursing roles. Each time students use one of these tools, they edge closer to reflection in action. Such reflection allows students to identify what they know and what they still need to learn. The use of such tools contributes to enhanced self esteem, a base of knowledge transferable to a variety of situations, and practical insights related to the role of the nurse.

Organizing student actions through the use of such tools provides an efficient use of time because information is sought and disseminated in a clear, well-defined way. Students and faculty alike are less frustrated with hit-or-miss approaches to obtaining report, navigating charts, planning for client tests or procedures, assessing important aspects of a client's problems, and seeing the relationship among all these variables. The students have a plan of action for the day and they know exactly what it is. The tools guide their data gathering and provide cues for them to think about important aspects of care for their clients.

Sample Critical-Thinking Tools

The ultimate challenge for faculty is to design educational experiences so that they foster one of the most highly valued student outcomes: critical thinking. Critical-thinking tools may be devised in a variety of ways, and they may be easier to create than faculty suspect. The following tools are described so that faculty consider the value they offer to students. Faculty may wish to use some of these tools to spark development of their own, specialized tools that can be used to direct student learning with specific client populations.

Chart Explorer

Often, students have no idea what to glean from a chart. They do not understand how charts are organized, or where they might obtain specific information. The chart explorer tool was developed to foster successful chart navigation and enhance use of the chart. This tool is especially helpful when students begin their first clinical rotation. It is also helpful to use the tool on a daily basis so students have the necessary information to render client care. The tool contains questions that impact the plan and delivery of client care. Figure 19.3 presents the chart explorer; a printable version is included on the CD-ROM accompanying this book.

Figure 19. 3 - Chart Explorer

Chart Explorer

Please answer each of the following questions and indicate from which part of the chart you obtained the information.

1. What is the client's admitting diagnosis?
2. What medications does the client normally take at home, in an extended care facility, or elsewhere?
3. What do the progress notes indicate has transpired with the client in the past 48 hours?
4. Which, if any, laboratory or diagnostic tests reveal significant data relative to projected client needs or problems?
5. List five problems noted on the client's interdisciplinary plan of care (IPOC).
    a.
    b.
    c.
    d.
    e.
6. Identify two teaching strategies noted on the client's interdisciplinary patient education document (IPED).
7. When did the client last receive any medication to assist with pain control?
8. What is the client's last recorded intake and output?
9. What do you want to know but can't find in the client's chart?

Report Organizer

The report organizer is a tool that helps students understand what information should be shared during report. It also helps students focus questions to the person who is giving the report and the nurse with whom they will be working during their clinical experience. In addition, there is a section on the report organizer for students to note what they need to provide in their off-going shift report. Students may use this section to write notes in particular data categories, so they do not lose sight of any information that should be communicated to the next shift. If students are not on the nursing unit for an entire shift, they may use

Teaching Nursing: The Art and Science

this information when they report off. This tool is presented in Figure 19.4; a printable version is included on the CD-ROM accompanying this book.

Figure 19.4 - Report Organizer

Report Organizer	
Client initials:	Client diagnosis:
DNR status:	Allergies:
Your shift	**Oncoming shift**
Neuro status	
Orientation	
Pain control	
Respiratory status	
Oxygenation-pulse oximetry	
Lung sounds	
O_2	
CV status	
Vital signs	
Heart rhythm	
Edema	
Weight	
CMS	
GI status	
Diet	
Abdomen	
Bowel sounds	
Last BM	
Glucose checks: Times:	
GU status	
I & O	
Catheter/voiding	
Amount/color	
Frequency	
Activity/mobility status	
PT/OT	
Speech therapy	
Dressing change procedure:	
IV: Solution/Rate: Location: Site/tubing— due to change:	
Tests/Procedures:	
Other:	

Critical-Thinking Activity for Patient Tests or Procedures

Another critical thinking tool is one that outlines the details the student should address when a client undergoes a diagnostic test or procedure (see Figure 19.5). This tool is generic and therefore can be used with a variety of interventions. A 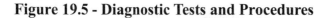 printable version of this tool is included on the CD-ROM accompanying this book.

Figure 19.5 - Diagnostic Tests and Procedures

Diagnostic Tests and Procedures

Pre-procedure
1. Client's diagnosis:
2. Test/procedure ordered:
3. Has consent been obtained for this procedure?
4. What is the purpose of the test ordered for this client?
5. How is the client being prepared for the test?
6. Resources used to provide client education:
7. Content of client education: What did you or what would you teach the client about this procedure/test?
8. What would you document before the client leaves for the procedure?

Post-procedure
1. What is the protocol of care for the client post procedure?
2. What is the first priority of care for this client post procedure?
3. Is there any aspect of care that is appropriate to delegate to the patient care technician? If so, what would you delegate?
4. What documentation would you make in the client's chart upon receiving the client post-procedure?

Intravenous Medication Administration and Monitoring

Often students are assigned to care for clients who are receiving medications via intravenous (IV) infusion. It is important that students understand the rationale, purpose, and nursing interventions for IV infusion as well as client care during administration of the medication. A critical thinking tool can provide the focus for these considerations. Figure 19.6 contains a sample tool for administering and monitoring IV drip medication; a printable version is included on the CD-ROM accompanying this book.

Figure 19.6 - IV Medication Administration and Monitoring

IV Medication Administration and Monitoring

1. What is the client's admitting diagnosis?
2. What medication is prescribed via IV infusion pump for the client?
3. What is the dose and infusion rate of the medication for the client?
4. What are you going to need to know prior to, or during administration of, this medication?
   a. Weight
   b. Vital signs
   c. Laboratory values
   d. Signs and symptoms
   e. Side effects
   f. Other
5. How will you know the drug is effective?
6. What are the nursing implications in the event of extravasation of the prescribed medication?

Client-Specific Tools

Several tools may be designed to focus students applying theory to practice. Students use information, such as noting clinical manifestations. The following tools highlight the relevance related to nursing care for clients with specific medical conditions.

The Client with Congestive Heart Failure

One focus for critical thinking might be learning how to recognize important manifestations of congestive heart failure and provide appropriate care for the client who is in congestive heart failure. This is especially helpful because students might not know how to put together all the facts to identify and monitor signs and symptoms of this condition, or what to do once the signs and symptoms are recognized. Given the task of identifying critical information and evaluating the client for particular manifestations of congestive heart failure, students begin to see the big picture. The tool helps relate theory to practice with questions that guide students' thinking and lead them to draw conclusions. The information students glean while completing such a tool is valuable on many levels and may be used to plan and provide client care. This information may be shared later in postconference.

Once students have written responses to the thinking tool, the faculty can examine the answers to determine how well students sought and understood information and determine whether the questions led to the desired outcome. Faculty may see a need to revise the tool or may simply gain an understanding of how students see a particular client situation or disease state. Figure 19.7 provides a tool to use with students caring for a client with congestive heart failure; a printable version of this tool is included on the CD-ROM accompanying this book. This tool may be modified for clients with various cardiac conditions.

Figure 19.7 - Critical-Thinking Tool for the Client with Congestive Heart Failure

---

The Client with Congestive Heart Failure

1. What was the client's admitting diagnosis and what effect does it have on the cardiovascular system?
2. What factors are of primary concern right now?
3. Does the client need or exhibit any of the following? If so, please describe.
   a. Oxygen
   b. Mobility limitations
   c. Edema
   d. Jugular vein distention
   e. Rales
   f. Dysrhythmia
   g. Dyspnea on exertion
   h. Daily weights
4. What lab values must be monitored for this client, and why?
5. What medications is the client currently prescribed?
6. What special teaching needs does this client have?
7. What concerns you most about this client? How do you plan to deal with this concern?

The Client with Renal Failure

A second client-focused activity is a tool for care of a client in renal failure. Figure 19.8 contains a sample tool for caring for a client with renal failure; a printable version is included on the CD-ROM accompanying this book.

Figure 19.8 - Critical Thinking Tool for the Client with Renal Failure

---

The Client with Renal Failure

1. What was the client's admitting diagnosis and what affect does it have on the renal system?
2. What factors are of primary concern right now?
3. Does the client undergo dialysis? How frequently?
4. What lab values must be monitored for this client, and why?
5. What medications are currently prescribed for this client?
6. If the client is to undergo dialysis, which if any of the medications listed in #5 may be given prior to dialysis?
7. What special teaching needs does this client have?
8. What concerns you most about this client? How do you plan to deal with this concern?

Two-Minute Assessment

Students report the two-minute assessment is fun and validates that they actually know more than they realized. Before assigning the client for assessment, the faculty procures the client's permission and explains that two students will come into the room, one at a time, to make some observations; the client should be unknown to the two students. It is important to reassure the client that there are no problems and this is simply an exercise to help students learn, and to thank the client for cooperating. The teacher may complete an assessment that is compared with the results obtained by the students. Figure 19.9 contains the two-minute assessment tool; a printable version is included on the CD-ROM accompanying this book.

Figure 19.9 - Two-Minute Assessment Tool

The Two-Minute Assessment

During this activity you will have two minutes to assess a client. You will be paired with a buddy who also will assess this same client.

Objective

Obtain as much information about the client as you possibly can by simply making observations. Your observations should begin at the door, as you enter the room. You should not touch the client.

Directions for the Buddied Pair

You may make notes during or after your two-minute assessment period, but you may not view the client or the client's room once your two minutes are up. Your buddy will time you while you assess the client. When your time has elapsed, your buddy assesses the client, and you time your buddy.

Once both partners have assessed the client, compare notes with each other and with the teacher, if the teacher also assessed the client. If there were findings that were abnormal, review the client's chart for possible answers or rationales for the noted abnormalities.

During postconference, the buddies will provide a brief report of their findings to the other students in the clinical group.

Reflective Practice

It is important for students to take responsibility for their own learning. To do this, students need to examine factors that either contributed to, or detracted from, their clinical performance and experience. For this reason, a tool was developed that students can use to evaluate their clinical experience so they can take pride in their successes and make improvements for the future. This tool is especially beneficial because it gathers objective information about the student's performance. Students assume responsibility for their actions by actively evaluating themselves and determining any need for improvement. Figure 19.10 contains the reflective practice tool; a printable version is included on the CD-ROM accompanying this book.

Figure 19.10 - Reflective Practice Tool

Reflecting on Your Practice

Consider for a moment how things went during your clinical day. Answer the following questions.

1. How did you prepare for this clinical day?
2. What was your main goal for care of assigned clients after you obtained report?
3. What resources did you use today? How were they helpful? Would you use the same resources again? If not, what would you do differently in your selection or use of resources?
4. How well did you communicate with others? Consider the following list of healthcare team members and your interactions with them during the course of your shift.
   a. Physicians
   b. Other nurses
   c. Patient care technicians on your team
   d. Unit clerk
   e. Respiratory therapists
   f. Laboratory personnel
   g. others
5. If I were your client, would I have been pleased with the care provided to me today by you or members of your team?
6. What did you do particularly well today?
7. What would you do differently if given the opportunity to begin the day and do it all over again?
8. Describe the single most important thing you learned today and how it will impact future nursing care that you provide.

Summary

With pre-planned critical-thinking tools, the teacher is better able to design instruction and evaluate student performance. When it is time to evaluate student learning, the faculty can access these tools and highlight areas of student progression or student need. The tool can be used to objectively assess a student's ability to gather data and put together facts.

Perhaps the biggest advantage of critical thinking activities is that students actually think about their thinking (Caputi, 2004). They are not just going through the motions, performing skills, or reading lecture notes, without really understanding why they are doing what they are doing. In addition, the exercises help students transfer the information from one critical thinking activity to new and different situations. Eventually students will function without the use of critical thinking tools and will be able to formulate patterns of thinking and responses that shape their approach to practice. Encouraging reflective practice helps ensure that students become practitioners who question and critically examine the answers they do have.

Learning Activities

1. Evaluate your clinical teaching-learning environment. Are there particular content areas that you would like students to better understand? Are there times when you feel students do not have a clue as to how to proceed? Are students lacking assessment skills? If you answered yes to any of the above:

    a. Design a critical thinking tool that fosters understanding of content or organizational skills.

    b. Design a buddy plan (such as the two-minute assignment) in which the first student performs an activity, the second student performs the same activity, and the two students compare their findings. Discuss your experience using the above with your colleagues.

2. Evaluate student learning in your classroom. Is there room for enhanced application of concepts? If so:

    a. Assign students to complete concept maps of selected topics and share the concept maps among students in the class.

    b. Design your own concept maps to use when you present topical content.

References

Alfaro-LeFevre, R. (2002). *Applying nursing process: Promoting collaborative care.* Philadelphia: Lippincott.

Caputi, L. (2004). Operationalizing critical thinking. In L. Caputi & L. Engelmann (Eds.) *Teaching nursing: The art and science, Vol. 1 & 2,* (pp. 696-719). Glen Ellyn, IL: College of DuPage Press.

Caputi, L., & Engelmann, L. (2003). *Teaching critical thinking at the grassroots level.* Paper presented at the National League for Nursing education summit, San Antonio, TX.

Couey, D. (2004). Using concept maps to foster critical thinking. In L. Caputi & L. Engelmann (Eds.) *Teaching nursing: The art and science, Vol. 1 & 2,* (pp. 622-633). Glen Ellyn, IL: College of DuPage Press.

Ignatavicius, D. (2004). An introduction to developing critical thinking in nursing students. In L. Caputi & L. Engelmann (Eds.) *Teaching nursing: The art and science, Vol. 1 & 2,* (pp. 634-651). Glen Ellyn, IL: College of DuPage Press.

Bibliography

Alfaro-LeFevre, R. (2001). *Critical thinking.* Handout from presentation at National League for Nursing faculty development institute. Retrieved March 23, 2004, from http://www.nln.org/ce/alfaro-handouts.doc.

Brookfield, S. (1987). *Developing critical thinkers.* San Francisco: Jossey-Bass.

Hamza, M., & Alhalabi, B. (1999). *Teaching in the information age: The creative way!* Paper presented at international conference of the Society for Information Technology & Teacher Education. San Antonio, TX.

Focus on Accreditation

Unit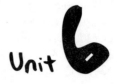

Chapter 20: The Nuts and Bolts of CCNE Accreditation
Kathleen Twohy, BSN, MPH, PhD, RN

Chapter 21: The Nuts and Bolts of NLNAC Accreditation
Gay Reeves, MSN, EdD, RN

Chapter 20: The Nuts and Bolts of CCNE Accreditation

Kathleen Twohy, BSN, MPH, PhD, RN

Commission on Collegiate Nursing Education (CCNE) accreditation is an option for baccalaureate and higher nursing education programs. Dr. Twohy takes us through this process from a faculty point of view. – Linda Caputi

Introduction

Specialized program accreditation has developed in the United States as a mechanism to assure quality in disciplines whose graduates are destined to interface with society members around critical issues such as education and health. It is a **voluntary** review of program quality, unlike "approvals," such as those required by Boards of Nursing, which usually focus on threshold safety.

The process of external accreditation is most strategically—and wisely—perceived as a snapshot in a larger, continuous process of program assessment and improvement. Use of selected systems, procedures, and resources by faculty can minimize duplication, gaps, workload, and stress in an institution's accreditation processes. An assessment process that simultaneously attends to all of the relevant approval or accreditation constituencies—such as institutional program review, state regulators, national specialty accreditors, and regional institutional accreditation—can produce efficiencies in time and effort. This chapter focuses on the accreditation process of the CCNE for baccalaureate

Educational Philosophy

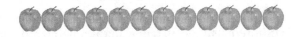

I believe teachers set the stage for learning, designing varied activities and environments that inspire learners to continue their journey of discovery about themselves and their world. Teachers are privileged to witness the excitement and growth as learners gradually or suddenly—and sometimes unexpectedly!—discover their own knowledge and power to improve the human condition. It is an awesome experience for both teacher and learner. – Kathleen Twohy programs, with particular emphasis on small schools and programs in curricular transition.

Overview

The U. S. Department of Education (DOE), through the Accrediting Agency Evaluation Unit, has recognized CCNE to accredit baccalaureate and higher degree programs in nursing in the United States and its territories (U.S. Department of Education, Accreditation in the United States). This recognition is subject to regular reviews by DOE to assure ongoing quality processes and procedures. Initial recognition was granted in 1996 and has since been renewed with no requirements for improvement (Commission on Collegiate Nursing Education, Annual Report 2002, 2003).

Like most voluntary accreditation agencies, CCNE requires membership of nursing programs and a stepped process toward initial accreditation (CCNE Accreditation, 2003).

The Commission on Collegiate Nursing Education is an autonomous accrediting agency, contributing to the improvement of the public's health. CCNE ensures the quality and integrity of baccalaureate and graduate education programs preparing effective nurses. CCNE serves the public interest by assessing and identifying programs that engage in effective educational practices. As a voluntary **self**-regulatory process, CCNE accreditation supports and encourages continuing self-assessment by nursing education programs and supports continuing growth and improvement of collegiate professional education. (Mission Statement and Goals, 2002)

The major elements of the accreditation process are:
- The preparation of a self study;
- An on-site verification by an evaluation team; and
- Determination of standard compliance and program quality.

The CCNE accreditation standards, process, and procedures are included in comprehensive web pages maintained by the organization. The reader is referred directly to the website http://www.aacn.nche.edu/accreditation/new_standards.htm for the most current information (CCNE Accreditation, 2003). This site can be launched easily from the CD accompanying this book. Simply launch your Internet browser, put the CD-ROM in the drive, go to Chapter 20 on the CD, and then click on the website address.

Four standards guide each of these elements of accreditation:
- Standard I. Program Quality: Mission And Governance
- Standard II. Program Quality: Institutional Commitment And Resources
- Standard III. Program Quality: Curriculum and Teaching-Learning Practices
- Standard IV. Program Effectiveness: Student Performance And Faculty Accomplishments

Each standard has five to six key elements that are evaluated to determine compliance. A key element for Standard I is:

A. The mission, goals, and expected outcomes of the program are written, congruent with those of the parent institution, and consistent with professional nursing standards and guidelines for the preparation of nursing professionals.

Each standard also includes examples of evidence that can be used to substantiate program compliance. The standards and key elements were recently amended and will be in effect in 2005.

CCNE provides superb assistance prior to, during, and after the accreditation process. Very able staff members willingly—and kindly—answer questions posed by e-mail, by telephone, or in person. Do not hesitate to take advantage of their expertise.

The Vital Signs: Perspective, Planning, Timing, and Ownership

Regardless of the accrediting agency, successful accreditation processes require perspective, planning, timing, and ownership. Each of these components is discussed below in relation to CCNE accreditation.

Perspective

Maintaining a meta-view of the accreditation process within the institutional and departmental assessment and review cycles helps to minimize duplication and gaps. This can sometimes require mental gymnastics but keeping the big picture in mind can save time in the end. At my institution, programs undergo institutional program review concurrently with external accreditation, minimizing duplication. The self study, visitors' report, and letter of final disposition together comprise program review; there are no additional institutional requirements related to program review. Institutions that have not yet adopted this practice would do well to take the same approach, as external accreditation requirements are generally more rigorous than those established by the institution. If an exact substitution is not possible, be sure to include collection and analysis of institution-required information in the self study to maximize the efficiency and efforts of department members participating in the review.

While institutional accreditation ordinarily does not require any special or additional efforts for nursing programs (other than to present program assessment evidence), state board of nursing approval requirements may present additional burdens. Whenever possible, it is best to fully integrate these standards and requirements into the program assessment and evaluation plan. For example, the Minnesota State Board of Nursing Program Approval Rules call for documented evaluation of more than 70 "nursing abilities." These abilities are worked into the course syllabi and course grading, and are aggregated in various sections of the assessment plan as methods for meeting expected outcomes. Since the Minnesota board has a 10-year maximum for approval, and requires a brief annual report, documenting and aggregating evidence of these abilities is not an onerous task. Regulators' requirements in other states may be more difficult to accommodate. Bundling accreditation and approval requirements into an integrated assessment and evaluation plan can help the institution maintain perspective on the accreditation process.

Planning

Planning for accreditation is essential to a successful outcome. CCNE provides procedures and guidelines (Procedures for Accreditation, 2001; General Advice for Programs Hosting, 2001) to help direct the accreditation process. Regular and repeated review of these documents by all faculty is strongly recommended. Preparation should begin a minimum of a year to 18 months before the site visit. The nursing faculty should thoroughly review and discuss the accreditation standards, key elements, and examples of evidence as an essential first step in planning the self-study and review process. Periodic review and refocus of these components should also enhance the process and outcome. The first discussion of standards by faculty may take one to two hours; subsequent reorientations can be briefer—15 to 20 minutes—and may be held every term.

At times it may be helpful to talk with people outside the school of nursing. It may be useful to retain a consultant for the planning process, but this is by no means necessary. Calling a colleague whose program recently completed CCNE accreditation can also be beneficial. Lastly, faculty can visit the AACN in Washington, D.C. and review reports from site visits of other schools. These schools can then be contacted and asked if they would be willing to share their accreditation documents. All these sources of information can be extremely helpful.

The educational process in a nursing program cannot, unfortunately, be put on hold while faculty and staff step out of their teaching roles to prepare the self study and organize an evaluation site visit. A written planning document, prepared at least 18 months in advance of the site visit, may help some institutions identify additional resources they need to support accreditation efforts. Academic administrators are better able to account for requests for release or reassigned time, supplemental staffing, and external consultation, with written requests prior to budget finalization. Since the accreditation schedule is seldom a surprise, advanced planning should be possible in almost every situation.

Timing

Given the ongoing activities of the institution and nursing unit, the timing of the accreditation process is not always convenient or ideal. The normal necessity for both general education and nursing curriculum redesign or improvement, or changes in significant personnel (eg, chief academic officer, chief nurse administrator, etc.) can add challenges to an already taxing process. If these types of institutional alterations are in process, additional time is needed in the accreditation plan.

Establish a written timeline for the entire accreditation process that allows time to:
- Write the self study;
- Organize the campus visit;
- Maintain order in the necessary activities; and
- Assure completion by established due dates.

Work backward from the earliest potential site-visit dates—since you will not have these dates confirmed at the outset of the process—and determine key target dates for writing, printing, and shipping self-study drafts and organizing the site visit. If planning is thorough **and** no significant crises occur, it should be possible to meet the established timeline. Early in the accreditation process, adapt the elements listed in Table 20.1 for your institutional and nursing-unit

Table 20.1 - Sample Timeline for Accreditation Process

Time	General	Self Study	Site Visit
12 to 18 months before visit	Send letter of intent to CCNE, requesting reevaluation. Review CCNE standards, key elements, examples of evidence (one to two hours). Visit a school that has had a recent CCNE visit.	Identify principal writer/editor and begin writing. Negotiate release time if indicated and financially feasible. Contract consultants. Alert key personnel in the system.	
6 months	Review standards, key elements, examples of evidence (20 to 30 minutes).	Complete first draft. Submit for review and editing by faculty teams.	Schedule visit dates with CCNE, review visitor. Reserve time on administrators' schedules.
5 months		Complete second draft. Submit for review and editing by faculty teams.	
4 months	Review standards, key elements, examples of evidence (20 to 30 minutes).	Complete third draft. Conduct final editing, collate appendices. Ensure final administrative approval for printing.	Identify preferred visit participants, clinical, and class visits
3 months	Publish third-party comment notification of CCNE review (eg, in area newspapers, on web pages).	Send self study to printer. Generate copies for CCNE, visitors, each faculty, president, chief academic officer, library, assessment office/program review, and students.	Schedule preparation meetings. Send invitation to participate in visit to students, non-nursing faculty, graduates, academic services, community of interest representatives. Begin collecting and organizing resource room materials. Negotiate mock visit if desired.

Teaching Nursing: The Art and Science

Table 20.1 - Sample Timeline for Accreditation Process, cont.

2 months	Visit student classes and explain accreditation process, its importance, and students' role in the visit. Meet with upper administration and explain the strengths of your program.	Distribute self study.	Finalize visit agenda with team leader Confirm visit participants meetings, clinical, and class visits Finalize visitor housing accommodations, local meals, and transportation. (Some visitors prefer to manage this themselves.)
1 month	Schedule post-visit celebration/relief party.		Send relevant self-study sections to visit participants. Hold meetings to prepare visit participants. Make housing arrangements for evaluators.
2 weeks	Conduct mock visit.	Reread before mock visit.	Finalize resource room materials.

culture. In addition to scheduling the time needed for writing the self study, other activities need to be planned. The dates of the site visit usually are scheduled by the chief nurse administrator and the staff at CCNE about six months in advance. Be sure to clear—and hold—the proposed dates of a site visit with the offices of the president of the college and chief academic affairs officer as these institutional officials are expected to meet with the site visitors. In addition to the president and chief academic affairs officer, evaluators ordinarily meet with other institutional and community stakeholders. It is necessary to include visit-preparation meetings in the timeline for students, nursing faculty, faculty representing pre-requisite or co-requisite courses, faculty representing general education courses, alumni, academic services staff (eg, computing, library, registrar), and representatives from the community at large.

Beginning six weeks to a month before the visit, the chief nurse administrator, in consultation with faculty, should identify which particular faculty, students, and staff will actually meet with the visitors. Class schedules may preclude some participation but needed participants usually cooperate willingly. While CCNE recommends not altering students' class schedules for the site visit, the importance of having all nursing faculty present for meetings with the visitors seems to outweigh maintaining the schedule. We took CCNE's advice on this and, in hindsight, some adjustments in the teaching schedules would have helped enhance faculty participation. Planning ahead for dropping or shortening a class period may be wise, though it may not be possible to decide which class, on which day, until shortly before the visitors arrive. It is even possible that the team leader will change the established agenda upon arrival at the school.

Ownership

Ownership of the nursing program as well as the self study is an expectation in any accrediting process. Ownership is manifested in the degree to which institutional and department or unit members understand and are committed to the success of the program and the self-study process. All faculty should know at which level and in which course major curricular concepts are initiated, developed, and applied. They also should be fully aware of any department- or unit-specific academic policies that have bearing on student performance and progression. This is particularly challenging if a program has several new, adjunct, or part-time faculty. Ongoing orientation and mentoring procedures can facilitate policy and curricular understanding, though a crash course may be needed if new faculty are hired shortly before accreditation. Even experienced faculty in a well-established curriculum may concentrate so intently upon their own courses and concepts that they may not be as knowledgeable as they should be about courses and content in other segments of the program. Review of course syllabi and exams may help remind faculty of which courses cover certain critical concepts.

All faculty should be very familiar with the information in the self study and have a sense of the types of materials available in the resource room, where site visitors will access these materials. **All questions about your program are fair**

game for any and all faculty when the evaluators are on-site. Some ideas for establishing ownership include involving faculty teams in the review and editing the sections of the self study, a mock visit, and a resource room "scavenger hunt." Or, conduct an all-day orientation for faculty and have faculty select which sections they would like to write.

A series of meetings can be scheduled in which small groups of faculty each review a written draft of a different standard and write comments and suggestions to the main editor. Another draft can then be generated and reviewed again, but by a different small group. The process is repeated until all groups have reviewed and edited each standard. Our faculty of about 15 has worked in teams of three or four, each group reviewing and editing each standard. This process resulted in each of us gaining a fairly basic knowledge about each standard and how our program was meeting each of the key elements.

A mock visit can be arranged with an outside consultant or conducted by the faculty members themselves. The consultant—preferably a current or former CCNE evaluator—reviews the latest draft of the self study and resource materials then asks the faculty questions that are likely to be asked by the visiting team. If budgets are limited, the mock visit might be conducted as a telephone conference call, though "live performance" generates more of the actual visit's anxiety and stress, which can, in turn, stimulate better preparation and ownership on the part of the faculty. Another low-cost strategy is to arrange a trade in which two institutions agree to conduct mock visits for each other. This works best if accreditation cycles are within six months to 24 months of each other.

Other members of the campus community must also demonstrate commitment to and knowledge of the nursing program. Student ownership can be enhanced through a number of methods. Our department has class representatives and student representatives, elected by their peers, on selected department committees. Since this was a diverse group of students and there was representation across classes, we invited this group of about 10 students to meet with the visitors. Three copies of the self study were made available for student use. An informational meeting was scheduled to answer students' questions and familiarize them with questions the visitors might ask. Once the time and dates of class and clinical visits were established, the students in those sections were made aware of the availability of the self study. Faculty helped prepare these students for the presence of visitors in classes or the clinical setting.

One problem that may occur during site visits relates to terminology. Sometimes the terminology a program uses can create some confusion for students during evaluation. For example, in clinical, our evaluators asked students and graduates questions about which practice standard they were implementing. Our curriculum uses nursing process terminology rather than practice standards terminology. The students appeared to lack knowledge about practice standards. In fact, they were very knowledgeable about implementing the nursing process but had not regularly referred to it as standards.

It is important to schedule preparation meetings with academic officers, particularly those new to their positions or those with limited knowledge about the nursing program. Our program was in the early stages of a complete curricular revision, and accreditation review was based on the new curriculum. While the department had informed the various campus offices about our curricular changes, we were only in the first year of curricular transition. Administrators and academic service staff needed a thorough reorientation to the revision. Preparation also included questions the visitors were likely to ask each of them.

Full ownership of the nursing program is critical to a successful accreditation process and outcome. Programs should work toward a culture of trust and individual and group accountability for the quality of the entire program. Full ownership is not full agreement; professional differences, resource constraints, and institutional goals can be at odds, but disagreements must be handled professionally.

The Self Study

The self study is a written report that organizes and analyzes a wide array of information that, together, substantiates the program's educational quality. It is a periodic self evaluation against a set of criteria (ie, the standards). While the self-study process is required as part of external accreditation, it has the strongest benefits internally. Without the cycle of external accreditation, how likely would we be to carefully examine our nursing programs for quality? We have all seen the answer to that question in our own institutions among departments, majors, or programs that do not participate in specialized accreditation. The pressure of competing demands takes over and faculty (or administration) does not commit time to self-analysis, reflection, and improvement.

Since the self study process focuses on a program at a point in time, it is unwise to try to make major program changes in the midst of the study process. Certainly, minor changes, involving minimal time and effort, can and should be undertaken. Minor changes might include updating a website or correcting small discrepancies in policies. This is not the time to begin big projects such as major curriculum revisions, significant changes in an assessment and evaluation plan, or restructuring a program. The need for major changes might be uncovered by the results of a self evaluation, but these would then need to be planned and implemented over a reasonable time period. Attempting to perfect a program during the self-evaluation process can distract faculty and staff from the task at hand and can cause unnecessary diversions of energy and delays in preparing the written document.

Writing the Self Study

The organization of the self study is up to the writer or writing team, though organizing according to the four standards and related key elements is simple and straightforward (Commission on Collegiate Amended, 1998; Amended 2003). Organizing the report according to the standards and key elements also provides a built-in mechanism to check that everything has been covered completely, clearly, and accurately. Use tables, charts, and graphs wherever possible. This allows density of information without exceeding the maximum 75 pages of narrative. Number the tables, graphs, and charts according to the relevant standard or key element and insert them in the report in numerical order. For example, Table II.D.3. is the third table related to Key Element D in Standard II. Do not split tables across pages. Include URLs for relevant department or unit websites such as those with curriculum plans or academic policies. Use appendices for key documents like the unit's mission, goals, or objectives, and the assessment and evaluation plan. Provide URLs for online access to lengthy documents or documents that provide context about the institution rather than including them in the self study.

The self study should be written with one voice; therefore, it is usually better to have one person designated as the primary writer or editor. In smaller programs this person is often the department chair. Programs with the resources to do so sometimes contract with a writer or editor for assistance, though this can decrease faculty ownership and responsibility for the endeavor. It is advisable to seek some reassigned time—possibly a course release—for preparing the self study, though it is not always feasible. Careful advanced planning can alleviate last-minute writing panic.

A few time-saving strategies in the writing process are suggested. First, keep self-study writing and materials organized during the self-study process to maintain the writer's sanity. Nursing faculty and administrators are busy people, often inundated with unexpected demands and challenges. Organization and planningcan preserve time and relationships. Some of these time-saving suggestions may seem time **consuming** in the beginning, but each can save many hours later in the process. Figure 20.1 lists some time-saving strategies.

On-Campus Visit

The purpose of the site visit is to verify and amplify information about the program that has been presented in written documents, including the self study, college catalog, handbooks, brochures, and web pages. Verification boils down to the question, "Is this institution doing what it says it is doing? It occurs through individual and group interviews, observations, and review of additional supporting materials.

Interviews are conducted with administrators, academic support services staff, students, faculty, graduates, clinical partners, and any other stakeholders that the chief nurse administrator and the team leader deem appropriate. Observations occur in classroom, clinical, and lab settings, and during campus tours. Additional supporting materials are organized in a designated resource room, which is often the home base for the evaluation team during the site visit.

The site visit culminates in a written report of the team's findings and a reading of a draft of that report before the team leaves campus. The report is the team's determination on each key element and a conclusion as to whether each standard has been met. The team also may request that the program submit additional information to its case to the visiting team and CCNE before a specified date. The deadline is usually a month before meeting at which the commission makes its final decision about the accreditation.

Preparation

Ordinarily the evaluation team is composed of three to four members, including a team leader, one or two faculty, and a master's-prepared nurse from clinical practice. The number of team members and the length of the site visit depend on the complexity of the program and the review. For an institution with more than one program—for example, a baccalaureate program, post-licensure program, and master's program—a site visit likely will last four days and include four

Figure 20.1 - Time-saving Strategies

1. For each standard, develop a template that includes a heading for the standard's name and lists each key element.
2. Keep each standard and each appendix in a separate electronic file until the very end of the study process.
3. Within each key element section, note the number and types of tables that could demonstrate that the program has met that element. For example, two tables might be appropriate for Standard I, Key Element A: one that compares institutional and departmental/unit mission statements, and another that evaluates the institution's expected outcomes with those of the nursing unit.
4. Label each table based on the standard and key element to which it is related. The examples in Strategy 3, above, would be identified as I. A.1. and I. A. 2., signifying the first and second tables for Standard I, Key Element A. This is actually most useful in tables related to Standard IV, as the information can then be used as part of ongoing internal and external assessment reporting. They can easily be slipped into place in subsequent self-study documents.
5. Use narrative to explain *conclusions* from the data; do not restate the data from the table in the body of the narrative.
6. As with any writing, use summary paragraphs at the end of a section. Include declarative sentences to state conclusions. For example, "We believe the evidence presented supports accomplishment of Key Element C" or "The available evidence related to Key Element C is inconclusive. A task force is reviewing the causes of the poor graduate survey response rates and exploring alternative methods for acquiring meaningful data."
7. Prepare a list of strengths and areas for improvement at the end of each standard. Be honest when developing this list.
8. Use the search feature of your word processing program to find references and materials that should be in the resource room. Generate an inventory of materials listed in the self-study that are in the resource room and add the materials recommended in CCNE's On-Site Resource File listing (Procedures for Accreditation, 2001). This will help assure consistency between the self-study body and references and the materials in the resource room.
9. Back up all work. Throughout the process, save copies of electronic files in multiple places.

evaluators; a visit to a baccalaureate-only program typically lasts three days and is conducted by only three visitors.

The site visit dates are negotiated between CCNE and the chief nurse administrator about six months in advance. Evaluators meet with the president and academic officers (eg, the provost and vice president for academic affairs) so it is wise to ensure that they will be on campus before finalizing the dates. The agenda is jointly organized by the chief nurse administrator and the evaluation team leader. The chief nurse administrator develops a draft agenda that is then shared with the team leader. The evaluators ordinarily divide up most of the meetings, conducting only a few as a team. The team leader helps determine which team member should meet with which person or group. Essentially, a schedule is designed for each member of the evaluation team and negotiated with the team leader.

In addition to meeting with institutional officials, the team tours the campus and selected clinical sites, observes classes and clinical settings, and meets with representatives of academic support services, the entire nursing faculty, and selected faculty from supporting and general education courses. These appointments are usually led by a team member; neither nursing faculty nor the chief nurse administrator attends. Nor does the chief nurse administrator attend the meeting with the nursing faculty.

It is wise to schedule informational meetings with team members for all individuals or groups who will meet with the visitors. For most participants these can be conducted in 20- to 30-minute sessions and scheduled in the same order as they will be scheduled to meet with the visitors. It is helpful to provide the relevant section of the self study to each participant for review prior to the meeting. The academic services meeting should include a representative from academic advising, the registrar, the director of assessment, a library representative, and a representative from information technology services. The non-nursing faculty group includes representatives from prerequisite or co-requisite courses and general education or core courses.

The team leader works with the chief nurse administrator to ensure appropriate accommodations are planned for the evaluation visitors. Air travel arrangements are usually managed by each team member individually. The nursing program should recommend ground transportation options and hotel accommodations and determine if the visitors need Internet access in the hotel. If the hotel does not have this service, it may be possible to arrange online connections through the school's information technology office. It is important to ensure the safety of the visitors in their hotel and while they are visiting the campus and other locations.

All necessary on-campus room reservations should be made well in advance to maximize convenience and save time. The resource room is often the home base for the evaluation team between tours and meetings. The room should be secure and keys should be provided to each team member. Stock the room with a few refreshments like hot and cold beverages and snacks. Copies of all materials mailed with the self study should be available in the resource room along with supplementary materials cited in the self study and those required by CCNE (see Procedures). Arrangements should be made for students or faculty to escort team members to their various meetings, classrooms, and clinical settings. It is important to always have someone available to escort the visitors until they leave campus each day. The chief nurse administrator should not try to be the escort as she or he will need to be available to attend to any last-minute details in the office.

They've Arrived!

If planning and lead time were sufficient, everyone should be ready for the evaluators. Still, the visit is often a stressful few days, particularly for the chief nurse administrator. Adopting a "learning perspective" might be helpful during the visit. Frame the evaluation visit as a time to learn, or for constructive critique, rather than a time to be apologetic or defensive. It is impossible to anticipate every eventuality that might occur during an evaluation visit, so both the evaluators and program faculty and staff need to be flexible and adaptable. Minimize all nonessential commitments—that is, clear the calendar except for the visit and essential teaching.

The initial meeting between the team leader and chief nurse administrator ordinarily takes place at the beginning of the first day. The team leader asks questions that were raised by team members in the review of the written materials and requests any supplementary materials he or she may want. The agenda may also be adjusted at this time.

The time for the on-campus visit is very limited and therefore must be used efficiently. While it may be tempting to show off a beautiful campus, a three-hour walking tour is not a good use of the evaluators' time. Team members are responsible for adhering to the schedule, though the escort returning evaluators to the resource room or taking them to the next meeting could rap on the door to let the team member know it is time to move on. Failure to adhere to the schedule can prove detrimental to a program as the evaluators may not have enough time in the resource room to verify self-study claims. Evaluators, it is hoped, will ask about documents they are unable to locate in the resource room but, as we discovered during our evaluation, that is not always the case.

Team members take notes as they gather data from interviews, observations, and resource room materials. In the evenings, back at the hotel, they draft their report. No social activities should be planned for the evaluators, though lunch meetings with various constituencies are often necessary to ensure all the essential contacts are made and issues discussed.

And They Leave

The program gets little sense of "how things are going" during the visit. While evaluators are pleasant, they are likely to reveal little in conversation or body language. By midday on the last day of the visit, the evaluators gather faculty and academic officers to read the draft of their report. **There is no opportunity for questions or comment on the report at this time.** Immediately after the report is read, evaluators leave campus to return home.

It is helpful to plan a debriefing session following the evaluators' departure. Faculty have worked hard and the tension is sometimes high during the site visit. A time to celebrate is appropriate if the outcome is positive. If one or more outcomes have not been sufficiently demonstrated, there is likely to be some degree of surprise and dejection.

The evaluation team has two weeks to submit its report to CCNE, which reviews the report before returning it to the chief nurse administrator. The program then has two weeks to correct errors of fact (eg, names and titles) and agree or disagree with the team's conclusions about each standard. If the program disagrees with any conclusions, it is advisable to craft the response carefully to avoid communicating a defensive posture. It may take several drafts and reviews by colleagues to write appropriate, impassionate responses.

CCNE allows additional materials to be submitted between the end of an evaluation visit and 30 days prior to the Accreditation Review Commission (ARC) meeting at which final determinations are made. The staff at CCNE is very helpful in guiding the program through this process. Once the program receives ARC's final decision, all official documents should be altered to reflect the new accreditation status.

The results should be shared within the institution, particularly with those who participated in interviews and meetings. Written or other acknowledgements of appreciation can be extended especially for exceptional assistance. We provided breakfast to the housekeeping department because they went well beyond our expectations, washing and repainting walls, replacing window screens, and shampooing carpets. Once internal notices have been sent, it may be appropriate to send a press release to local media.

At this point the accreditation process is complete. The self-study process and external reviewers have scrutinized the nursing program and reached conclusions about its quality. As with any review process, strengths and areas for improvement have been uncovered. It is important for the program to claim and celebrate its strengths and make plans for improving those areas that need attention. Incorporate improvement objectives into the program's strategic planning documents so these issues will be addressed and progress made toward ever-higher program quality.

Accreditation During Curriculum Transition

Timing an accreditation process to avoid periods of curriculum change may no longer be possible. Nursing education has been criticized for taking an unacceptable amount of time to make essential and significant curriculum revisions, particularly given the pace of change in health care. Some criticism is justified and some is not. Our department finished a thorough curricular revision in May 2004 that was initiated with a revision in the department's mission in 1999—a five-year span. While the pace of change in health care dictates more frequent and pervasive revision in curricula than now occurs, curriculum change is still difficult and time-consuming work. Ensuring inclusion of concepts essential for nursing in the future, building vertical and horizontal integration and consistency, avoiding duplication, and achieving faculty consensus—including slaying sacred cows—all while operating at least one existing curriculum makes it incredibly challenging to change curricula at a rate that keeps pace with change in health care. Curricular revision needs to be a continuous process. Nursing needs flexible curricula that can be redesigned quickly but maintain their core essence and not create obstacles for students working to complete their programs.

Accreditation issues will arise in a continuous curricular change process. These might include concerns about which curriculum should be discussed in Standard

III and designing and implementing an assessment process that is generic enough to provide meaningful information yet flexible enough to build patterns of evidence during curricular adaptations and improvements. The accreditation process our program experienced in 2002 occurred in the first year of the curriculum transition. CCNE advised that we report on the **revised** curriculum in Standard III and the **previous** curriculum in Standard IV. Only two courses in the revised curriculum were offered in 2001-02. While the curriculum structure and skeletal course syllabi had been approved in the department and the college, implementation of the planned senior-level courses was three years away so course development was planned in order of implementation. Visitors expected to see more fully-developed courses for the **entire** curriculum and tracking of the teaching/learning practices and essential concepts across all courses for us to meet Standard III.

The site visit also presented some challenges. Having only two new courses being offered made the visitors' observation impossible or inadvisable. One course was a two-credit offering that had ended and the other was a four-credit interdisciplinary health promotion course that was being team-taught by a nursing faculty and a dietetics faculty; the dietetics faculty was teaching during the time of the visit. Consequently, evaluators observed class and clinical courses that were part of the previous curriculum. They also met with graduates of the previous curriculum and with clinical partners who were familiar with the previous curriculum but less knowledgeable about the revised curriculum.

The timing of our CCNE accreditation process during that stage of the curriculum transition was unfortunate but unavoidable. The infancy of the CCNE accreditation process and the evaluators' inexperience with application of accreditation standards in such an early stage of an extensive curriculum transition resulted in a review of Standard III that was less than favorable. The program was invited to submit additional materials, so 10 faculty spent a full month rapidly completing the curriculum-development work, a project that was originally planned for the entire following year. The final outcome was full initial accreditation with no recommendations.

Summary

If nursing programs are to rise to the challenge of more adaptable curricula, undergoing more frequent change in response to healthcare transformations, nursing programs accreditors will need flexibility in the interpretation and application of accreditation standards. While it is desirable to address the curriculum of the future in Standard III, there must be some leeway for examining both the existing curriculum and the new program if the stage of transition warrants. Quality education efforts in the previous curriculum are unlikely to be totally abandoned in a revision. If needed, a program could submit a subsequent report on curriculum progress. This would ensure continuous application of standards throughout a curriculum development process.

Specialty accreditation is a valuable asset to any educational program. It requires internal and external examination of program quality against pre-established criteria and leads to program improvement. While it may cause some angst, the CCNE accreditation process is not unduly painful—and the angst can be reduced by a strong assessment and evaluation program. The value of the support of the CCNE staff and available resources cannot be overstated. They are true professionals who hold quality nursing education at the core of the process.

CCNE Websites

The list of references at the end of this chapter includes several CCNE websites. These sites can be launched easily from the CD accompanying this book. Simply launch your Internet browser, put the CD-ROM in the drive, go to Chapter 19 on the CD, and then click on the website address.

Learning Activities

1. Review CCNE accreditation websites cited in the references.
2. Ask a local nursing program if you can review their most recent self study for CCNE accreditation.
3. Interview a dean or department chair and nursing faculty about their most recent experience with CCNE accreditation. Ask:
   - What the preparation process and the actual experience was like for them;
   - What they view as the strengths and weaknesses of the accreditation process; and
   - What they learned about their program from the accreditation process.

4. Interview a CCNE evaluator and gather his or her perspective about accreditation.
5. If a local nursing program is undergoing a CCNE review, ask if you can attend some of its meetings in preparation for the site visit.
6. Compare and contrast the CCNE's accreditation standards, processes, and procedures with those of the National League for Nursing Accrediting Commission.

References

Commission on Collegiate Nursing Education. (2003, March). *Annual Report, 2002*. Retrieved January 10, 2004, http://www.aacn.nche.edu/accreditation/annualreport02.pdf.

Commission on Collegiate Nursing Education. (2003). *CCNE accreditation*. Retrieved January 10, 2004, from http://www.aacn.nche.edu/accreditation/index.htm.

Commission on Collegiate Nursing Education. (2001, March). *Checklist of activities in a CCNE accreditation review*. Retrieved January 10, 2004, from http://www.aacn.nche.edu/accreditation/cheklist.htm.

Commission on Collegiate Nursing Education. (2002, July 24). *Commission on Collegiate Nursing Education retains its status as a nationally recognized accrediting agency by the U.S. Department of Education*. Retrieved January 10, 2004, from http://www.aacn.nche.edu/accreditation/july02release.htm.

Commission on Collegiate Nursing Education. (1998). *Standards for accreditation of baccalaureate and graduate nursing education programs*. Retrieved January 10, 2004, from http://www.aacn.nche.edu/accreditation/standrds.htm.

Commission on Collegiate Nursing Education. (2003, October). *Standards for accreditation of baccalaureate and graduate nursing programs (effective January 2005)*. Retrieved Jan. 10, 2004, from http://www.aacn.nche.edu/accreditation/new_standards.htm.

Commission on Collegiate Nursing Education. (2001, March). *General advice for programs hosting an on-site evaluation by CCNE*. Retrieved January 10, 2004, from http://www.aacn.nche.edu/accreditation/advice.htm.

Commission on Collegiate Nursing Education. (2002). *Mission statement and goals: Commission on Collegiate Nursing Education*. Retrieved January 10, 2004, from http://www.aacn.nche.edu/accreditation/mission.htm.

Commission on Collegiate Nursing Education. (2001, May). *Procedures for accreditation of baccalaureate and graduate nursing education programs*. Retrieved January 10, 2004, from http://www.aacn.nche.edu/accreditation/procrevd.htm.

United States Department of Education. (n.d.). *Accreditation in the United States: National Institutional And Specialized Accrediting Bodies*. Retrieved January 10, 2004, from http://www.ed.gov/admins/finaid/accred/accreditation_pg6.html#nurse.

Chapter 21: The Nuts and Bolts of NLNAC Accreditation

Gay Reeves, MSN, EdD, RN

Accreditation of a nursing program by an outside body provides valuable feedback to the faculty of the nursing program and ensures to others that the program does as it says it is doing. These two rationales form the basis for accreditation by the National League for Nursing Accrediting Commission (NLNAC). This chapter discusses accreditation by the NLNAC from a faculty perspective, providing valuable information for faculty preparing for accreditation. – Linda Caputi

Introduction

National accreditation is a voluntary peer review process. However, some state boards of nursing require national accreditation for any school wishing to maintain state approval (Blais, Hayes, Kozier & Erb, 2002). The NLNAC and the Commission on Collegiate Nursing Education (CCNE) are the only two national accreditation agencies recognized by the Department of Education as national accrediting bodies of nursing education programs. The CCNE grants accredited status only to baccalaureate degree and higher nursing programs. The NLNAC accredits programs at all levels of nursing education.

Educational Philosophy

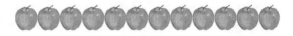

I believe every student deserves the opportunity to obtain an education and that every adult deserves the opportunity to pursue an educational career that will afford a quality lifestyle. It is the teacher's responsibility to nurture the student and provide the best education possible so the student can be successful in his or her chosen career. The nursing educator is challenged to be innovative and creative, and take intellectual risks to assure the students' learning needs are met. The educational environment needs to be learner-centered, foster mutual trust and respect, and encourage lifelong learning and student success for people of all ages and cultural backgrounds. – Gay Reeves

Overview

The NLNAC is separate from, but related to, the National League for Nursing (NLN). The NLN had been the official professional accrediting organization for all levels of nursing programs since 1952. Beginning in 1997, to meet Department of Education requirements, the NLNAC assumed the accrediting responsibilities (Ellis & Hartley, 1998).

NLNAC accreditation goes beyond the minimum required state approval and offers a method for providing prospective students and the public with verification that the nursing program has met prescribed criteria. The NLNAC compares the educational quality of the program with established standards and criteria (Chitty, 2001). According to the NLNAC (2003, p. 3), the accreditation process also fosters a nursing program's ongoing self-examination, re-evaluation, and long-term planning. The focus of NLNAC accreditation has shifted from evaluating the educational process to evaluating the outcomes a program identifies for each of the NLNAC criteria. Areas for which criteria have been established for the accreditation review process include:

- Administration and governance;
- Finances and budget;
- Faculty;
- Students;
- Program outcomes; and
- Resources.

When a nursing program first seeks accreditation and demonstrates compliance with all accreditation standards, the program is granted initial accreditation for a five-year period. Thereafter, continuing accreditation is granted for an eight-year period once the program demonstrates compliance with all accreditation standards. There are varying levels of accreditation status for programs that do not meet all accreditation standards. Accreditation can be withdrawn from a program for continued noncompliance with accreditation standards (NLNAC, 2003, p. 45-46). The different types of commission action on applications for accreditation are discussed in detail in the NLNAC Accreditation Manual Interpretive Guidelines, which is available through the NLNAC. For more information on these guidelines, visit the NLNAC website at www.nlnac.org. This URL also can easily be launched from the CD-ROM accompanying this book. Simply launch your Internet browser, put the CD-ROM in the drive, go to Chapter 21 on the CD, and then click on the website address.

Accreditation Process

The Self Study

Nursing programs applying for accreditation must first complete a self study to determine whether the program meets the accreditation standards and criteria (NLNAC, 2003, p. 21). This process takes from 18 months to two years to complete. The NLNAC notifies the nursing program director approximately one year prior to scheduling a site visit. The program should write a schedule for completing each aspect of the self-study process. The self-study report is due six weeks prior to the on-site visit.

Unless a member of the nursing program has extensive current experience in developing a self study, it is recommended that the program hire a consultant who has current knowledge of the NLNAC accreditation process. The consultant can review the nursing program in relation to the NLNAC criteria and help the faculty outline their plans for addressing each criterion. At this time the consultant can make recommendations to the nursing program for correcting areas of weaknesses. The consultant should visit the program to review supporting documentation that will be used to support the self study. During the visit, the consultant may chair a mock meeting with the nursing team to prepare the team members for their meeting with the NLNAC reviewers. The consultant can review and make recommendations for improving the rough draft of the self study. Upon request, the NLNAC will provide names of faculty who have previously served as peer reviewers and are available for consulting. The staff of the NLNAC is also available to answer questions about the self-study process.

Assembling the Team of Faculty

All members of a nursing team need to be active on the self-study committee and participate in preparing the self-study report. The nursing program director or a faculty member should be selected to chair the self-study process to ensure that the study is conducted in a timely manner and that there is continuity among the sections of the written report. It is beneficial for the chairperson to attend

NLNAC's annual Self Study Forum to ensure that the program uses current information for the self study. In fact, it is recommended that a member of the nursing team attend this forum annually so changes in the criteria can be incorporated into the program's evaluation process as they occur.

Each criterion is assigned to either an individual faculty or a nursing committee for development, or individuals may be asked to volunteer to develop the criteria that is of interest to them. Criteria should be assigned according to content and complexity. For example, the nursing program evaluation committee would be assigned all the criteria that deal with educational effectiveness and the plan for systematic program evaluation. The director of the program could develop those portions of the criteria that address the mission, governance, and faculty.

If there are only a few members of a nursing team, it is more practical to have the chairpersons of the appropriate nursing committees develop the related criteria. For example, the chair of a budget committee has the information needed to develop the program resources criterion. Dividing the criteria among subcommittees is an efficient way to handle this work.

The chair of the self-study committee needs to ensure that all members of the program equally share the workload and that work is then distributed to faculty. Some criteria are more complex than others and require more time to develop. The two criteria that are the most challenging to develop are those for curriculum and instruction, and educational effectiveness. These two criteria require collection of data from students, faculty, and employers; therefore, creating data collection tools and analyzing data are inherent parts of developing these criteria. The educational effectiveness criterion includes the Plan of Systematic Program Evaluation, which is the most detailed and time-consuming criterion in the self study. There is a strong emphasis placed on these two criteria because this is where the nursing program explains the program outcomes and describes how it is meeting them.

Time Commitment

Developing the self study is very time consuming, but with about two years' lead time, the process can be completed by faculty along with their other regular educational responsibilities. Faculty need to plan to spend two to three hours per week developing the criteria. The chair of the self-study committee may be granted one course release time during the last year of the process to finalize the self study. If this is not feasible, another option is to excuse the chair from all other program committee work while the report is being developed.

Collecting and Evaluating Data

The nursing program establishes outcomes for each NLNAC criteria. Data are then collected, analyzed, and documented to demonstrate how each outcome has been met.

Instruments need to be developed for collecting the data that support the outcomes of each criterion. For example, instruments to collect student and faculty evaluation of the different aspects of the program will be needed. This may include students' evaluations of courses, college facilities, and clinical sites. Faculty also will need to evaluate college facilities and clinical sites.

Some instruments used to collect data will need to have validity and reliability established. This can be accomplished using a statistical software package like SPSS. The graduate version of SPSS contains all the programs needed to analyze data and establish data collection tools' reliability and validity.

Once these tools are developed, data collection responsibilities and deadlines should be assigned. This information will be included in the Plan for Systematic Program Evaluation, which is also included in the self study.

The NLNAC team site visitors will review all supporting data collected for each criteria, as described in the Plan for Systematic Program Evaluation in the self study, and the team will request data from the previous two to three years. Therefore, the program should make sure data is easily retrievable. Minutes of all nursing program committee meetings should be made available to support criterion outcomes. It is important that meeting minutes reflect how the outcomes of the data were used to enhance the effectiveness of the program. Student input that resulted in program revisions should be included in the appropriate committee minutes. For example, if a textbook change was made as a result of student input, the minutes of the nursing curriculum committee meeting should reflect this.

Continuous Program Self Study

The program evaluation process should be ongoing to facilitate continuous program evaluation. Continuous data collection and evaluation of each individual criterion greatly decreases the work of developing future NLNAC self-study reports. To facilitate this process, at the beginning of each academic year, the chair of the systematic program evaluation committee should review the faculty criteria assignments and make any necessary assignment changes. At this time, the faculty responsible for each criterion may provide the nursing evaluation committee with the previous year's outcome data and the plan of systematic program evaluation is then updated. If established outcomes have not been met, appropriate changes need to be implemented. The plan of systematic program evaluation should reflect these changes. The SPSS data package can be used to save all collected data for future data trending; at least five years of data is needed for reliable data trending. The data analysis and trending should be completed annually by a member of the nursing evaluation committee. Social studies or math faculty may help set up formats for:

- Inputting data;
- Establishing reliability and validity of instruments; and
- Analyzing and trending data.

Meetings of the Self-Study Committee

At the beginning of the process, the entire self-study committee will need to meet for three to four hours at least monthly so all faculty can help shape the development of each criterion. The committee should meet at least twice a month during the last six months of the development process.

The first draft should be submitted to the chair of the self-study committee for review and editing at least six months before the study's due date. The final draft should be submitted at least six weeks before the study is due to the NLNAC. Time must be allowed for final editing, typing, and copying. The NLNAC Interpretive Guidelines lists the maximum number of pages for the finished document—including the main body and the appendices—and it is important to keep writing succinct so the self study does not exceed the page limit.

Funding for Completing the Self Study

Programs generally need to set aside funding for the self study. At a minimum, the budget should cover the cost of the NLNAC accreditation, a consultant, and printing and binding of the finished study. Funding also may be needed for typing the report, depending upon the program's available clerical assistance. Whether the typist is on staff or a hired hand, additional clerical assistance will be needed for typing the self-study. The typist will need to review the typing and formatting instructions in the NLNAC Interpretive Guidelines; word processing software generally makes this easier. The completed criteria can then be merged into a final copy and edited by the chairperson of the self-study committee. With the large volume of revisions that typically occur during the last month of the self-study, it may be a good idea to have a typist available for four to five hours a day.

The On-site Visit

Getting Ready

When planning for the site visit, be sure to assign someone to meet the visitors at the airport and provide transportation between the hotel and college each day. The reviewers also will need to be returned to the airport at departure time, and at least one of the reviewers will need to be transported to the pre-selected clinical site during the visit.

Most on-site visits last two or three days. The visitors will have an assigned chairperson. The chairperson typically provides the nursing program director a list of ancillary people they wish to visit. Minimally, this list includes the college president, director of finance, and library director. At least one clinical site visit is made, preferably when a nursing faculty and students are present. The agenda for the visit will be finalized with the chairperson of the site visitors. Time must be scheduled for the reviewers to read and review available support documents.

The nursing program director may be asked to make hotel reservations for the reviewers. Ideally, the hotel should be close to the college campus and should have a restaurant on-site or nearby. Reviewers generally appreciate having adjoining rooms. The chairperson may request Internet access in the hotel rooms and may ask to borrow a laptop computer from the school for use in the evening. Because the reviewers will spend much of their evening hours at the hotel compiling their findings, the school should provide fruit baskets, additional snacks, and drinks for their rooms.

The nursing program director should escort the visitors to meetings with ancillary people and to the clinical site. The reviewers likely will request additional information as needed to support the self study; the program chairperson or director should be readily available to provide this information to them for the duration of the visit. The visit will progress more quickly and smoothly if it is convenient for the reviewers to confirm that a program is doing what they say it is doing in the self study. It can be time-consuming and frustrating for the reviewers to repeatedly wait for documentation they request, so it is critical to the evaluation process for the documentation to be easily accessible in the reading room.

It is important to meet with students, charge nurse, and other hospital staff before the NLNAC reviewers conduct their clinical site visit. They should be prepared to answer questions about how faculty and staff address students' needs, how students select their clients, and other questions that will help the reviewers evaluate how effectively the clinical site meets student needs. A short meeting between the hospital director of nurses and the reviewers should be scheduled to help demonstrate the institutional support of the nursing program.

The Visit

The reviewers meet with nursing team members, students, the college president, and other school officials. Faculty who teach support and core courses also may be interviewed. In addition, the reviewers may choose to meet with members of the community who support the nursing program. Community supporters can include members of the nursing advisory committee, hospital CEOs, and healthcare consumers who can attest to the competence of the nursing program's graduates. Recent graduates of the program also can be included in this meeting. This is a time for the program to "show and tell" and may provide the reviewers with a sense of the community's support for the program.

Reading Room

The program should designate one secure, on-campus room as a reading room for the duration of the visit, and each site visitor should be given a key during their stay. Documents that will provide information to support the self study can be housed within this room. They include:

- Nursing committee meeting minutes;
- Samples of students' work;
- Student handbook;
- Faculty handbook;
- Budget report;

- Summaries of program evaluation data;
- Copies of syllabi;
- Recent letters verifying state accreditation; and
- Any other related information.

It is especially important to have available student work samples that demonstrate critical thinking. These can include written case studies, reports, concept maps, and care plans.

The reading room also should have computers, a printer, and a telephone for the reviewers to use. Because the reviewers will spend much time there, keeping snacks, juice, and coffee in the room is recommended.

Wrapping Up

At the end of the visit, the reviewers meet with all members of the program, and other invited guests including the college president and instructional dean. The reviewers will present a preliminary report of their findings, including recommendations and commendations for each criterion. This is an opportunity for nursing team members to clarify any findings with which they disagree. If there is evaluation data that the nursing program faculty believe is incorrect, they can discuss this information and offer additional supporting evidence to the reviewers. These are the findings that the site reviewers will present for review to the NLNAC staff.

After the Visit

After the reviewers have completed the evaluation process and given the nursing program a preliminary report of their findings, members of the nursing program should meet to analyze the findings. If necessary, plans can be made to implement immediate program revisions to align with the NLNAC criteria requirements. This is also a good time to review the entire self study and on-site visit to determine if changes can be made that would enhance the evaluation process in future accreditation visits. If a consultant was hired to assist with the process, the program should inform that person of the reviewers' findings. This information can be used to provide better consultation services during subsequent visits.

Final Report

After reviewing the findings, the NLNAC staff refers its final recommendations to the NLNAC Commission. The commission makes the final accreditation decision. The nursing program may appeal the decision if it disagrees with the commission's ruling. The director of the nursing program should attend the reviewers' presentation to the commission, either by telephone or in person, although the director's presence at the meeting suggests stronger interest and support from the program.

Summary

The NLNAC accreditation process provides the nursing program faculty an opportunity for ongoing self-examination, re-evaluation, and long-term planning. Preparation of the self study requires the participation and commitment of all team members. A well-defined plan for developing the self study and preparing for the NLNAC reviewers' site visit can bolster the chances for accreditation success. The peer preview process contributes to a program's ability to consistently meet the graduate nurse's educational needs.

Learning Activities

1. Review the accreditation standards at the NLNAC's website, www.nlnac.org.
2. Ask a local nursing program if you might review their most recent NLNAC accreditation self study.
3. Interview a dean or department chairperson and nursing faculty about their most recent experience with NLNAC accreditation. Ask:
   - What the preparation process and the actual experience was like for them;
   - What they view as the strengths and weaknesses of the accreditation process; and
   - What they learned about their program from the accreditation process.
4. Interview an NLNAC evaluator and gather his or her perspective about accreditation.
5. If a local nursing program is undergoing a NLNAC review, ask if you can attend some meetings as that program prepares for the site visit.

6. Compare and contrast the NLNAC's accreditation standards, processes, and procedures with those of the Commission on Collegiate Nursing Education.

References

National League for Nursing Accrediting Commission. (2003). *Accreditation Manual Interpretive Guidelines*. New York: Author.

Bibliography

Blais, K. K., Hayes, J. S., Kozier, B., & Erb, G. (2002). *Professional nursing practice: Concepts and perspectives* (4th ed.). Upper Saddle River, NJ: Prentice Hall.

Chitty, K. K. (2001). *Professional nursing—concepts and challenges* (3rd ed.). Philadelphia: W. B. Saunders

Ellis, J. R., & Hartley, C. L. (1998). *Nursing in today's world: Challenges, issues, and trends* (6th ed.). Philadelphia: Lippincott.

Faculty Support and Development

Unit 7

Chapter 22: Nursing College Evaluation Systems and Their Legal Implications
Marilyn Frank-Stromborg, MS, Ed D, JD, RN, ANP, FAAN,
and Bob Morgan, BA

Chapter 23: Action Research to Develop Evidence-Based Teaching
Enid A. Rossi, MSN, Ed D, RN

Chapter 24: Starting an Email Discussion List
Doug Heaslip

Chapter 25: Empowering One Another
Lynn Engelmann, MSN, Ed D, RN,
and Janice A. Miller, BSN, MSN, RN

Chapter 22: Nursing College Evaluation Systems and Their Legal Implications

Marilyn Frank-Stromborg, MS, EdD, JD, RN, ANP, FAAN, and Bob Morgan, BA

As with any professional position, faculty are evaluated. It is imperative that all faculty understand the system used to conduct their evaluation. When all parties are informed, the faculty evaluation can be used for professional growth. Dr. Frank-Stromborg and Mr. Morgan explain the different types of faculty evaluations and provide insights into their legal implications. – Linda Caputi

Introduction

With a greater emphasis on increasing educational standards, the quality of faculty has become a significant issue on college campuses. A century ago, professors in higher education had few protections from the arbitrary hiring and firing decisions of administrators. Today, professors generally find themselves with job security through negotiated contracts and statewide tenure systems.

To better understand the impact of higher standards for faculty, one must look no further than the expansion of faculty evaluation programs. Public and private colleges today evaluate their faculty in myriad ways, trying to achieve the appropriate balance between academic freedom and the public's desire for more accountability in higher education. Many universities employ both external and internal evaluations of their faculty, including peer review, administrative observations, self evaluations, student evaluations, and external observers. Evalu-

Educational Philosophy

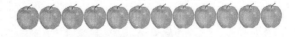

Effective teaching is based on the personal interaction and caring between teacher and student. This interaction can occur anywhere, anytime, can last a lifetime, and has the potential to significantly change the student's life for better or worse. The role of teacher thus is a serious responsibility that should not be entered into lightly. – Marilyn Frank-Stromborg

ation of faculty in nursing education is unique because clinical expertise, national certifications, and the professional nature of nursing must be taken into consideration along with classroom performance. In any assessment of faculty, several legal issues must be considered to protect the rights of each faculty member as well as the college and the students. How much influence can a faculty evaluation have on employment decisions? Are faculty losing protections for academic freedom as administrators initiate more rigorous evaluation systems? What state laws protect the faculty member or college during this process? How can faculty protect themselves against illegal discrimination while their superiors develop evaluation guidelines?

AAUP Standards for Faculty Evaluation

Although there is no federally mandated standard for faculty evaluations, the American Association of University Professors (AAUP), a highly regarded, national body of college educators who pass nonbinding guidelines, created a Statement on Teaching Evaluation (AAUP, 1990). When a faculty evaluation plan is developed, it is important that the expectations the institution places upon the teacher be known to all. The university then has the obligation to provide the conditions and support necessary for meeting these institutional expectations. AAUP identified areas for schools to focus on when developing a faculty evaluation plan. First, AAUP advocates that institutions declare their values and communicate them clearly to enable colleges and departments to set forth specific expectations related to teaching, research, and service, and to make clear any other faculty obligations. "Too often, even at the simple point of numbers and kinds of students taught, departments and institutions operate on value assumptions seldom made clear to the faculty" (AAUP, 1990). The AAUP continues that an appropriate faculty evaluation system would recognize the broad spectrum of teaching, be sensitive to different kinds and styles of instruction, and be useful in distinguishing superior teaching from merely competent teaching.

Different Types of Faculty Evaluation

Faculty evaluation has developed in recent years, with many different techniques being used in colleges across the country. Nursing programs increasingly use faculty evaluations and place greater value on these evaluations than they have in the past. The National League for Nursing includes "creating environments that promote ongoing faculty development" as a primary category in its list of criteria for a school to be identified as a "Center of Excellence in Nursing Education" (NLN, 2004). In the last 30 years, teaching evaluation has evolved from its primary reliance on a chairperson's informal assessment to a formal, comprehensive, and systematic approach (Ory, 1991). Though evaluation can take place outside of the classroom through lesson plans and individual meetings with administrators, most of the process of evaluation takes place inside the classroom. It has become rare for a college to not employ some method of faculty evaluation. A study of 450 nursing schools (Crawford, 1998) found 79 percent used classroom observation as a method of faculty evaluation.

Developing a successful faculty evaluation system can be difficult. There is constant tension between administrators and faculty related to how evaluations are structured and utilized. A systematic evaluation plan that is realistic, philosophically driven, and focused on data of interest to all stakeholders (ie, faculty, employers, and students) results in program improvement (Hammer & Bentley, 2003). But there can easily be confusion about faculty evaluations. Faculty tend to take the position that evaluations should not be a part of the process of hiring, firing, and promotion, but instead should provide a basis for constructive criticism with the sole focus on improvement of teaching and sharing of different teaching styles. On the other hand, administrators often use professor evaluations as a primary basis for tenure decisions, wage changes, and disciplinary action. In the 1998 study by Crawford, there was an significant difference between the perceptions of administrators and faculty about the purpose of classroom observation. Administrators used classroom observation most frequently for annual reviews and promotion considerations. In contrast, faculty expected that classroom observation would be used to provide feedback for improvement of teaching.

To minimize the conflict between administrators and faculty, administrators need to communicate the goals of the evaluation process and explain how the results will be used. Faculty should know the evaluation criteria well in advance, and they should be confident in administrative assurances that the criteria will be applied equitably. The evaluation criteria should allow for flexibility to serve varying faculty roles including full- and part-time faculty, clinicians, and adjunct instructors. "If faculty are to believe the evaluation process is effective and helpful, the data collected should serve a purpose for the individual faculty member as well as for administration" (Bobbitt, 1985). Evaluations can be a valuable tool for attaining excellence in academic instruction, but they must be done with respect to all parties that are involved.

Also important when developing faculty evaluations are determining what criteria are to be most highly valued in the process. Depending on the location, academic area, and composition of the student body, administrators might place greater value on multicultural sensitivity, success in preparing students for professional careers, or the ability of the faculty member to work well with their teaching colleagues. Still, some criteria are more common than others when preparing a faculty evaluation system. The most common criteria deemed important in judging overall teaching effectiveness are whether the teacher:

- Presents material clearly;
- Answers students' questions;
- Treats students in a courteous and professional manner; and
- Appears to be well prepared for each class (Tang, 1997).

But every school is different, and the formation of a faculty evaluation system should be a collaborative effort among students, faculty, and administrators. Therefore, the process of developing a faculty evaluation system involves both the technical requirement of good measurement and the political process of gaining the confidence of the faculty (Arreola, 2000).

Administrators need to be cognizant of faculty differences based on gender and race when conducting faculty evaluations. Faculty apprehension about their evaluation system must not be ignored. The three most common concerns of faculty are resentment of the implied assumption that they may not be competent in their subject area, suspicion that they will be evaluated by unqualified people, and anxiety that they will be held accountable for performance in an area in which they have little or no training or interest (Arreola, 2000).

Peer Review

Faculty evaluations often include a component of peer review, which is a long-standing academic practice. This method involves other faculty evaluating a teacher's performance through classroom observation, review of instructional materials, and course design (Arreola, 2000). Typical areas of focus of peer evaluation include content and organization of material, communication style, questioning skills, critical thinking skills, rapport with students, learning environment, and teaching materials (Naumann, 2004). Administrators tend to prefer peer faculty review because it is:

- Cost-efficient;
- An easily managed process; and
- Conducive to an atmosphere of mutual cooperation among the faculty.

Faculty also have positive feelings about peer review systems. In the 1998 Crawford study of nursing faculty and administrators, the majority of faculty (70 percent) agreed evaluation data from peers might be more meaningful than student input because faculty have broader perspectives. An evaluation from a peer can lead to accurate and beneficial results because the peers are generally highly educated, are attuned to the specific needs, uniqueness, and personality of an institution, and similarly benefit from the productive and honest peer review they receive in turn.

Peer review can be a positive approach for a nursing education program, but it must be done carefully and correctly. In the Crawford (1998) study there was a consensus (79 percent) among faculty that "more than one or two observations are necessary to evaluate teaching effectiveness." It is recognized that everyone has a bad day and it is unfair to base an entire evaluation on that one particular bad day. Having more than one observer would also safeguard against animus between teachers having a strong effect on another teacher's employment. Successful development and implementation of a program of peer review in a nursing program is directly related to at least four factors:

- The program should be voluntary.
- The peer review should be designed in a way that reflects the unique characteristics and culture of the nursing program.
- The implementation and development of the peer review system should have strong administrative sanction and support.
- The timing of the peer review process should be considerate of the schedules of both the faculty and the administrator (Martsolf, 1999).

There are criticisms regarding peer review of faculty. One criticism focuses on the possibility of infighting among faculty, which might reflect unfairly in the evaluation. Another criticism is that faculty may not have expertise in conducting peer evaluations, so they must be internally prepared through training seminars that explain the criteria to be used and how best to judge a given classroom. It is plausible that a faculty member could even consider giving negative evaluations to peers with the hope of improving his or her own chances for retention and promotion. In other words, peer evaluations are not a perfect method.

Administrators, too, are sometimes skeptical of peer evaluations. The 1998 Crawford study found administrative opinions toward peer review to be measured. For example, one respondent stated, "rarely do faculty give constructive suggestions" (Crawford, 1998), implying that faculty are either unprepared for such a process or simply hesitant to criticize peers with whom they work closely on a regular basis. Other challenges to the establishment of a program of peer review include the amount of faculty time involved in the activity and the cost of releasing faculty to participate in reviews. Lastly, administrators must find faculty who are willing and able to participate in peer evaluation. Faculty who acknowledge the importance and benefits of placing value on the scholarship of teaching are more likely to be willing to allot time to review their own and colleagues' teaching (Martsolf, 1999).

While there will always be uncontrollable variables, there are several ways to ensure that the peer evaluations are as productive as possible. The success of a peer evaluation system depends primarily on positive faculty involvement, short but objective methods, trained observers, constructive feedback for faculty development, and open communication and trust (Brown, 1994).

Administrative Evaluation

In an administrative evaluation, the professor's supervisor, department head, or dean serves as the observer. Administrative evaluation integrates all the other methods of faculty evaluations: peer, self, student, and external evaluations. Though administrators are ultimately the ones putting the professor evaluations to use, this method involves an administrator throughout the entire process. This system saves faculty time by limiting peer and self evaluations, leaving faculty more time to perform their work. As with other faculty evaluation systems, there are problems. The administrator evaluation system can produce a power struggle between administrators who may have the discretion to fire teachers they do not like and faculty hesitant to be involved in a process where administrators have total control over firing faculty. Information from administrative evaluation of faculty is most appropriate when it guides the professional growth and development of faculty, not when it is used for personnel decisions (Arreola, 2000).

Self Evaluation

Another method of professor evaluation, less common than peer evaluation, is self evaluation, also known as reflective inquiry and portfolio. In self evaluation the professor spends time evaluating him or herself in teaching, organization, and course preparation. The professor generally uses a variety of methods during the self-evaluation process, filling out self-descriptive paperwork and journals, looking back at past teaching practices to better assess where to go in the future, and identifying personal strengths and areas requiring improvement. Faculty study both themselves and the act of teaching in self-study evaluations, resulting in a clearer understanding about who they are as teachers. "For college professors, self study is about improving teaching through greater understanding of teachers' identities, developing relationships with colleagues and exploring inconsistencies between teaching beliefs and practices" (Drevdahl, 2002).

Self evaluation can be an advantageous process, but it is not undertaken very often in nursing evaluation systems. For those schools that have chosen to incorporate self evaluation into their professor evaluation system, the three phases of self evaluation are "enlightenment (ie, helping practitioners understand who they are), empowerment (ie, taking the necessary steps to change), and emancipation (ie, freeing practitioners from their prior ways of practicing to be reconstituted as new practitioners)" (Drevdahl, 2002). Though a self-evaluation system may not provide the extensive, objective results of a peer evaluation, it is a process that may improve the quality of the faculty teaching. The act of writing descriptive and reflective self evaluations helps a writer to get a holistic view of his or her teaching (Ory, 1991). The weaknesses of self evaluation include:

- Results that are not necessarily consistent with other raters' assessments;
- Faculty may be unwilling to collect and/or consider data relative to their own performance; and
- Faculty tend to rate themselves higher than students do (Arreola, 2000).

Objectivity concerns are valid when professors have a tangible way to influence their own employment, but this risk should not prohibit exploration of this evaluation method.

Student Evaluation of Faculty

Another common method for evaluating faculty is student portfolios or student evaluations. This system calls for students to rate a teacher's performance, often near the end of a course, through structured or unstructured questionnaires or interviews (Arreola, 2000). Student evaluations have become very popular in recent years and are used by universities more than any other system. Student evaluations are the most ubiquitous source of faculty evaluation data, used by nearly 90 percent of academic administrators as a basis for improving teaching and judging faculty performance (Appling, 2001). What began as a student activity aimed at helping students select courses has become a powerful source of information that is widely used by administrators to make personnel and program decisions (Ory, 1991).

Student evaluations can be one of the strongest indicators of a professor's teaching skills, or they can be a waste of time. Indeed, student evaluation data can be used for summative evaluation—to make administrative personnel decisions—and for formative evaluation—to improve teaching effectiveness (Appling, 2001). Student evaluations can be a surprisingly accurate depiction of a professor, since students see the professor teaching on a regular basis, while other observers will be judging the professor based on a small window of classroom observation time. Further, students tend to give constructive feedback, often producing an insightful opinion about the professor's ability to teach well.

However, student evaluations must be viewed with caution. Students seem to be generous in their ratings, and often include factors in their decisions that do not coincide with administration-identified factors—eg, class size and time of day (Arreola, 2000). Student evaluations often show more of the students' opinion about the teacher, rather than the course, so their ratings may have little to do with what they learned (Marsh, 1981). There is a concern about gender bias, with most students assumed to prefer male professors. Moreover, students do not always take professor evaluations seriously, leaving a possibility of skewed results. Great care should be taken to guarantee that students participating in this form of evaluation fully understand the criteria to consider, and be aware their opinions may be used, in conjunction with other data, to make important employment decisions. Another consequence of placing significant value on student evaluations is that professors may shift to teaching only what is politically correct, focus on entertainment rather than instruction, and cater to what brings a positive response from the students. This could allow for easier grading, avoidance of any controversial discussions, and stifling of analytical debate. Alternatively, knowing students will be evaluating them, faculty may be encouraged to introduce more lively class discussions, prepare more interesting lectures, and expend a higher energy level in the classroom.

Peer, self, and student evaluations are most successful when used in conjunction with one another to form a triad and, in fact, a triangulation of sources. A faculty evaluation system that incorporates all three sources is more balanced and fair than a system based on only one or two of these sources (Appling, 2001).

External Observers

External observers also can be used in a faculty evaluation system. This would involve qualified teams of observers from other schools or professional evaluation committees observing faculty performance and evaluating student learning data (Arreola, 2000). The use of external evaluators is relatively rare for evaluating teaching effectiveness (Bialik, 1994). The obvious benefit to bringing in external observers is that they have no connection to the faculty—unlike student, peer, and administrator evaluators—so there is little chance of an evaluation that is predisposed. Additionally, external observers have expertise in evaluating faculty. It is possible that there may be bias, since many external observers have a broad agenda, and may be from rival schools or agencies that value different criteria. But overall, external observers provide a distinct benefit to the faculty evaluation plan when combined with other methods.

Unique Nursing Considerations

As a professional curriculum, nursing education integrates clinical work into an otherwise typical course progression. This distinction requires that professor evaluation systems developed by administration take into account the impact a clinical has on a student's education. Employing faculty who are excellent classroom teachers as well as expert clinicians is integral to producing competent and qualified nurses.

The unique nature of nursing education, as compared to most other higher education departments, can become an issue when statewide, regional, or even college-wide faculty evaluations systems are developed. For instance, councils of higher education usually determine classroom student-to-faculty ratios. However, that formula may not take into account the large number of contact hours involved in clinical teaching (Bobbitt, 1985). Similarly, any time a faculty evaluation system is established beyond the jurisdiction of the nursing program, as happens at many large colleges, the value of nursing clinicals rarely are factored into the process. When clinical hours are taken into account, clinical teaching environments are evaluated with many of the same criteria listed for peer evaluations—with the exception of content (Naumann, 2004). Nursing programs must also take into account the national licensure examination and national nursing certification examinations, and the role these play in the excellence required of nursing faculty. Since passing NCLEX is a necessity to practicing nursing, the abilities of faculty to prepare students for the state licensing examination should be a criteria for any nursing evaluation system. Students in graduate programs must also pass an examination—the national certification examination. The ability of graduate faculty to prepare students to successfully pass this examination should be part of the evaluation system.

Legal Concerns

The legal protections for administrators, faculty, and students depend on whether the college is public or private. Public universities are covered by the protections of the United States Constitution, while private universities are governed by contract law. Nonetheless, both public and private nursing programs have legal considerations when creating and implementing faculty evaluation systems.

Due Process

Due process is used in many contexts and has several meanings. For the purpose of faculty evaluations, "procedural due process" refers to the right to notice of an action being taken against the teacher, the reasons for it, and an opportunity for a hearing where the teacher can make a case against the action (Poskanzer, 2002). Due process is a constitutional privilege granted to faculty at public colleges, but as a matter of public policy, courts will weigh this privilege against the legitimate concerns of the academic institution. The Supreme Court has stated due process should balance the private interest at stake—and the erroneous deprivation of liberty or property—versus the college's interest (*Matthews*, 1976). Professors often claim that a property right has been taken when they lose their academic position. This claim stems from an implied tenure or implied contract provision protecting their employment. Due process also plays a role when a professor's continued employment is determined by questionable means. Whether it is excessive reliance on student evaluations, or peer evaluations from other faculty with vendettas, there is little reliability when it comes to professor evaluations.

When evaluation data is used to determine employment changes, there may be legitimate grounds for a reversal of an administrator's decision as a tangible result of a required due process hearing (U.S. Constitution, Art. 14). If a college fires or demotes a professor, the professor is entitled to a hearing on the matter. Once a due process hearing is scheduled, the professor may not be able to gain access to all the records that led to the administrative action. Most of the time, the college will provide the professor with all the evaluation documents when requested in the course of a due process hearing. Still, a college sometimes will refuse to submit confidential peer review documents in order to protect the anonymity of the peer reviewers. The Supreme Court has found this to be generally unacceptable, finding that a professor's due process rights extend to access to all relevant documents (*EEOC*, 1990).

Academic Freedom

Once faculty are placed in a situation in which what they say and do has an increased effect on their employment, academic freedom becomes a serious concern. Generally, academic freedom is defined as faculty's entitlement to full independence in research and in publication of the results, in the classroom in discussing their subject, and to speak and write as citizens free from institutional censorship and discipline (AAUP, 1990). Accountability is a positive pursuit, but if an institution fails to appropriately balance their administrative mission with the freedom of the professor to teach as he or she wishes, there may be an implied discouragement of independent thinking and innovative teaching.

There is some concern that academic freedom has insulated faculty teaching from scrutiny by their peers (Martsoff, 1999). Academic freedom has been strongly protected by the courts, allowing professors to present their opinions, even to the extremes, and be exempt from reprimand. Fear of litigation is real and justified in today's litigious society, and any peer or administrator who attempts to restrict the words or actions of a professor, no matter how absurd that professor's performance might be, is likely to be vulnerable to a lawsuit (*Sweezy*, 1957).

With the increasing use of professor evaluations, concerns about the proper storage or disposal of those sensitive documents have arisen. If a professor is negatively evaluated based on harsh and discrediting comments by peers, what happens to those comments if the professor is promoted or leaves the position to work elsewhere? When professor evaluations are completed, the data is kept in administrative files and considered confidential information. However, these records are often easily obtainable by the public through state open-records laws. In other words, peer and student evaluation documents are accessible in many states that have no exceptions to state laws that allow the release of all faculty personnel records (Arreola, 2000).

Tenure and Post-Tenure Considerations

Laws about tenure become relevant when devising faculty evaluation systems. In the last half century, state tenure laws have developed a web of protection around faculty who have:
- Worked at the college for an predetermined period of time;
- Published scholarly articles;
- Received positive teaching evaluations; and
- Earned tenure.

But what happens once a tenured professor's performance deteriorates? What if a teacher begins to receive poor student and peer evaluations? What if the material taught in class borders on racism, sexual harassment, or support of terrorism? Should there be a distinction made between classroom teaching and clinical teaching when evaluating senior faculty? Post-tenure review is being instituted in a number of academic settings because of these issues. The primary purpose of the post-tenure review is to gather data on which to base the termination of tenured faculty whose performance no longer meets accepted professional standards (Arreola, 2000).

Post-tenure review is quickly becoming the norm as tenure itself is being challenged as a roadblock to achieving faculty excellence (Arreola, 2000). According to a 1996 (Licata) survey of 680 colleges and universities, 61 percent had post-tenure review policies in place and another 9 percent were considering imposing such a requirement. A similar survey in 1989 (Licata) showed only 3 percent with post-tenure review.

Tenure itself is at risk, as the process once acclaimed for protecting professors from arbitrary employment actions is now criticized for keeping "dead-wood" faculty on the payroll. In response to intense societal demands for accountability, there is a growing movement in the direction of a tenure-free academic environment among colleges and universities (Arreola, 2000). The idea behind this movement is that absent tenure protections, faculty will be more apt to abide by administrative changes and professor evaluation recommendations.

Once post-tenure review is established, what role should it play in the faculty evaluation process? This question is still largely unanswered, with some universities using post-tenure review purely as a method for giving constructive criticism. Others universities are finding post-tenure review to be a useful method for putting pressure on faculty who are performing poorly or at least failing to join the effort to improve the quality of education at the school. There is a noticeable trend in public institutions to attempt to build sanctions into newly formulated post-tenure review programs (Seldin, 1999). There are many advantages to post-tenure review; particularly reshaping a teacher who is failing to meet established teaching standards. Yet, post-tenure review will generally not lead to firing the employee. Tenured professors are usually only fired for cause, such as incompetence, breach of academic integrity, moral turpitude or reprehensible personal conduct, sexual harassment, or civil rights violations (Poskanzer, 2002). Alternatively, advising a professor that he or she is not performing as anticipated may lead that professor to seek employment elsewhere, thus avoiding the loss of face and potential damage to reputation associated with the non-renewal, or the denial, of tenure (Poskanzer, 2002).

Defamation is another claim that can arise when a professor is disciplined as a result of faculty evaluations. A professor may feel his or her name is being tarnished if negative evaluations are leaked and used in unintended ways. However, courts have generally protected administrators from defamation charges resulting from performance evaluations, absent some gross misconduct such as intentional leaking of confidential information (Zirkel, 1996).

Summary

American society is struggling with the issue of improving its education system. As a country, we have increased student testing, allocated more money for schools in impoverished areas, and demanded more from our students, faculty, and administrators. Professor evaluations have become a common and expected form

Table 22.1 - Methods of Evaluating Faculty Performance

	Peer Review	Administrative Review	Self Evaluation	Student Evaluations	External Observers
Description	Other college faculty members observe classroom of peer professor.	Supervisor or department head observes classroom of professor.	Professor evaluates self through journals and reflective observation.	Students use questionnaires and are interviewed to evaluate their professor's performance.	Trained, external observers visit classroom for short time to evaluate quality of instruction.
Strengths	Cost-efficient, manageable, attuned to specific needs of the college, mutual benefit.	Saves faculty time, administrators understand the scope of the evaluation system and have broad academic perspective.	Beneficial for professor to spend time identifying their own strengths and weaknesses, the teacher knows him or herself best.	Surprisingly accurate ratings, students have most time to judge professor's talents and areas for improvement, provides candid responses.	No predisposed feelings toward individual professors, evaluators are trained for such evaluations, can often identify larger themes to improve upon.
Weaknesses	Significant faculty time used, may require several observations, may cause animus among teachers, faculty untrained in proper evaluation.	May give administrator dangerous amount of discretion, any existing animus could harm a professor's evaluation.	Difficult to be objective, tends to result in higher ratings, observations will be limited to obvious skills and weaknesses.	Possible gender bias, focus on insignificant factors, students could take the process too lightly.	May lack understanding of unique character of college, short period of classroom observation, may have ulterior agendas.

Teaching Nursing: The Art and Science

Table 22.1 - Methods of Evaluating Faculty Performance, cont.

	Peer Review	Administrative Review	Self Evaluation	Student Evaluations	External Observers
Overall	One of the easiest, most effective methods, can improve relations among faculty, is a strong component of any evaluation system.	Adds another dimension to the evaluation, could disturb delicate professor-administrator balance.	Can only be a positive experience for a professor, and the resulting difference is dependent on the effort and time given.	Most common system, can produce very accurate description of the quality of teaching but can fail to evaluate proper factors.	Another positive method in coordination with other evaluation methods, can bring new ideas for innovative teaching.

of maintaining faculty excellence and progress. Table 22.1 summarizes the methods of faculty evaluation discussed in this chapter.

Teaching evaluation in higher education is no longer a "shifting and ambiguous activity" conducted by the seat of the pants wherein "casual praise from a single student or a casual impression of a public performance could pass as substantial evidence" (Ory, 1991). Colleges now use complex and varied methods to evaluate professors, and improvements have been realized in discharging stagnant and complacent professors, even those faculty who are tenured. There is a shift in educational priorities as colleges move away from the time that tenured professors were never seriously evaluated. It is increasingly common for a tenured professor to be evaluated every three years. Innovative peer review systems are being integrated into nursing colleges.

With this new wave of professor evaluations, faculty are fighting back in the courts to protect their positions and their freedom to teach what and how they want. Administrators must use prudence in stripping faculty of their jobs, or discouraging individual methods of teaching, based on the results of professor evaluations. Today's administrators face the ever-present threat of litigation and must be able to support their decisions with tangible and objective evaluative information (Ory, 1991). Moreover, colleges will continue to adapt to the many ways that faculty evaluation can be used to improve the quality of nursing education.

Learning Activities

1. Interview one professor who teaches in a public institution and one who teaches at a private school to learn about the type of evaluation systems used in their institutions. Compare and contrast the two.
2. Think about your personal experiences with evaluation. What types of evaluation were used? Which did you like the most? Which did you like the least? Why?

References

American Association of University Professors. (1990). *1940 Statement of principles on academic freedom and tenure*. Retrieved Feb. 11, 2004, from http://www.aaup.org/statements/redbook/1940stat.htm.

American Association of University Professors. (1990). *Statement on teaching evaluation*. Retrieved Feb. 11, 2004, from http://www.aaup.org/statements/redbook/rbeval.htm.

Appling, S. E., Berk, R., & Naumann, P. A. (2004). *Crouching professor, hidden peer evaluator*. Retrieved Feb. 11, 2004, from Johns Hopkins Nursing Institute website: www.son.jhmi.edu/newsandmedia/files/crouching_prof.pdf.

Appling, S. E., Berk, R., & Naumann, P. A. (Sept./Oct. 2001). Using a faculty evaluation triad to achieve evidence-based teaching. *Nursing and Health Care Perspectives, 22*(5), 247-251.

Arreola, R. A. (2000). *Developing a comprehensive faculty evaluation system* (pp. xix, xxii, 48-49, 62, 93). Bolton, MA: Anker Publishing.

Bialik, D., Dilts, D. A., & Haber, L. J. (1994). *Assessing what professors do: An introduction to academic performance appraisal in higher education*. Westport, CT: Greenwood Press.

Bobbitt, K. C. (1985). Systematic faculty evaluation: A growing critical concern. *Journal of Nursing Education, 24*(2), 86-88.

Brown, B., & Ward-Griffin, C. (1994). The use of peer evaluation in promoting nursing faculty teaching effectiveness: A review of the literature. *Nurse Education Today, 14*(4), 299-305.

Crawford, L. H. (1998). Evaluation of nursing faculty through observation. *Journal of Nursing Education, 37*(7), 289-294.

Drevdahl, D. J., Stackman, R. W., Purdy, J. M. & Louie, B.Y. (2002). Merging reflective inquiry and self-study as a framework for enhancing the scholarship of teaching. *Journal of Nursing Education, 41*(9), 413-419.

Hammer, J. B., & Bentley, R. W. (2003). A Systematic Evaluation Plan that Works. *Nurse Educator, 28*(4), 179.

Johns, C. (1999). Reflection as empowerment? *Nursing Inquiry, 6*(4), 241-249.

Licata, C. M., & Morreale, J. C. (1997). *Post-tenure review: Policies, practices, precautions* (AAHE New Pathways Working Paper Series No. 12). Washington, DC: American Association for Higher Education.

Marsh, H. W. (1981). The use of path analysis to estimate teacher and course effects on student ratings of instrument effectiveness. *Applied Psychological Measurement, 6*, 47-60.

Martsolf, D. S., Dieckman, B. C., Cartechine, K. A., Starr, P. J., Wolf, L. E., & Anaya, E. R. (1999) Peer review of teaching: Instituting a program in a college of nursing. *Journal of Nursing Education, 38*(7), 326-32.

Matthews v. Eldridge, 424 U.S. 319 (1976).

National League for Nursing (2003, Sept. 17). *Centers of excellence in nursing education: Criteria.* Retrieved Feb. 11, 2004, from http://www.nln.org/profdev/excellence.htm.

Ory, J. C. (1991, Winter). Changes in Evaluating Teaching in Higher Education. *Theory Into Practice, 30*(1), pp. 30, 32, 34.

Poskanzer, S. G. (2002). *Higher education law: The faculty.* Baltimore: Johns Hopkins Press.

Seldin, P. (1999). *Changing practices in evaluating teaching: A practical guide to improved faculty performance and promotion/tenure decisions.* Boston: Ankler Publishing.

Sweezy v. State of New Hampshire by Wyman, 354 U.S. at 250; 1957 (Supreme Court reaffirming the importance of academic freedom and the strong protection it will receive from the courts).

Tang, T. L. (1997). Teaching evaluation at a public institution of higher education: Factors related to the overall teaching effectiveness. *Public Personnel Management, 26*(3), 379.

University of Pennsylvania v. EEOC, 493 U.S. 182, 1990.

U.S. Const. Amend. Art. XIV. There are minimal requirements to fulfill a public university professor's due process rights; namely "some form of notice of the action being taken against the faculty member and the reasons for it, and some kind of opportunity for a hearing at which the faculty member can make a case against the proposed action." (Poskanzer, p. 244, 2002).

Zirkel, P. (1996). *The law of teacher evaluation.* Bloomington, IN: Phi Delta Kappa Educational Foundation.

Chapter 23: Action Research to Develop Evidence-Based Teaching

Enid A. Rossi, MSN, EdD, RN

Nursing faculty, like all professionals, must strive to become the best they can be. One way is to adopt a continuous quality improvement program using evidence-based practice. Dr. Rossi suggests reflective action research as a useful tool for gathering information for a quality improvement program. Once this process is learned, it can be incorporated into the teacher's daily life, providing insights and feedback to improve teaching. The ultimate goal is to incorporate the process as a natural part of one's practice so it becomes transparent and painless. It also will become infinitely helpful in improving one's teaching!
– Linda Caputi

Educational Philosophy

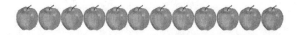

I have a deeply held belief in an individual's abilities and potential. The individual has the ability to participate in the process of learning within an interactive learning environment and to develop personally relevant knowledge. I value self-awareness, self-efficacy and self-choice and assume these will contribute to learning. My role as a teacher and facilitator of learning is to stretch learners beyond what they would learn by themselves, but not so far as to cause a high level of stress. The teacher creates an environment for such learning to occur and facilitates that process. – Enid A. Rossi

Introduction

Individual, reflective action research is a method for identifying and using components of best practices that fit each unique practice situation. Nursing faculty are constantly confronted with changing role expectations and contexts. Schools' professional development programs often do not allow nurse educators to determine best practices for themselves because nurse educators' special knowledge is learned through inquiry and participation in their unique practices (Fullan, 2001; House & Lapan, 1988; O'Toole, 1995). Action research involves a systematic study of a practice situation carried out by professionals involved in these situations so they may improve both practice and quality of understanding.

Burbules and Callister (2000), Privateer (1999), Skiba (1997), and Carnevale and Descrochers (1997) wrote that faculty are facing challenges presented by increasing class size, burgeoning financial burdens, and the changing student populations of colleges and universities. Market pressures for new communication technologies and vocational education also have changed the educational environment.

Studies of university nursing faculty (Coleman, 1994; Hannah, 2000) describe pressures associated with the multiple roles required of nursing faculty. Professional identity issues and time constraints are identified as major factors contributing to these pressures. Other factors include ever-changing role expectations, faculty restructuring, unfamiliarity with new technology, and difficulty balancing personal and professional lives. Nurse educators perceive themselves as underprepared to fulfill all these roles. Inadequate preparation for the teaching role leading to role strain for nursing faculty is well documented. In addition to their teaching responsibilities, nurse educators also need to maintain their clinical competence (Bachman, Kitchens, Halley & Ellison, 1992; Choudhry, 1992).

New faculty have an additional sources of stress. Discovering the nature of teaching and making the transition from practitioner to educator were identified as major contributors to role strain for new faculty (Bachman, Kitchens, Halley & Ellison, 1992; Choudhry, 1992). An example illustrates this: After teaching one semester, two new university nursing faculty decided to write an article about their introduction to their new teaching roles. Both had been highly respected clinical experts when they became nurse educators. However, in their new setting, both faculty experienced culture shock when they found they lacked some of the knowledge and skills needed for teaching at a university. The title of the article summarized their experience: *From Expert to Novice.*

Teaching is a complex and intensely social art that "demands knowledge, skill, self-reflection, intuition, empathy, caring, and self confidence…. Teachers need the capacity to think about many different things all at once and must act thoughtfully under pressure, often without time to stop and ponder what to do next; they must stand apart from and assess their own teaching…." (Lagemann, 1991, p. 1).

Action research provides a vehicle for faculty to stand apart from and assess their teaching. It is a useful, contextually relevant approach for nursing faculty to learn knowledge and skills for teaching in today's climate of changing faculty roles, limited resources, and demanding workdays. This chapter presents the use of self-directed, group-supported action research to help faculty deal with these types of challenges. It discusses a program of ongoing awareness and direction for one's teaching practice through a self-study process that focuses on adjusting how faculty engage students in learning (Rossi, 2002).

Explanation of Action Research

How can nursing faculty use action research to improve their teaching and understanding? In brief, action research is accomplished through practical actions, personal reflection on the effects of those actions, and then adjustment of practice to improve teaching effectiveness based on the results.

Educational action research is the systematic study of a teaching situation carried out by the teachers involved in that situation to improve both their practice and the quality of their understanding. This is accomplished through practical actions, personal reflection on the effects of those actions, and adjustments to practice to maximize effectiveness. The process incorporates ongoing, recursive reflection with focusing, planning, observing, acting, and revising during short-term cycles, as quickly as a single class session (Ebbutt, 1985; Kemmis & McTaggart, 1988; Lapan, 1999; McLean, 1995; Winter & Munn-Giddings, 2001).

Key characteristics of action research include:

- **Systematic.** This is an ongoing approach for learning effective teaching strategies for the teacher's current students.
- **Carried out by the teacher.** The teacher decides the focus of inquiry (the problem to be addressed) and direction of the investigation. The action research is conducted based on individual interests and level of comfort

with the process.

- **Teacher-focused.** With the emphasis on improving teaching practice and quality of understanding, the focus is on what the teacher does, not what the students do—although the two are related.

A complete understanding of how to use action research requires actual participation in the process; it cannot be learned intellectually alone. Haggerson and Bowman (1992) use the metaphor of a running stream to explain the multiple viewpoints of inquiry. The metaphor describes one path to inquiry as analogous to sitting on the edge of the stream and making generalizations and predictions about the flow of the water. A second path is to experience the stream by being a participant-observer, investigating the mutual impact the stream and the investigator have on each other. A third path is to become the stream as a total participant. The final path of inquiry is to cross to the other side of the stream, bringing all the previous experiences along.

Ongoing reflective practice is inherent in the action research process. Such a practice involves a spiraling-cyclic, recursive process of reflecting on concrete practices in conflicted and complex situations for the purpose of enhancing understanding and changing practice. A spiraling cycle is used to designate growth and change. The focus of attention in reflective practice includes "how phenomena fit together into patterns, how events flow and unfold over time, and how patterns shift and change" (Baxter & Montgomery, 1996, p. 11).

Steps in the Action Research Process

There are five steps in the action research process:
1. Focusing on an initial inquiry question;
2. Planning;
3. Implementing the plan and observing effects;
4. Re-planning and re-implementing; and
5. Reflecting with revised focus.

An example describes in detail how the five steps are used. (Hopkins, 1993; Kemis & McTaggart, 1988; McLean, 1995). The example demonstrates how action research incorporates interrelated components in mini-loop cycles that focus the teacher on the aspects of teaching practice to change and those related to the initial focus of inquiry.

Step One: Focusing on an Initial Inquiry Question

The teacher focuses on something that is important to that teacher's situation, such as exploring a promising new approach or a skill that teacher wants to improve. Completing the following statements can help the teacher identify a focus:

- I am perplexed by…;
- I have an idea I would like to try out in my class…;
- I would like to change…; and
- I would like to improve… (Hopkins, 1993, p. 63).

Example: My discussion questions are disrupted by my need to keep control in class.

Step Two: Planning

Planning involves making a decision about:

- What aspect(s) of the approach to try first; and
- How to obtain student feedback.
  Giving students a few specific questions to answer anonymously is a useful approach to obtaining feedback. Audio or video recordings of class sessions also may be good ways to obtain feedback.

Example: I am going to audiotape questions and responses for one class session and see what is happening.

Step Three: Implementing the Plan and Observing Effects

Implementing the plan and using students' feedback to observe its effects is the next step. The teacher reflects on student responses and attempts to determine the effectiveness of the intervention. The teacher then makes revisions based on the lessons learned.

Example: I learned that students think the nursing process means recalling facts rather than engaging in exploration. How can I stimulate exploration in my students? I should shift my questioning to encourage students to explore answers to their own questions.

The teacher now has identified another inquiry focus to investigate. This demonstrates the cyclical nature of action research.

Step Four: Re-planning and Re-implementing

The findings from step three are used to redesign instruction. The new instruction is then implemented.

Example: I will try to formulate and use questions that encourage students to say what they mean and what interests them.

Step Five: Reflecting with Revised Focus

The purpose of this step is to reflect on the revised instructional strategies implemented in step four. A focused approach is then planned and implemented.

Example: Based on my observations, I have noticed that my discussion questions were improving but students were still unruly. How can I keep them on track? I am going to make a greater effort to listen to students as they attempt to answer their questions.

The teacher may then decide to audiotape revised questioning and control statements.

The action research process continues through interrelated mini-cycles that facilitate ongoing growth for the teacher. Action research is a practical approach. Week-by-week action research provides specific feedback about teaching strategies and stimulates changes for improvement during the next contact with students. The nurse educator keeps refining this process until the **best practice** for the current group of students is achieved.

Difficulties of Action Research

Rossi (2002) found that nursing faculty in a study evaluating an action research program had difficulty narrowing their initial inquiry focus. The best way to overcome this is just to start. Using the stream analogy, the teacher needs to get in the boat and become a participant-observer and a full participant in this experience. The process begins by jumping in.

Rossi (2002) also found that some faculty had difficulty knowing how to word questions that would generate the student feedback they needed, but minimize a sense of vulnerability associated with the consciousness-raising aspect of action research. Nurse educators who participate in action research need to be willing to risk seeing their teaching practice in new ways that may not support their current professional self-concepts. Rossi also found that when certain questions were asked—for example, "What in this course is working so far?" and "What is not working?"—student feedback often was a laundry list of general complaints, including aspects of the course that were not under control of the faculty. Wording the questions carefully can helps minimize these issues.

The questions should be about what the teacher does, not what the students do. They must not contain evaluative words, like **best** or **worst**. Also, the questions must be focused on issues the teacher controls. The following questions can be adapted for the reader's own classroom use:

- What part of the theory content I have presented have you used in your clinical setting?
- How did the clinical conference contribute or not contribute to your understanding of what I taught in class?
- What did I do or not do in class to help you connect theory with practice?
- What is the main thing you learned by participating in the role play (or case scenario, or activity)?
- What do you still wish to learn more about?

After feedback is obtained, the nurse educator reflects on the student responses. This reflection is likely to stimulate a change. Students can be asked through another written, anonymous question whether changes are working to address the issue.

Group Supportive Component

It may be helpful for faculty who are using action research to meet regularly in small groups to reinforce each other's commitment to the practice. Several collaborative action research projects indicated that ongoing group-support meetings encourage persistence throughout the action research process. Also, sharing the endeavor with others was found to be crucial for addressing teachers' concerns and satisfying their needs (Baird, 1991; Baird, 1989; Baird, Mitchell & Northfield, 1987; Baird & Mitchell, 1986; Kemper & McKay, 1996).

Group support can be incorporated into the action research program to explore teachers' concerns and issues about focused-inquiry options and to encourage their persistence through the process (Rossi, 2002). Participants can schedule a series of meetings; six such meetings is a typical number used. During the meetings, participants learn the action research process and share their questions, concerns, and progress. They also explore teaching strategies and propose solutions for each other's classroom situations.

All nursing faculty in Rossi's study (2002) indicated that they greatly valued having group meetings every other week to share and discuss their common struggles, successes, and questions. The group meetings were essential for learning how to use action research and for enjoying the process. Often, one person's question would stimulate a need for clarification from others.

The same nurse educators shared that they liked meeting in a social environment, such as a restaurant, away from the college or university (Rossi, 2002). They also enjoyed meeting with faculty from another college or university to discuss common, cross-college issues in a supportive climate. Two of their comments follow:

- "The best aspect of this experience is working with other educators who are struggling to find the same answers."
- "I learned that my frustrations regarding teaching are real and shared by my colleagues, and that we all have a passion to do what is best for our students."

Results of an Action Research Program in Nursing Education

Rossi (2002) reported that all the nursing faculty who participated in an action research program said that the experience had been an educational eye-opener. They believed their teaching had improved and planned to continue the process. The nurse educators said the concrete feedback from students was important and useful, and provided the basis for changes. Participants reported that they developed can-do attitudes and that their teaching skills improved during the program. Some of their comments were:

- "It's interesting: You think you know what you're doing, and then it turns out not to be exactly what [students] need so you do an about-face. It takes the students to help update us and improve our practice."

- "We can change anything if we start listening to each other... back-and-forth listening and then modifying our innovations in the classroom."

Of particular interest to some faculty were interactive teaching approaches that engage students in learning yet do not require major time commitments from teachers and students. Another area of interest was adapting teaching approaches for diverse student profiles, aptitude levels, and expectations. Questions related to those issues included:

- "How can I encourage students to answer to their own questions instead of the instructor answering?"
- "When I see somebody putting forth a lot of extra effort [but they] can't get it, what do I do?"
- "What do you have to do to modify teaching for different generational groups?"

Best Practices in Teaching

Best practices in nursing education often apply learning strategies from research outside of the nursing profession. Observers may believe that what works in one setting will work in another. However, Haddon and Rossi (2003) define best practices as "a careful study of teaching processes and the use of this knowledge to improve practice; an ongoing search for the best example of teaching for a particular situation."

Nurse educators in an action research program conducted by Rossi (2002) used outside best practices only as they were related to their teaching situation. At the conclusion of the action research program, these educators believed that what they had learned was the best practice for their immediate situation. The impetus for learning about teaching and best practices originated from their current teaching practice issues. A comment from one participant demonstrated this: "I've learned that you can't take as gospel truth what the so-called experts tell you. I thought what I was doing was current. However, I've come to find out that for my students, it has not been helpful."

Nursing Faculty Stories

Following are stories about four nursing faculty (Rossi, 2002). These stories are provided to enhance understanding of the action research process and demonstrate that each nurse educator's experience is unique.

Shelly: Teacher in an Accelerated Baccalaureate Program

Shelly taught medical nursing in an accelerated baccalaureate program for students getting their second bachelor's degree. Shelly incorporated a variety of interactive teaching approaches, including using case scenarios and teaching clinical skills concurrently with related theory. She particularly focused on how to incorporate her students' life and educational experiences into her teaching strategies by asking students to share their expertise during class sessions. While most of her students' feedback was positive, some made suggestions—for example, speaking slower and making copies of PowerPoint slides to help students taking notes—that Shelly implemented.

Theresa: First-Year Teacher at a Rural Community College

Theresa taught leadership and maternal nursing. She kept a personal diary and reflected extensively about her teaching practice as she moved through the program. She investigated two interactive approaches:
- A bingo game to review key concepts; and
- Complex clinical scenarios to stimulate critical thinking related to leadership issues.

Her students shared very positive feedback about these strategies.

Sally: Experienced Medical-Surgical Teacher at a Rural Community College

Sally progressed through several mini-cycles of action research propelled by negative feedback from frustrated students. She reported: "They want me to be able to answer questions immediately and correctly in class and not refer to other students and they don't want me to contradict anything in the book. This is my life; welcome to it."

Sally said her participation in the action research program provided her with structure and support to work on these issues. She initiated changes in her teaching each week, obtaining student feedback about each change and making adjustments accordingly. Some examples are provided:

- Sally thought students preferred lectures using PowerPoint slides, but found they did not. Sally plans to use PowerPoint slides for her next class, however, because she believes each class has its own preferences.
- Sally lowered the level of her exam questions because this group of students had not been exposed to questions as difficult as the ones she used. However, she did incorporate higher-level questions for practice during lecture. Students offered much positive feedback about this change.
- Sally used a standard lecture format because this group of students seemed highly stressed and not open to changes during the last course of the program. Students requested a traditional format for lectures. She reported that students' satisfaction increased.

An Approach to Action Research

Introduction

Action research focuses on identifying the area of inquiry, obtaining useful feedback from students, and using their reaction to make changes in teaching strategies.

The learning experiences help the nurse educator discover how, where, and when to question the effectiveness of a teaching strategy. While these activities can be accomplished individually, regular meetings among faculty is an essential component to facilitate learning and commitment to the action research process. Therefore, learning experiences may be organized around group meetings to allow nurse educators sufficient time to work through the process.

Rossi (2002) recommends that the faculty group meetings be limited to four or five members to encourage all faculty to participate, and that groups be composed of college nursing faculty and graduate nursing education students. Group meetings should be held regularly so participants can practice and clarify the action research process and share questions, concerns, and details about their progress.

Planning for Groups

Initially, one person needs to take responsibility for arranging for the group sessions. For graduate students, the nursing faculty is the obvious choice. For practicing nurse educators, one person familiar with the group process and/or action research may serve this role. However, after sessions begin, the leadership role should be shared among members. Participants need to jointly decide the location and times of the meetings. Should they be held for two hours every other week for 12 weeks or weekly for six sessions during one academic term?

First Group Meeting

The first group meeting should be held the within the first few weeks of the term. Each participant should prepare for the session by carefully reviewing this chapter.

Facilitator

The group organizer should initially serve as the group facilitator. However, the facilitator's role then becomes a shared endeavor. At each session, a person is identified to initiate the session and provide a summary and closing comments. The facilitator for the first session explains this idea of sharing the facilitator role.

The facilitator provides a brief summary about what will occur during the meetings as each member progresses through the action research process. This process proceeds as follows:

- First meeting: Establish norms and clarify the research process.
- Second meeting: Establish the focus of inquiry, plan the changes in instructional strategies, and determine how feedback will be obtained.
- Third, fourth, and fifth meetings: Reflect, revise, and refocus the research.
- Sixth meeting: Discuss successes and struggles and develop a plan to incorporate active research into ongoing practice.

All the participants are likely to go through the same general process but they may follow slightly different sequences or have different teaching focuses.

Members

At the first meeting, members set standards for group sessions and agree on the norms that fit their group. The following guidelines can be used to facilitate trust among members and ensure their control over the extent of their sharing and participation (Rossi, 2002):

- During the group sessions, participants will share only at the level at which they feel comfortable.
- The facilitator and participants will support each participant's choices, challenges, and discoveries at his or her own level and pace.
- Each participant will have the freedom of choice in the focus and selection of teaching-related issues.
- Each participant will freely make decisions about the sources of data and methods he or she wishes to use.

All members initiate, seek, and provide information. Members also clarify and explore alternatives or deeper meaning to the focus queries that members seek to explore. Members encourage and support each other and harmonize to reduce tensions and assist others to explore differences. Each member helps maintain the flow of communication among the group.

Clarifying What Action Research Is All About

The facilitator reviews and discusses with the group the definition of educational action research and its interrelated components. The facilitator emphasizes that regular meetings are held to teach and clarify the action research process and for participants to share questions, concerns, and sense-making as they progress.

Identifying a Focus of Inquiry

The facilitator leads a discussion to facilitate development of a focus of inquiry for each participant to study. Each participant individually focuses on a question of concern related to their own practice. This becomes their **focus of inquiry**. Getting started is often the hardest step in action research, so the group members can help each other identify a personally meaningful first focus for their action research. The following statements may be used to spark ideas:

- I am perplexed by…;
- I have an idea I would like to try out in my class…;
- I would like to change…; and
- I would like to improve… (Hopkins, 1993, p. 63).

For the next group meeting, participants are asked to provide one question or concern they wish to use to conduct a mini-cycle of action research. They bring printed copies of their focus and study questions to share with the other members of the group.

Each person then plans to implement a small change in their teaching, collect data for observation, reflect on the feedback, and re-plan. The feedback findings are likely to stimulate further short loops of inquiries, actions, and reflection.

Second Meeting

A facilitator or co-facilitators are identified at the beginning of this session. During this meeting, participants are asked to discuss their inquiry focus and the questions they developed. Each inquiry focus should:

- Relate to what the teacher does, not what the students do;
- Not contain evaluative words, such as **best** or **worst**; and
- Relate to something the teacher has control over.

The second purpose of this meeting is planning. Participants discuss how to obtain student feedback or observations after their planned teaching strategy changes are implemented. Possible sources of student feedback are:

- Interpretive evidence or data obtained during teaching practice from students and colleagues;
- Audio or videotape recordings of teaching sessions;
- A report from a colleague observing students' responses; and
- Short questionnaires for students.

Using a student questionnaire to obtain feedback is called the **class check-up**. Participants in the action research group can discuss and work together on developing these questions. Remember, the questions should be about what the teacher does and must not contain evaluative words. Also, each question should address a specific, planned change in teaching. Be careful to word questions to obtain specific information from students rather than a laundry list of general complaints. One way to do this is to adapt the following questions to the participant's unique inquiry focus:

- What part of the theory content that I have presented have you used in your clinical setting?
- How did the clinical conference contribute or not contribute to your understanding of what I taught in class?
- What did I do or not do in class to help you connect theory with practice?
- What is the main thing you learned by participating in the role-play situation (or case scenario, or activity about setting priorities, etc.)?
- What do you still wish to learn more about…?

The responses are compiled anonymously and can be shared with the students at a later time to jointly make decisions about the identified teaching and student learning issues. Each participant keeps personal records of student feedback and shares aspects with the group.

Before the next group session, participants implement one teaching change and obtain written feedback from students through the class check-up. Remember to let students know their responses will be anonymous.

Third, Fourth, and Fifth Meetings

During the next three group meetings, participants share what they have learned about their teaching strategies from their students' feedback. These meetings should emphasize:

- Reflecting, to interpret the effects of their teaching changes;
- Revising, based upon what was discovered with reflection; and
- Refocusing on other related issues that may become the focus of future action research mini-cycles.

The participants are encouraged to move through related cyclic loops and/or two to three short mini-cycles.

Sixth Group Meeting

The final group meeting continues with the process described. The facilitator for this session leads a focused discussion about what has been meaningful and what has been frustrating about their experiences with action research. A discussion about the steps faculty can take to continue their action research on their own may also be helpful (Rossi, 2002).

The facilitator should pose the following questions to address continued use of action research: What factors would lead you to consider making this action research process a part of your ongoing practice? Is colleague or group support needed? What kind? What reasons would guide your decision to not incorporate action research in your practice?

Summary

Once learned, action research can be implemented intuitively throughout a teacher's career. It can be a valuable tool for improvement. Consider the parallel of the action research process with the nursing process. They both represent an ongoing process for improvement.

Resources

The following Internet resources provide more information about action research. These websites can be accessed from the CD-ROM accompanying this book. Simply launch your Internet browser, put the CD-ROM in the drive, go to Chapter 23 on the CD, and click on the website address.

- **Action Research Electronic Reader**
  www2.fhs.usyd.edu.au/arow/o/m01/m01.htm
  Collection of readings and information.

- **Action Research International**
  www.scu.edu.au/schools/gcm/ar/ari/arihome.html
  A refereed online journal.

- **Action Research Mailing List**
  To subscribe, send the following message with your first and last name to listproc@scu.edu.au
  subscribe arlist-1 firstname lastname.
  For help, contact Bob Dick, bd@psy.uqq.oz.ua.

- **Best Pick Resources on Action Research**
  http://www.aera.net/divisions/k/knews/sum99/internet-sum99.html

- **Mid-continent Research for Education and Learning (McREL)**
  www.mcrel.org/connect/action.html

- **Networks: An Electronic Journal of Teacher Research**
  www. tortoise.oise.utorontoo.ca/~gwells.journal.hthml

- **University of Bath School of Management Center for Action Research in Professional Practice**
  www.bath.ac.uk/carpp
  Includes links to doctoral and masters theses and other publications.

Learning Activities

1. Identify an area of your teaching that you would like to investigate using action research methodology.
2. Gather four or five colleagues and establish an action research group. Share what you have learned about the effectiveness of action research with your colleagues.
3. Visit one of the websites listed in the Resources list. What kind of information did you find? Was it helpful?

References

Bachman, J. A., Kitchens, E. K., Halley, S. S., & Ellison, K. J. (1992). Assessment of learning needs of nurse educators: Continuing education implications. *The Journal of Continuing Education in Nursing, 23*(1), 29-33.

Baird, J. R. (1991). Individual and group reflections as a basis for teaching development. *Teachers' Professional Development* (95-113). Melbourne: ACER.

Baird, J. R. (1989). Peer appraisal and school development. In J. Lokan & P. McKenzie *Teacher appraisal: Issues and approaches*. Hawthorn, Victoria: Australian Council for Educational Research.

Baird, J. R., & Mitchell, I. J. (1986). *Improving the quality of teaching and learning: An Australian case study—The Peel Project*. Melbourne: Monash University Printery.

Baird, J. R., Mitchell, I. J., & Northfield, J. R. (1987). Teachers as researchers: The rationale; the reality. *Research in Science Education, 17*, 129-138.

Baxter, L., & Montgomery, B. (1996). *Relating: Dialogues and dialectics*. New York: Guilford Press.

Boyden, K. M. (2000). Development of new faculty in higher education. *Journal of Professional Nursing, 16*(2), 104-111.

Bradshaw, M. J. (1992). *Teachers' practical knowledge in a nurse educator*. Unpublished doctoral dissertation, University of Texas, Austin.

Burbules, N. C., & Callister, T. A., Jr. (2000). Universities in transition: The promise and the challenge of new technologies. *Teachers College Record, 102*(2), 271-293.

Burton, L. (1997). *Overcoming the inertia of traditional instruction: An interim report on the social work faculty development program at Andrews University*. Berrien Springs, MI: Andrews University, College of Arts & Sciences.

Carr, W., & Kemmis, S. (1986). *Becoming critical: Education, knowledge and action research*. Brighton, Sussex: Falmer Press.

Carnevale, A. P., & Desrochers, D. M. (1997, April-May). The role of community colleges in the new economy. *Community College Journal,* 26-33.

Choudhry, U. K. (1992). New nurse faculty: Core competencies for role development. *Journal of Nursing Education, 31*(6), 265-272.

Coleman, J. F. (1994). *The lived experience of veteran nurse educators teaching in selected baccalaureate or higher degree programs in nursing: A study of professional development*. Unpublished doctoral dissertation, University of North Carolina, Greensboro.

Ebbutt, D. (1985). Educational action research: Some general concerns and specific quibbles. In R. Burgess (Ed.), *Issues in educational research* (pp. 152-174). London: Falmer Press.

Fullan, M. G. (2001). *The new meaning of educational change* (3rd ed.). New York: Teachers College Press.

Haddon, R. & Rossi. E. (2003, July). *Developing teacher strategies that engage the learner through reflective action research*. Paper presented at the annual Nurse Educators Conference in the Rockies, Breckenridge, CO.

Haggerson, N. & Bowman A. (1992). *Informing educational policy and practice through interpretive inquiry*. Lancaster, PA: Technomic.

Hannah, C. A. (2000). *The relationship between nursing education reform factors and undergraduate nursing faculty role strain*. Unpublished doctoral dissertation,

Hopkins, D. (1993). *A teacher's guide to classroom research* (2nd ed.). Philadelphia: Open University Press.

House, E. R., & Lapan, S. D. (1988). The driver of the classroom: The teacher and school improvement. In R. Haskins & D. MacRae (Eds.), *Policies for America's public schools: Teachers, equity, and indicators* (pp. 70-86). Norwood, NJ: Ablex.

Kember, D., & McKay, J. (1996). Action research into the quality of student learning: A paradigm for faculty development. *Journal of Higher Education, 67*(5), 528-554.

Kemmis, S., & McTaggart, R. (1988). *The action research planner* (3rd ed.). Burwood, Victoria: Deakin University Press.

Lagemann, E. C. (1991). Talk about teaching. *Teachers College Record, 93*(1), 1-5.

Lapan, S. D. (1999). *A selected glossary of terms.* Unpublished manuscript, Flagstaff, AZ: Northern Arizona University.

McLean, J. E. (1995). *Improving education through action research: A guide for administrators and teachers.* Thousand Oaks, CA: Corwin Press.

O'Toole, J. (1995). *Leading change: Overcoming the ideology of comfort and tyranny of custom.* San Francisco: Jossey-Bass.

Privateer, P. M. (1999). Academic technology and the future of higher education. *The Journal of Higher Education, 70*(1), 60-79.

Rossi, E. (2002). *Evaluation of a self-directed, group-supportive action research approach for nursing faculty teacher development.* Unpublished doctoral dissertation, Northern Arizona University.

Skiba, D. (1997). Transforming nursing education to celebrate learning. *Nursing and Health Care Perspectives, 18*(3), 124-148.

Winter, R., & Munn-Giddings, C. (2001). *A handbook for action research in health and social care.* London: Routledge.

Bibliography

Gay, L. R., & Airasian, P. (2000). *Educational research: Competencies for analysis and application* (6th ed.). Upper Saddle River, NJ: Merrill.

Hart, S. (1995). Action-in-reflection. *Educational Action Research, 3*(2), 211-232.

Jones, A. Sterling, H., Pollack, D., Doshier, S., Yeknic, C. Falls, D., et al. (1999). *Action research and educational practice.* Paper presented at the Arizona Educational Research Organization annual conference, Flagstaff, AZ.

Kemper, D. (1998). Action research: Towards an alternative framework for educational development. *Distance Education, 19*(1), 43-63.

Schon, D. A. (1983). *The reflective practitioner: How professionals think in action.* New York: Basic Books.

Skerritt-Zuber, O. (1992). *Action research in higher education: Examples and reflections.* London: Kogan Page.

Chapter 24: Starting an Email Discussion List

Doug Heaslip, Technical Advisor to Nurse Educator's email discussion,
an Online Discussion List for Nursing Educators since August 1994

As nurse educators we need to know we are not alone. We need a way to discuss issues, ask questions, and find out what others are doing. An international email discussion list like the Nurse Educator's email discussion provides just that. When I joined the Nurse Educator's email discussion list years ago, my first impression was: "It's like being at a nursing educators' conference from the comfort of my own home! The networking is wonderful!"

I still experience that same excitement when I read the daily postings. In this chapter Doug Heaslip gives us a behind-the-scenes look at what it takes to put together such a discussion list. As you will see, it is not for the weak, but it is well worth the effort! – Linda Caputi

Editors Note: To join NRSINGED, email listserv@uvvm.uvic.ca with the message: Subscribe NRSINGED *(Your name)*.

Educational Philosophy

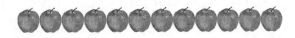

I believe teaching should focus on ways to complete solutions, not just ways to complete one task. Providing a methodology for learning to an eager apprentice provides that learner with research tools that contribute to an incremental education for the entire community. A teacher's greatest reward is seeing a student become a teacher. – Doug Heaslip

Introduction

The decision to create and manage an email discussion list is not one to be taken lightly by those wishing to succeed in such a resource-demanding, long-term, all-consuming project. Before committing to the creation of an email discussion list, you will need to:

- Evaluate, very critically, your motivation for starting a discussion list;
- Evaluate the amount of uncommitted time available daily for such a project;
- Evaluate your level of computer experience and associated skills; and
- Evaluate your level of patience and understanding of group behaviors.

This list implies that such a project requires a broad knowledge base and skill set, not necessarily typical of one individual. You do not have to launch this adventure alone. You may be able to form a list management team composed of directed volunteers to share the duties of list operational functions, such as:

- Overseeing subscriptions and member email delivery options;
- Moderating the list and editing postings;
- Handling mail server delivery errors; and
- Emergency control and corrective list functions.

Remember there is no efficient substitute for relevant, individual knowledge and experience for providing the list membership with a stable discussion platform. This chapter provides a wealth of technical knowledge needed to develop an email discussion list, but an additional goal is to encourage and inspire those interested in completing such a project.

Three Interest Objectives for Starting an Email Discussion List

There are basically three interests that motivate a person to consider establishing an email discussion list. These are:

- Professional (educational);
- Business (for profit); and
- Personal (hobby).

Following are specific issues that should be intellectually explored for each type of interest before making the decision to go forward. This initial work is very important to the success of an email discussion list.

Professional Interest

If your motivation for creating an email list is to facilitate a community for a group of students or a professional association—of nurse educators, for example—then you will need to search the Internet for available lists of lists (see the websites listed at the end of this chapter and on the accompanying CD-ROM) related to your subject of interest. This search would verify whether there is a need for a new discussion list on your topic or whether sufficient resources already exist. Join one of these existing lists so you can better evaluate the resources already available to subscribers. Ask yourself whether there is a stable supply of potential subscribers that would sustain the posting levels of your list.

Members join an email discussion list to interact with others who have a common interest. They have a desire to discuss topics of mutual interest. This requires a reasonable number of posts to the list. However, an overabundance of messages posted to the list can be detrimental. A nice mix of topics with a reasonable amount of activity is the ideal.

Since most of the professional or educational lists are hosted through institutional or association-related computer centers, the startup and hosting costs usually are negligible.

Business Interest

A business-oriented discussion list may be created for several reasons. Perhaps you would like a forum for your customers to discuss your product or service. The list provides an avenue for addressing issues your clients may have. However, prior to creating this email list, it is important to answer the following questions:

- What are the startup costs, including costs for purchase or rental of electronic hardware, software, and communication methods?
- What is the projected cost of managing and maintaining the list during its extended operating life?
- Is this method of communication the most efficient and cost-effective medium available to reach and interact with your clients?
- Are there other, more direct, communication channels available to improve your business plan?

A business email discussion list may be better focused on product service and technical support rather than exclusively on a direct, interactive discussion group.

Personal Interest

The final area of interest for establishing an email discussion list is for personal interest. Be very careful when considering the possibility of establishing a personal-interest list because it is highly likely you will be duplicating an already established list. Personal interests and hobbies usually flow into other areas of interest for both the list owner and subscribers. Ask yourself whether the mortality level of such lists is simply too high to justify the time commitment to creating the list and adhering to a maintenance schedule. Consider very carefully your motivation for creating this type of list.

Determining Your Resources

Assuming your personal motivation in creating an email discussion list is still valid, you will next need to determine the amount of time available to commit to the daily chores required of a list owner. Even on a day of moderate email traffic you can expect to spend from two to six hours dealing with posting delivery errors. Some of the most common errors are caused by:

- Host connection failures, such as host off-line, too many hops, MX (mail exchange) record errors, and unknown hosts;
- Invalid subscriber email addresses such as domain level changes, unknown user, forwarding delivery errors, and user alias errors;
- Email accounts over quota of disk drive-allocated storage space;
- Spam software program rejection of list postings, either by domain address, keyword selection listing, or false-positive selection;
- Incorrectly configured Internet service provider (ISP) and subscriber programs, usually due to incorrect path statements during rehosting of domains, and from not correctly updating email client mail server (SMTP and POP3) address assignments; and
- Failed Internet linking connections, caused by virus or spam attacks overloading relay mail servers, or by hardware-software failures and intermittent power supply issues.

You must also always be available for the following list duties:
- Accept, process, and set options for any new subscriptions;
- Complete email address change requests from list subscribers;
- Address subscription change requests (eg, stop or restart delivery, change mail to digest format);
- Assist with email client (eg, Eudora, Express, Pine) information to change addresses, formatting, expanded headers, attachment access, and line wrap;
- Assist with personal computer, word processor, or antivirus software settings, or special formatting required for any event announcement postings; and
- Correct editing or storage concerns within your public or private list archives.

Regardless of the frequency of postings, there always will be daily maintenance expected and required of the list owner to ensure the smooth, efficient operation of the many essential components of an email distribution or discussion list.

Technical Skills

To continue your inventory process, relevant current experience and technical skills do make it easier to provide efficient, independent, middle-of-the-night solutions to list emergencies that seem to arise only on holidays or weekends. These problems include virus infections, spam attacks, hackers, spoof artists, address harvesters, and denial of list control access for the list owner. If you have any level of experience with even some of these issues, then you have reserves of experience that will allow you to control the system and manage the list. If you have less technical experience, then you must be prepared to tap into any available resources to protect and defend your list and its subscribers.

It is most definitely your duty and responsibility as a list owner to defend your membership against invasions of privacy and personal information harvesting for non–list-related purposes. These offenders could send spam, spyware, or a virus, or solicit you with offers to purchase subscriber information. To defend your membership you must:
- Control the subscription process by verifying members' email addresses.
- Restrict initial posting access if you are even slightly suspicious of the identity or motives of a new subscriber by temporarily using the review command.
- Restrict access to the membership email distribution list.

- Restrict access to the archive email addresses.
- Restrict access to the list header configuration by using the "hidden" commands.
- Restrict posting access by using "nopost" and "edit-moderate" commands.
- Password protect all list owner command functions.
- Regularly scan with the most current definition files for viruses.
- Be prepared to instantly change any list header or its keyword configuration.

Managing Human Behavior within Groups

Although it is not absolutely essential, it is usually important for list owners to have a keenly developed ability to manage group behavior. List owners capable of assisting subscribers with their queries without creating confusion and misunderstanding or negative, emotional comments can greatly improve the quality of their own experience and that of subscribers. Tact and an ability to accept constructive criticism can be valuable assets for a list owner.

It is a good idea to gain list management experience before you create or assume ownership of a list. Subscribe to a list or volunteer to help the owner of an existing list. Working with a successful list owner is an excellent way to gain insight and experience handling:
- Subscriptions;
- Posting and delivery errors;
- Header configuration changes;
- Moderation and editing changes; and
- Spam and virus control configurations.

Email List Management Software

List management distribution software is required to establish an email discussion list. There are basically three different types of list distribution software that allow independent management: Majordomo, Listproc, and Listserv.

Majordomo

Majordomo is easily available via unlicensed copies for list creation and use. The program source code is written in pearl script, with many additional pearl script patches available online. The software is an accumulation of improvements contributed by volunteer programmers. Therefore, the program is not very user-friendly for the novice list owner. There are Internet help sites that provide information about Majordomo and assistance with questions about using the software, but list owners should remember that free software does have limited documentation and technical support.

Listproc

Listproc, the second option, is also easily available as free, unlicensed software for list creation and use. Like Majordomo, it offers only limited technical support resources, which may translate into hidden costs given the extra time list owners can spend looking for technical support.

Listserv

All Listserv list software is marketed by L-Soft International, which provides technical support for the programs. L-Soft offers three variations of list software; prices are dependent on the number of lists per host site, the number of subscribers per list, and the features required by the licensed host site. Listserv, Listserv Lite, and Listserv Lite Free are sold under license to a host site. There also are free-access subscriptions available to Listserv technical support lists for list owners, maintainers, and administrators.

Additional Considerations

Cost should never be the sole factor that determines the appropriate software for your list. You must also consider the whether the list host site is compatible with your operating system. The list software also must be accepted and efficiently supported by the host site technical staff.

Selecting a Host Site

A decision equal in importance to the selection of list management software is the choosing a host site. It is important to select a stable, efficient site that has proven online reliability and helpful technical support. Avoid choosing a host site whose problems could put your list out of business.

Three options for host sites are available to the list owner. They are:

- An existing business, work, or educational institution host site already hosting email distribution lists;
- A commercial host that charges a weekly, monthly, or annual fee based on the total number of subscribers and the total email volume generated by the list; and
- Your own personal computer. If you host the list yourself, the machine you use should be hardware-capable to serve a fast list and email server, and should have a constant Internet connection through an ISP cable modem.

Worksite Host

Hosting a list at your work site has some benefits to the list owner. Although it is usually not possible to select which software your new list will use, adding your list to the existing software license probably will not add any appreciable cost for the host site or yourself. The institution's existing computer services staff can help you set up and configure your new list and may use the existing lists' configuration as a template for yours. You may benefit from the host relationship by receiving prompt, cooperative technical service. However, this close relationship may pose serious challenges for the list owner. Employers may perceive conflicts between your assigned job responsibilities and the time spent on list maintenance, which could eventually develop into personal conflicts that affect your productivity and job security. Also, list postings must always meet the content approval guidelines of your hosting site staff, so list owners should clearly understand the host site's usage guidelines. You should be careful not to disclose any sensitive work through the list postings.

You should always strive to improve your technical diagnostic skills. Do not rely on technical staff to solve your list-related problems because emergencies may develop after midnight or on holiday weekends, when support may not be available; or technical staff can be reassigned, transferred beyond convenient access, or laid off, so it is best for the list owner to be able to solve these problems. Get in the practice of gleaning your own solutions by:

- Submitting questions to relevant technical lists;
- Performing searches of technical archives; and
- Using Internet keyword searches.

Some of the possible disadvantages of hosting the list through an employer can be avoided—usually at a larger expense to the list owner—by using a commercial host site.

Commercial Host

The second hosting option is an agreement with a company offering Internet list hosting for a weekly, monthly, or annual fee. Commercial hosting of your list allows the list owner more autonomy in determining acceptable discussion postings.

Since you are now paying for service, you can expect technical assistance whenever it is required. With a commercial host, if you are not satisfied with the costs or service, it is easy to transfer your list configuration and membership files to another commercial hosting business anywhere on the Internet without any negative implications for your employment.

The one obvious disadvantage of a commercial host is the expense, which might reduce your budget for additional technical services such as:

- Increased storage space for archive services;
- Premium cost, prime CPU demand time functions; and
- List software upgrades and patches.

List Owner as Host

As the list owner, you may want to privately host the list. However, if you have no software and computer skills, this option should be your last choice. Hosting on your own equipment requires you to use your own Internet connection, select your own software, and use one of your own computers as your list server.

However, this scenario offers a tremendous opportunity to build and to operate your list your way, and allows you to select:

- List management software to meet your needs;
- Other software; and
- Operating system and hardware configuration to upgrade your PC list server.

Just imagine not having to email technical support staff requesting assistance with a simple problem or document facts to diagnose problems. You can solve problems at any time that is convenient for you, even during holidays and weekends. What a rejuvenating opportunity!

Getting Started

Once a host is chosen, the list owner must configure the list type defaults, subscriber defaults, and list archive defaults. The default software options for list management, subscriber options, and archive options establish operational character of the list. An extensive review of software configuration is not included in this chapter because each discussion list management program has its own unique characteristics. But websites that provide the needed information are listed at the conclusion of this chapter. These websites provide information about list management software, program documentation, manuals, guides, feature patches, and list subscription information and other tips to help you survive and succeed as a list owner.

A Sense of Character:
Public, Private, Moderated, Unmoderated

List management default configuration options determine the operational character of your list—the face presented to the public and subscribers. The list owner must first decide whether access to the list will be public or private.

Public List Configuration

A public list may or may not require the user to have an email subscription before posting to the list membership. The subscription address may or may not require confirmation by the list owner, and postings usually are distributed without any editing or content moderation by the owner. Usually, if an archive is created, it also is open to the public. The public list configuration is usually open to any topic of discussion.

However, it is also open to spam attacks, email harvesters who use custom programs to scan the Internet for archived email addresses, and other fraudulent usage where the valid address is used by others without permission or knowledge of the owner.

Private List Configuration

Private list configurations usually require a subscription and confirmation of the subscriber's email address. This type of configuration may require the list owner to moderate or edit the postings. Public unsubscribed access to the archives may be restricted or not allowed. These restrictions provide security and privacy for the membership. The private list configuration requires active involvement by the list owner to actively moderate the list postings. Monitoring postings is justified for limiting content to only valid topics, deterring unacceptable behavior, and limiting virus infections to the membership.

Non-Interactive versus Interactive

In terms of list configuration and supervision, the announce-only, non-interactive list demands the fewest resources; facilitating the two-way communications between posting subscribers for an interactive, unmoderated list require more resources. The interactive, moderated list is the most secure against spam, virus, hackers (unsubscribed email), and inappropriate content being distributed to list members. The additional resources required for the interactive, moderated list monitoring may be justified under special conditions such as a wave of new virus or spam activity, inappropriate list content, and verifying subject lines are submitted properly.

Listserv software offers the option of using "topics: terms" by the "Subject:" line to actually create as many as 23 separate sub-lists. These topics: term sub-lists are able to sort subscriber postings through the subject line scanning for qualified "topics: terms" entered at the very start of that line, and to support individually separate subscription-mailing lists within the main list.

Subscribers: The Final Step

Perhaps the most important part of running a list is creating and maintaining an active membership. Promoting a newly created list is critical to generating frequent interactive postings. Professional associations, work groups, and related lists or interest groups are potential sources for new members.

Although the list owner sets list option defaults, mail delivery options—mail, nomail, digest, headers, and acknowledgments—can be selected and changed by each subscriber. These options should be outlined in a welcome message to each new subscriber.

List Security and Delivery Errors

In the list configuration, you must always be prepared to re-evaluate the appropriate level of security required for your list and your subscribers' privacy. Remember that security measures can never be implemented retroactively to protect your list. Security considerations must include list system files, membership lists, virus and spam protection, postings to the membership, and review of past postings.

List Security

List system and membership files can be secured by:
- Password-protecting access rights;
- Setting file attributes to hidden and/or read-only access;
- Making the configuration header file visible only to the list owner by setting configuration keywords with hidden header (HH) commands;
- Increasing the required level of validation necessary for list commands from the list owner and the membership;
- Verifying new subscribers' email addresses. The list owner can send a confirmation email notice to prevent address spoofing, which is the illegal, unauthorized use of another person's address as the return address of one's own email message.
- Setting list owner email addresses to the "nopost" default option level to prevent impostor access to the list;
- Limiting list access for unknown or suspect new subscribers using the "review" posting option until their posted messages verify that they are appropriate for membership; and
- Using a default option of "review" or "moderated-edit" mode if there is any

hint of membership posting attempts from spoofed addresses.

Protecting against virus email infections and spam is quite similar. Security is most effective if the anti-virus or anti-spam software's options and definition file updates are installed and active at all six repeated access points. These critical access points are:

- Subscribers' computers;
- Subscribers' ISP mail (SMTP) servers;
- List host computer system;
- Subscribers' ISP incoming mail (POP3) servers;
- Subscribers' own computers; and
- List owner's access to the list host, and also privately to the list members.

Additional security protection can be provided by:

- Allowing only the list owner to use the "review" membership list command function.
- Disabling the "attachment" option for postings to the list. This prevents virus and spam within attached files from infecting the list.
- Limiting the length of any single post using the "linesizelimit" function. This reduces the possibility of receiving large script sized virus code. As an added benefit, it also prevents members from posting messages that include past quoted messages that often are included in reply emails.

Remember that your list email postings must always be welcomed by your subscribers and their mail servers. This is especially important today, given industry estimates that 65 percent of email traffic is unwanted spam. This plague of useless mail is overtaxing the patience of systems staff and the physical capacity of the Internet delivery system. Therefore, list owners must accept some responsibility for controlling spam over their lists by reducing unauthorized access to list posting, membership files, and list archives.

Decisions related to the list's archives are also part of the owner's management responsibilities. The archive should become an accurate, historical record of all daily postings through the list, so security must be taken into consideration. Access options for the archive can be set to:

- Open to the public;
- Open only to list subscribers; or
- Open only to the list owner.

A list owner who wishes to provide access to subscribers or the public but also wants to retain a secure archive site can create a second off-site archive. The off-site archive could help foil email harvesters by storing archived list postings without the original email address header information.

Delivery Errors

List subscription delivery errors must always be corrected by analyzing the cause of the delivery failure and creating a way to restore delivery to the member. If it is not possible to restore delivery, the subscription must be deleted from the list. To analyze the error cause, the list owner should:

- Validate the email address in the error report as a correctly subscribed address using the "query" command, or by searching a recent copy of the membership list.
- Send a test email to the subscriber using your list-hosting email address without using any possible spam-blocking protection.
- If the first test message is returned to you as undeliverable, send another test email message from your private email account. Successful transmission of the **second** message would indicate the subscriber's server is blocking email from the list domain. If both test messages fail, either the subscriber's account is invalid or the subscriber's ISP is offline.
- Check the subscribed email address with an online email test tool (eg, www.dnsreport.com or www.samspade.org).
- Check the subscribed domain DNS at www.dnsreport.com.
- Use the WHOIS Lookup at www.dnsstuff.com to find the technical contact for the subscriber's email domain.
- Communicate your relevant evidence regarding the delivery error failures to the indicated technical contact, and to postmaster@*(the offending domain)*.

You Are Not Alone

The problems or concerns you encounter as a list manager are not unique. If you need answers, remember that someone else has probably already asked the same questions. You can find answers to most list-related concerns through:

- List software companies (either by emailing technical support or finding answers on company websites);
- Professional organizations that sponsor the list;
- Discussion lists that support your software; and
- Technical staff who have helped you in the past.

An Email Discussion List Can be Fun!

Managing an email discussion list does not have to be all work and no play. For example, the Nurse Educators list's Friday File is a humorous weekly posting that gives subscribers a chance to laugh at the end of the week. Occasionally, the Friday File serves as a catalyst for a playful exchange of email. One example follows.

The Friday File from February 20, 2004

One edition of the Friday File included Handy Latin Phrases. Entries on this list included:

- *Non calor sed umor est qui nobis incommodat.* Translation: It's not the heat, it's the humidity.
- *Lex clavatoris designate rescindenda est.* Translation: The designated hitter rule has got to go.
- *Neutiquam erro.* Translation: I am not lost.
- *Sic hoc adfixum in obice legere potes, et liberaliter educatus et nimis.* Translation: If you can read this bumper sticker, you are very well educated and much too close.

The list prompted a subscriber to post, "Thanks for bringing back memories of Latin class with Sister Theresa!" This message is typical of the postings that have been sent in response to the Friday File.

Additional Advice for Prospective List Owners

Following is a list of tips gleaned from years of experience as the list manager of the Nurse Educator's email discussion list:

- Create separate email folders in your mail client inbox for daily list postings, discussion list mail, and sent mail.
- Password protect and/or encrypt any electronically saved or stored list passwords.
- Install effective anti-virus software on your computer.
- Install anti-spy software that will auto-scan on startup, and ensure the software is updated frequently.
- Use separate discussion list sub-folders on your computer hard disk.
- Maintain logs of temporary changes to any subscriber options.
- Maintain valid copies of backup list headers for edited-moderated and unedited modes.
- Send discussion list commands only in plain text, and do not send signature files or attachments.
- Maintain a current backup list of your membership and their options in a separate location.
- Continue to enjoy learning your craft.

Resources

The following URLs provide sources for list management software; program documentation; manuals, guides, and feature patches; and list subscription information for list software tips. These URLs can be accessed from the CD-ROM accompanying this book. Simply launch your Internet browser, put the CD-ROM in the drive, go to Chapter 24 on the CD, and click on the website address.

Majordomo
www.visi.com/~barr/majordomo-faq.html
www-uclink.berkeley.edu/major/major.admin.html
www.wilsonweb.com/articles/majordomo.htm
www.greatcircle.com/majordomo

Listproc
www.cren.net/listproc
www.cren.net/closing_faq.html

Listserv
www.lsoft.com
www.mail-list.com

Internet Information Sources
www.llnl.gov/llnl/lists/listsc.html
www.lsoft.com/catalist.html
www.thefrontpage.com/search
www.cknow.com/ckinfo/list_a.htm

Summary

The heavy emphasis on the technical aspects of managing a discussion list may leave you with the impression the job is all work and no play. This is not the case. The list owner and technical adviser can inject their personalities into the list in many ways. The lesson is that this may seem like a lot of work, but it also can be fun!

Learning Activities

1. Join an email discussion list of your choice. Over the course of several weeks consider the following:
   - The number of postings per day;
   - The topics discussed; and
   - The tone of the postings.
2. Identify a person who manages an email discussion list. Ask to work with that person for several weeks. Identify:
   - The positive aspects of being a manager;
   - The negative aspects of being a manager;
   - The time involved in maintaining the list; and
   - Typical problems and how they were solved.

3. Compare and contrast the three email discussion list management software programs.

Chapter 25: Empowering One Another

Lynn Engelmann, MSN, EdD, RN,
and Janice A. Miller, BSN, MSN, RN

We often teach students how to empower themselves and their clients. We do not often think of empowerment in terms of nursing faculty. This chapter takes a look at faculty empowering each other. What a refreshing idea! – Linda Caputi

Educational Philosophy

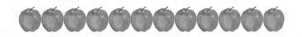

The teacher who artfully engages students in an atmosphere rich in trust, rapport, and resources is well on the way to developing a climate that is just right in which to learn. Students need to feel safe to explore and question, in order to gain meaning from their experiences. Students also need focus and perspective. In a collaborative atmosphere, both teacher and student are learners. It is equally important for teachers to be well ensconced in a positive working environment—one that fosters personal growth and enhancement. – Lynn Engelmann

Teaching has the power and ability to transform lives. The paradigm that guides my practice is humanistic: Provide a climate that fosters mutual respect and trust, support, openness, and authenticity. This atmosphere sets a premise that provides guidance, encourages independent decision-making, enhances learning, and assists students in realizing their potential. – Janice A. Miller

Introduction

The nursing faculty shortage has arrived (Trossman, 2002). One of the many factors that has contributed to the shortage is master's programs' focus on educating clinical practitioners rather than preparing nurses to be teachers (AACN, 2003). The new faculty entering academia have limited experience teaching. These nurses need mentoring and empowerment to survive their initial years of teaching and grow into skillful teachers and facilitators of learning.

This chapter explores the concepts of mentoring and empowering. First, thoughts on developing one's personal educational philosophy are explored. This is followed by a discussion of mentoring and empowering and a discussion of the authors' experiences working together as mentor and protégé.

Developing an Educational Perspective

Reflection is an important first step toward empowerment. Reflecting on past professional development provides insight into one's current behaviors. In this section, we share certain experiences that we feel have empowered us to be the nurse educators we are today.

Janice's Miller's Thoughts

I believe we build on experiences from many role models and life-changing situations. I can say I was blessed to have an array of teachers who contributed to my personal philosophy of teaching. The many individuals key to my development have modeled different facets of the human spirit, qualities that embellish the character of a teacher. All these individuals played a role in empowering me to become who I am; however, it was Professor Nancy Diekelmann who most impacted my development as an educator.

It was through her class that I felt—for the first time—a desire to teach. Dr. Diekelmann is an accomplished professional. She exuded respect, acceptance, simplicity, and trust. Her teaching methods were non-traditional. During discussions with her students, she listened intently with care and sensitivity. We walked away from her classes desiring to show that same caring attitude to someone else. In a chapter of the book *Extraordinary Teachers* (2001), Reiff wrote the following, which also describes my experience with Dr. Diekelmann:

The best compliment educators can receive from students is that we model not only what we teach but how to teach. We need to be able to practice what we preach and live the ideals we purport. A teacher committed to excellence will model high standards and expectations for self and for others but will exhibit flexibility while valuing learning differences (p. 166).

Dr. Diekelmann introduced me to the world of Heideggerian thought and philosophy. Martin Heidegger was a German philosopher whose teachings involved hermeneutics, the science of interpreting texts. Dr. Diekelmann has done extensive research on his work and has applied principles of Heidegger's interpretive pedagogy to the science of nursing. Dr. Diekelmann developed a narrative pedagogy, which calls upon the lived experiences of students, teachers, and clinicians in nursing education. This approach utilizes phenomenological, critical, and feminist pedagogies, along with postmodern discourses that create new possibilities for schooling. These practices provide a new language for contemporary nursing education. Our graduate class engaged in journaling or storytelling exercises, a form of interpretative study in narrative pedagogy. This teaching method allowed us to be reflective and thoughtful about what we heard in the classroom. As we listened to each other share nursing experiences, we found common themes, such as caring, embedded in each story. I was impressed with how Dr. Diekelmann taught us how to interpret stories in a common, nontechnical manner and brought out new meaning in mere conversations. I was in awe of the simplicity of this phenomenon. There was something profound in what we learned from one another through sharing stories.

Dr. Diekelmann also gave me the courage to teach and the willingness to learn. Thanks to her, the virtues of caring and courage are deeply embedded in my personal philosophy of teaching nursing.

Lynn Engelmann's Thoughts

There are two individuals who have had a tremendous impact on the nurse educator I am today. When I first entered graduate school, I had the good fortune to be in a nursing theory development class taught by Dr. Rosemary Ellis. This particular professor impressed me with her precision of speech and clarity of thought, as well as her perseverance; she had suffered a stroke long before I met her, yet met the physical and mental challenges of each day with fortitude and energy. As it happened, we often walked together to the classroom, and engaged in some excellent discussions. Dr. Ellis modeled the meaning of elegance in simplicity, and exemplified qualities that all nurse educators should emulate: intelligence, perspective, wisdom, and insight. She challenged us, rewarded us, and moved us forward to accept the charge of professional nursing.

One of Dr. Ellis' class assignments involved developing our own **personal nursing theory**. I was not looking forward to the assignment and I cannot recall what I decided to do for my theoretical rendering. But I do remember that one student in the class simply drew a flower in a pot. It was conceptually simple, but powerful at the same time. The idea of taking root and growing was symbolic of my time with Dr. Ellis. I now realize that my knowledge of nursing theory development grew out of the learning process Dr. Ellis led us through rather than the nursing theories created during her class.

The second faculty who made a tremendous impact on my development was Dr. Jerald Apps. His was the second class I attended in my doctoral program in adult and continuing education. At the time I began his class, I was not certain whether I would pursue a doctorate in education or nursing. Dr. Apps' class, which involved developing one's **philosophy of education**, determined the path I would take for the next several years. He had fabulous, relevant stories, my favorite of which involved Maynard the Frog, a unique frog who could see what was happening in the community of frogs, but could not effect a change for the better. In this story, Apps (1985) describes how Maynard, a leader within a society of frogs, tried to get the other frogs to pay attention to warming water trends in their pond. However, the frogs were too busy with their day-to-day activities to pay attention to Maynard, and chastised him until he retired. His pleas to consider what was happening to the water temperature went unheeded, and an earthquake struck, causing the pond water to boil. The community of frogs was lost. The story challenges us to think about the big picture while attending to day-to-day activities. This story illustrated to me the importance of setting goals and the meaning of perspective.

Dr. Apps provided a springboard from which to leap. He made sure we knew as much as possible about the waters into which we would enter. He structured class so that it was personable but not superficial. We discussed everything from Aristotle to the hippie generation of the 1970s. Ultimately, we developed our own personal philosophies. Dr. Apps' class fostered soul searching and gave me new ways to apply my knowledge.

Building on One's Educational Perspective

Most new nursing educators arrive in academia with a formal education and extensive clinical experience. Reflecting on one's experience and developing a perspective, as discussed in the previous section, provide a foundation for developing a personal educational philosophy to guide one's teaching. For new faculty, this process can be facilitated through the mentoring and empowerment of a collegial relationship.

Developing a Collegial Relationship

For new teachers, assimilating into the structure of the school is a major task. Developing a mentoring relationship with an experienced educator can help smooth the process. In this section, we describe how Janice and Lynn worked together after Janice joined the faculty at College of DuPage and why both were empowered by the relationship.

Janice's Thoughts

After meeting Lynn and the other faculty in the nursing program, I was excited to work with a team of experienced educators. Like many new faculty, I was changing careers, moving from a comfortable clinical practice into academia. It was indeed frightening, but I was up for the challenge. Lynn and I were assigned to work in the skills laboratory together and I was honored to be working with her. Over a cup of coffee, we discussed our professional nursing philosophies and areas of expertise. In a short time, we developed a mutual trust and respect. When discussing our plans to teach together, I told Lynn about my need for guidance in my new role as educator. I needed to learn how to conduct a skills laboratory class. Lynn suggested that we work together as a team. We planned to alternate teaching the class. The first week I would observe how she conducted the class, and the next week I would present the content.

Throughout the following weeks, Lynn's presence was reassuring and comforting, especially when I was confronted with questions from students. Managing classroom dialogue was a skill for me to learn. Lynn could skillfully articulate responses to an array of questions. I wondered how long would it take me to reach that level of comfort and knowledge.

I was concerned about the impression I was giving the students. I felt I should be real and honest with myself, Lynn, and the students. When I did not know something, it was alright to acknowledge my limitation because I, too, was learning. Lynn had the sensitivity and insight to give me what I needed, never embarrassing me for my lack of teaching expertise. Instead, she prodded and guided me as I developed my teaching approach.

During the weeks of team teaching, I learned how to prepare for a laboratory session. As Lynn modeled a teaching method, I observed how she conducted the class. I, in turn, tried to incorporate content I felt was important for the class. Lynn supported me, chiming in with updates on the content. She provided immediate feedback after class. The experience was the beginning of my transition to educator. Lynn's mentoring allowed me to observe the role of teacher and modeled ways of presenting content. But more importantly, I walked away from the experience empowered to develop and create my own methods for teaching.

Lynn's Thoughts

When Janice and I met, I sensed she was willing to work diligently to succeed in her new role. Janice was candid about the fact she had previously taught only in a clinical setting, but never in a classroom or skills laboratory. I thought it would be helpful for Janice to observe how laboratory sessions were conducted, then talk about possible approaches for leading the session. I took the lead organizing and planning the course, highlighting several important points. For example, I explained the laboratory sessions would be primarily hands-on. This meant that as faculty we should be comfortable demonstrating and performing the skills we presented to students. Didactic content would be succinct and limited to allow students ample time for practice and feedback. Janice planned and developed her laboratory session and I was available to answer questions. I then observed as Janice conducted the laboratory session. During class I helped her respond to student questions.

I highly regarded Janice's efforts in preparing for the skills laboratory classes as we worked together throughout the term. We spoke twice weekly about equipment needs, our approach to the content, and our plan for the learning experience. We were both willing to plan in advance, and we both valued a standard of excellence in teaching.

Janice demonstrated attributes of a prepared educator. She wrote salient points on note cards to organize her presentations. We soon developed a comfortable rhythm for working together, and created an environment wherein we respected one another and used our combined talents to provide sound instruction for the students.

There were times while Janice was teaching when I sensed her anxiety, but I just nodded my head and encouraged her to continue. Soon Janice became more comfortable, and her spirit, caring, concern, and knowledge of the content carried her. I had gained a colleague who was on her way to establishing skillful teaching techniques. It may have been easier to have taught all the classes myself with Janice observing, but I would have missed all that Janice had to offer.

In a speech to accept the presidency of the Illinois Nurses Association on October 16, 1999, Ann O'Sullivan included a quote on empowerment from Stephen Covey:

The gardener knows that life is within the seed. Effective leaders must cultivate conditions in which empowerment can grow. To empower means to spark the power within, to enable or magnify potential capacity. We must be enablers. Now, that word has gotten a negative meaning recently, but I am talking about encouraging, supporting and cheering for one another. In working with each other, we must bring out the life in each other (the seed) and nurture our growth (p. 2).

A Closer Look at Empowerment

Empowerment has been defined as "the interpersonal process of providing the resources, tools, and environment to develop, build, and increase ability and effectiveness of others to set and reach goals for individual and social ends" (Hokanson-Hawks, 1992, p. 610). The goal for the individual is to develop a sense of autonomy and accountability in professional practice. Lee (2000) wrote:

Historically nurses have been cast in positions of subservience, bereft of power. It has only been in recent years that nurses have been successful in asserting themselves by recognizing, developing, and using their own strength as a source of empowerment. Power may seem like a dissonant companion to a nurse's dedication to serve others. But power through empowerment fits comfortably with the nurturing that is central to the nursing identity. Empowerment is a logical strategic goal for nurses' professional development (p. 25).

Porter-O'Grady (1998) wrote that empowerment is recognizing the power that already exists in a role and allowing or expecting a person to express it. The emphasis is on recognizing the power in a role, not generating power from somewhere outside the role.

The authors' earlier story described a relationship based on mutual respect and trust. More importantly, the relationship gave rise to a framework for collegiality, empowerment, partnership, and respect. Our working together facilitated personal and professional growth and inspired educational excellence for both parties in the relationship.

When Mentoring Leads to Empowerment or The Power in Mentoring

Empowerment is the expression of trust between two partners who are equally committed to a process. Each recognizes in the other an essential contribution that neither could achieve alone (Porter-O'Grady, 1998). These attributes of trust, partnership, and commitment define an empowering relationship. However, extensive literature explains that these same attributes are present in a mentoring relationship (Ashton, 2003; Thorpe & Kalischuk, 2003; Owens & Patton, 2003; Shelton, 2003; Bess & Associates, 2000). This section examines the relationship between mentoring and empowerment.

Mentoring has been described as a potentially powerful partnership (Shaffer, Tallerico & Walsh, 2000). The mentor-protégé relationship can be likened to that of a master craftsman and apprentice. It is a journey that is guided by experience where knowledge is transformed from theory to practice (Dragoo, 1998). According to Anderson, Kroll, Luoma, Nelson, Shemon & Surdo (2002):

The mentoring relationship is a dynamic relationship that develops from the needs of the mentee and the abilities of the mentor. A healthy mentor relationship is a "win-win" situation for both the mentee and the mentor. The purpose of the relationship is to help the mentee adapt to the new role. Through the relationship, the needs of the mentor/mentee must be identified. A mentor is not a friend, nor a boss, but a colleague with the expertise that the mentee desires to attain (p. 25).

Mentoring promotes all of the following:
- Career advancement;
- Work satisfaction;
- Improved productivity;
- Increased self-worth;
- Preparation for leadership positions; and
- Strengthening of the profession (Herbert-Ashton, 2004).

The process of mentoring exposes the reality of empowerment. Empowerment, in turn, enhances motivation and stimulates individuals' need to succeed (Lee, 2000).

Empowerment gives individuals freedom to use their creativity and turn their ideas into action. They become role models for others and enrich themselves by teaching and sharing their ideas. See Figure 25.1.

Figure 25.1 - Mentoring, Empowering, and Role Modeling

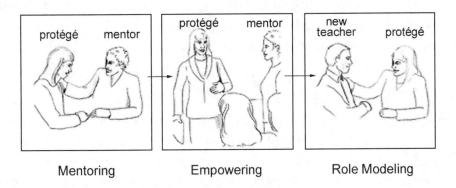

Mentoring   Empowering   Role Modeling

Empowerment in Action

Worell, McGinn, Black, Holloway, and Ney (1996) proposed a model for empowerment that comprises four critical elements:
- Collegiality;
- Communication;
- Autonomy; and
- Accountability.

This section addresses each of these elements.

Collegiality

A collegial relationship is one based on cooperative interactions and mutual respect for individuality (Worell et al, 1996). Balsmeyer, Haubrich and Quinn (1996) clarified the meaning of collegiality within academia as:

> an attitude about professional relationships that leads to genuine collaboration, potentiated individual endeavors, and mutual respect. With collegiality there is a willingness to serve, to provide guidance, to conduct one's life without prejudice, and to demonstrate respect for the ideas of others (p. 265).

When colleagues take the time to connect with one another and mutually share concerns, they set the stage for enhancing their general well-being. This synergy enables new insights about personal and professional roles and responsibilities. Collegiality replaces competition (Thorpe & Kalischuk, 2003). The results of collegial relationships are increased productivity and creativity, contributing to personal and professional growth.

Communication

Communication is the exchange of information and its meaning among individuals (Worell et al, 1996). In a collegial relationship individuals can participate in open and honest dialogue. A safe environment allows people to connect and care for one another. Caring is reflected in attitude and approach toward the other individual. Caring means encouraging and supporting one another. Communication, connecting, and caring are inseparable processes, each contributing to the success of a relationship (Thorpe & Kalischuk, 2003).

Autonomy

Autonomy is the ability to be independent, self-directed, and self-governed (Worell et al, 1996). In collegial relationships, boundaries should be established. Zerwekh & Michaels (1989) stated that allowing others to have their own thoughts and think independently indicates intellectual boundaries are intact.

In a mentor-protégé relationship, the end goal is for the protégé to become independent. Empowerment fosters independence by encouraging decision-making (Lee, 2000). Autonomy addresses the conflict often felt by empowered individuals. When a person is autonomous, that person not only is free to make decisions, but also is obligated to accept responsibility for those decisions. There is definite risk associated with accepting the consequences of one's actions. But responsibility is assumed in an environment of empowered individuals. Therefore, if a teacher can say, "I can accept autonomy and will behave in an autonomous fashion," the teacher is ready for empowerment (Milner, 1995).

Accountability

Accountability is an assumption of responsibility for one's actions (Worell et al, 1996). In nursing education, accountability is a significant value. It means assuming responsibility for one's own learning (Espeland & Shanta, 2001). Accountability through empowerment demands affirmation of one's own strength and sharing this strength with others (Mason, Costello-Nickitas, Scanlan & Magnuson, 1991). These elements allow empowerment to evolve in a meaningful manner.

Factors that Impede Empowerment

Health care is constantly changing and unity of professions is crucial to empowerment. Campbell (2003) conducted a qualitative study of the processes related to empowerment and disempowerment among 16 faculty, administrators, and students from a baccalaureate nursing program. Although nurses embraced the concept of empowerment and teamwork, the concept of **individuality** permeated their discussion. Campbell concluded that "faculty tended to gravitate away from group efforts and center on individual goals that might benefit their own careers and were more likely to experience personal empowerment than group empowerment" (p. 425).

Mentoring programs can foster empowerment. These programs help new faculty understand the organizational culture and facilitate orientation to and socialization in their roles in specific academic settings. However, successful mentoring relationships require time and directly impact the mentor's workload. If the mentor's workload is perceived to be overwhelming, the protégé may feel reluctant to initiate meetings (Lewellen, Crane, Letvak, Jones & Hu, 2003).

Another potential barrier to empowerment is enabling. Enabling has been defined as "behaviors by others that perpetuate dependent behaviors" (Haber, Krainnovich-Miller, McMahon & Price-Hoskins, 1997, p. 516), and as a component of codependency (Espeland & Shanta, 2001). According to Caffrey & Caffrey (1994), in codependent relationships, participants often attempt to control and disempower one another, impeding self-actualization. In academia, enabling may allow or encourage irresponsible behavior or foster dependence.

Reflections on One Year of Mentoring

Janice's Thoughts

My first year of teaching was a year of growth. Placing myself in a new career in education took courage, vulnerability, and humility. I experienced some successes and made many mistakes along the way. But I was not discouraged from continuing to place myself under fire, because I know the profession is worth it. The outcome was a story of success in teaching and empowerment. The process of empowerment brought forth my desire to master the role of educator. Through peer reviews and personal and professional dialogue, I was challenged to refine and expand my knowledge base. Through the guidance I received from Lynn and other faculty at the college, I feel confident that in time I can become a competent nurse educator. I will be forever grateful to Lynn for the opportunity to learn how to teach and foster student learning. She allowed me to take control and make my own decisions, which nurtured the confidence and comfort in teaching that I feel now. This is the outcome of an empowered relationship.

Lynn's Thoughts

Although Janice and I no longer teach the same course, we still share thoughts and teaching perspectives. For example, during Janice's first year, she taught the topic of fluid and electrolytes in a conventional lecture format. Although I had reviewed the lecture materials and test items, Janice's students did not achieve the results she had hoped for. We talked about possible solutions and an instructional design that applied the content to client situations. I did not give explicit directions for accomplishing this task; I merely made a few suggestions, such as using case studies to present select medical-surgical problems. I also directed Janice to some resources for guidance on writing test items. Janice willingly received this feedback and created a presentation that used animation to illustrate the relationship among fluids, electrolytes, and client conditions. Learning improved, as evidenced by higher test scores.

Why was my relationship with Janice empowering for me? I felt satisfied that I had been helpful to Janice, and all it took was a little time. It was a pleasure to work with her, as she demonstrated all the attributes of an ideal protégé. Together we were able to meet students' needs. I also grew in my professional practice as I modeled and revisited my own teaching philosophy.

Empowerment of Students

Nurses are challenged to disseminate knowledge to students and share best practices starting at the grassroots level. Diekelmann and Ironside (2002) encourage us to share practices that we know are effective. This is what we do with students on a daily basis: share best practices from our repertoire of knowledge and explain the constructs that shape nursing. Knowledge is perhaps the most obvious element for empowering future nurses. Students need knowledge about empowerment, and empowerment of faculty has the potential to translate into empowerment of students. Just as critical thinking must be demonstrated for students (Caputi, 2004), so must empowerment be demonstrated. Mentoring, at its best, serves to empower and to provide an avenue for those who teach to share their nursing knowledge with current colleagues and with their future colleagues, the students of today.

Before mentoring and empowerment can occur, the attributes and characteristics discussed in this chapter that are prerequisites for mentor and protégé must be in place. If faculty are to actively engage one another and their students, the environment in which faculty work must also be conducive to, and value, empowerment.

Faculty who hold students responsible for their own learning communicate a confidence and trust in students. Once this trust is communicated, students are motivated to formulate and achieve educational goals. Ultimately, these are the educational goals that faculty strive to effect as they foster learning climates that empower students. In this way, power is used as a positive and energizing force (Forrest, 2004).

Ultimately, the profession of nursing seeks graduates who have the self-confidence and ability to think critically and take charge. These are the nurses of the future who will seek, and revel in, autonomy and accountability in their professional practice (Espeland & Shanta, 2001).

Summary

What does it take to become a nurse educator? According to National League of Nursing (NLN) (2002), master's and doctoral nursing programs designed to prepare nurse educators saw a decline in enrollment from 1993 to 1999. NLN emphasized that the cadre of experts in nursing education are aging and there is a need to prepare future nursing educators. (For more on this topic, see the chapter in this book, *The Nursing Faculty Shortage*, by Linda Caputi). The academic community should not assume that individuals learn to be teachers, advisors, curriculum developers, and educational leaders through on-the-job training or trial by fire, but rather by a thorough, deliberate preparation for such roles and responsibilities (Kelly, 2002).

The NLN (2002) made the following recommendations for nurses and nursing faculties:

- Nurses should seek out and take advantage of opportunities that prepare them for a nurse educator role.
- Faculty should promote careers in nursing education through the early identification of talented neophytes and the encouragement of experienced nurses who have demonstrated nurse educator skills.
- Senior faculty who themselves are expert educators should mentor novices and foster professional growth in the role.
- Faculty should partner with colleagues in other disciplines to explore the implementation and implication of a heightened focus on educational excellence, pedagogical research, and innovative program design (p. 269).

This chapter explored one avenue for educators to answer the charge of preparing new educators for the task of teaching nursing. We ask you to think about what this means to all of us, as we strive to prepare both those who would teach and those who would enter the profession of nursing.

Learning Activities

1. Think about the benefits of mentoring. Consider the faculty with whom you teach. Would you be willing and able to mentor any of these individuals? If so, in what capacity? Consider actively mentoring a colleague for six months. Keep a journal of the experience. Include this information in your self-evaluation.
2. Identify a teacher who you think might help you in your role as a nurse educator. Approach that individual, and ask if he or she would be willing to mentor you. Think about what you would like to gain from the relationship, and outline what you would like to learn. Think about what you might offer as the protégé in the relationship.

References

American Association of Colleges of Nursing (2003). White paper: Faculty shortages in baccalaureate and graduate nursing programs. Washington, DC: Author.

Anderson, M., Kroll, B., Luoma, J., Nelson, J., Shemon, K., & Surdo, J. (2002). Mentoring relationships. *Minnesota Nursing Accent, 74*(4), 24-29.

Apps, J. (1985). *Improving practice in continuing education: Modern approaches for understanding the field and determining priorities.* San Francisco: Jossey-Bass.

Balsmeyer, B., Haubrich, K., & Quinn, C. (1996). Defining collegiality within the academic setting. *Journal of Nursing Education, 35*, 264-267.

Bess, J. L., & Associates (2000). *Teaching alone, teaching together: Transforming the structure of teams for teaching.* San Francisco: Jossey-Bass.

Caffrey, R., & Caffrey, P. (1994). Nursing: caring or codependent? *Nursing Forum, 29*(1), 12-17.

Caputi, L. (2004). Operationalizing critical thinking. In L. Caputi & L. Engelmann (Eds.), *Teaching nursing: The art and science, Vol. 1 & 2.* Glen Ellyn, IL: College of DuPage Press.

Campbell, S. L. (2003). Cultivating empowerment in nursing today for a strong profession tomorrow. *Journal of Nursing Education, 42*(9), 423-426.

Diekelmann, N., & Ironside, P. M. (2002). Developing a science of nursing education: Innovation with research. *Journal of Nursing Education, 41*(9), 379-380.

Dragoo, J. (1998) Mentoring a novice chief nurse executive. *Journal of Nursing Administration, 28*(9), 12-14.

Espeland, K., & Shanta, L. (2001). Empowering versus enabling in academia. *Journal of Nursing Education, 40*(8), 342-346.

Forrest, S. (2004). Personal power and conflict resolution. In L. Caputi & L. Engelmann (Eds.), *Teaching nursing: The art and science, Vol. 1 & 2.* Glen Ellyn, IL: College of DuPage Press.

Haber, J., Krainnovich-Miller, B., McMahon, A., & Price-Hoskins, P. (1997). *Comprehensive psychiatric nursing* (5th ed.) St. Louis: Mosby.

Herbert-Ashton, M. (2004). Mentoring new faculty. In L. Caputi & L. Engelmann (Eds.), *Teaching nursing: The art and science, Vol 1 & 2.* Glen Ellyn, IL: College of DuPage Press.

Hokanson-Hawks, J. (1992). Empowerment in nursing education: Concept analysis and application to philosophy learning and instruction. *Journal of Advanced Nursing, 17,* 609-618.

Kelly, C. M. (2002). Investing in the future of nursing education: A cry for action. *Nursing Education Perspectives, 23*(1), 24-29.

Lee, L. (2000). Buzzword with a basis. *Nursing Management, 31*(10), 24-27.

Lewellen, L. P., Crane, P. B., Letvak, S., Jones, E., & Hu, J. (2003). An innovative strategy to enhance new faculty success. *Nursing Education Perspectives, 24*(5), 257-260.

Mason, D. J., Costello-Nickitas, D. M., Scanlan, J. M., & Magnuson, B. A. (1991). Empowering nurses for politically astute change in the workplace. *The Journal of Continuing Education of Nursing, 22,* 5-10.

Milner, S. (1995). An ethical practice model in the age of empowerment. *Mississippi RN, 57*(5), 16.

National League of Nursing. (2002). NLN position statement. *Nursing Education Perspectives, 23*(5), 267-269.

Owens, J. K., & Patton, J. G. (2003). Taking a chance on nursing mentorships: Enhance leadership with this win-win strategy. *Nursing Education Perspectives, 24*(4), 200-204.

O'Sullivan, A. (1999). President's message. Empowerment, synergy and unit. *Chart 1999, 96*(9), 2-3.

Porter-O'Grady, T. (1998). The myths and reality of empowerment. *NursingManagement, 29* (10), 5-6.

Shaffer, B., Tallerico, B., & Walsh, J. (2000). Win-win mentoring. *Educational Dimensions, 19,* 36-28.

Shelton, E. N. (2003). Faculty support and student retention. *Journal of Nursing Education, 42*(2), 68-69.

Stephenson, F. (2001). *Extraordinary teachers: The essence of excellent teaching.* Kansas City: McMeel-Andrews.

Thorpe, K. & Kalischuk, R. G. (2003). A collegial mentoring model for nurse educators.*Nursing Forum, 38*(1), 5-14.

Trossman, S. (2002). Who will be there to teach? Shortage of nursing faculty a growing problem. *American Nurse, 34*(1), 22-23.

Worrell, J., McGinn, A., Black, E., Holloway, N., & Ney, P. (1996). The RN-BSN student: Developing a model of empowerment. Journal *of Nursing Education, 35,* 127-130.

Zerwekh, J., & Michaels, B. (1989). Co-dependency: Assessment and recovery. *Nursing Clinics of North America, 24,* 109-120.

Index

Academic freedom 29, 423-424, 433

Academic program review 336-352

Academic support 195, 204, 402, 404

Accreditation 86, 146, 318, 320, 331, 336-339, 343, 351-352, 356, 391-421

Action research 440-456

Active learning 15, 125-141, 298, 302, 364

Active learning approaches 125-141

Administrative evaluation 29, 87, 428

Adult learners 8, 27, 150, 194, 296-297

Adult learning theory 126, 133, 300

Affective domain 283-286, 290, 294, 299

Affective learning 138, 282-295

Affective strategies 284, 294

American Association of Colleges of Nursing (AACN) 3-5, 7-8, 14, 17, 20-21, 283, 316, 318, 395, 478

American Association of University Professors (AAUP) 424, 433

American Nurses Association (ANA) 8-9, 17, 81, 265, 278, 315, 320

Americans with Disabilities Act 209, 212, 216, 223, 226

Approval 73, 279, 318, 324-325, 328-329, 336, 391, 394, 411-412, 466

APRNs 5

Arousal 94, 127, 140

Arousal activity 127, 140

Assessment 10, 13, 15, 17, 27, 61, 77, 87, 102-103, 122-123, 127, 137-138, 150-151, 158, 163-177, 180-191, 204, 217-218, 220, 232, 234-235, 243, 256, 259, 261, 287, 293, 304-305, 337, 339-343, 377, 385-386, 388, 391-394, 401, 404, 407, 409, 424-425, 429

Asynchronous 148, 153, 158, 216, 358, 361-363, 365-366

Author guidelines 38-39, 43, 46, 53

Author information page 38, 47

Barriers to Writing 34-35

Benchmarking 314-332

Benchmarking for progression 314-332

Bloom's taxonomy 246, 254, 277

Boilerplate 65, 67

Caring 30, 97, 132-134, 139, 171, 173, 186, 243, 256-257, 267, 282-283, 288, 291, 293, 304, 314, 384-385, 442, 478-479, 483, 486

Case study 11, 18, 129, 133, 197, 208, 373, 376

Case-based learning 132

Center of Excellence in Nursing Education 425

Charting 27

Chat room 195, 201, 204, 358, 362, 364

Chief academic nursing officer 71-75, 85

Clinical assessment 163-191

Clinical decision making 129, 166

Clinical faculty 75, 151, 163-165, 171, 173-174, 176, 180, 234

Clinical judgment 131, 133, 166, 169

Clinical reasoning 125, 132-133, 166

Clinical setting 33, 78, 148-149, 151, 163-166, 173, 177, 180, 283, 285-286, 288-289, 291-292, 306, 316, 367-388, 399, 404-405, 446, 454, 482

Clinical skill performance 131

Clinical teacher 147, 153, 164-167, 171, 173, 175

Clinical teaching 3, 5, 33, 317, 326, 388, 432, 434

Clinical-track appointment 71, 79

Clock hour 5, 73

Cognitive domain 138, 254, 283-284, 299

Cognitive learning theory 126-127, 131

Cognitive retention 284

Collaborative learning 137, 139

College Classroom Environment Scale (CCES) 134

College evaluation system 423-438

Commercial host 466-467

Commission on Collegiate Nursing Education (CCNE) 146, 318, 320, 336-337, 343, 352, 391-410, 411, 421

Community of learners 167

Community reflexive scholarship 169

Computer literacy 203-204

Computerized adaptive testing (CAT) 245, 249, 261-262, 273

Computerized nursing exams 315

Concept map 18, 44, 131, 368, 376-378, 388, 419

Concept mapping 18, 131, 368, 377-378

Constructivist learning theory 299

Consulting grants 63

Contact hour 5, 432

Continuous quality improvement 320, 338, 440

Cooperative learning 126, 137-138, 140, 167

Core competencies 10, 278

Course management software 152

Critical thinking 8, 15, 128, 132-133, 138-139, 147, 152-153, 157, 159, 161, 166, 170, 177, 181, 197, 204, 207, 212, 254, 284, 296, 298, 301, 304-305, 311-312, 328, 355-366, 367-388, 426, 449, 489

Critical thinking online 355-366

Critical thinking skills and strategies 371-373

Critical thinking tool 368-373, 378-379, 382, 384-385, 387-388

Conventional pedagogies 167

Cultural awareness 243-244, 267, 275, 290

Cultural competence 105-106, 114, 122

Cultural immersion 101-123

Cultural immersion experience 101-123

Culture shock 112-113, 441

Curricular benchmarks 326

Curriculum development 11, 34, 36, 193, 408-409

Debate 136, 358-359, 365, 431

Disabilities 172, 209-229, 232-236, 270

Disability awareness activities 213

Teaching Nursing: The Art and Science

Discussion 11, 18, 20, 28, 61, 72, 77, 92, 94, 108, 112, 126-128, 132-133, 135-136, 146-162, 164, 167-168, 170-172, 174, 176-177, 180-191, 195, 197, 201, 204, 215-216, 235, 251, 286, 289-290, 293, 299, 341, 358, 362-364, 370, 378, 394, 431, 444-445, 452, 454, 459-476, 478, 480, 487

Discussion board 156, 159, 195, 197, 201, 204, 358, 362-363

Distance Education 15, 33, 203

Diversity 5, 8, 102, 209, 215, 259, 297, 312

Drawings 131

Due process 432-433

Education for all Handicapped Children Act of 1975 217

Educational perspective 478, 481

Educational research 7, 238

Electronic forum 150, 216

Email 35, 39, 47-48, 72, 152, 156, 195, 201, 204, 222, 459-476

Email discussion list 459-476

Email list 461, 464

Empowering 9, 477-491

Empowerment 429, 477-478, 481, 483-485, 487-489

Endowment grants 63

Entry-level nursing competencies 250

Essential functions 212

Evaluation 10-11, 14, 16, 18, 29, 33, 36, 46-47, 65, 71, 80, 86-87, 123, 133, 135-136, 140, 150-152, 154, 157, 164, 166, 169, 206, 217, 232-233, 236, 251, 256, 267, 285, 287, 291-292, 298-300, 304, 306, 312,

315, 317, 319-322, 324-325, 328, 330-331, 337, 346-348, 363, 377, 392, 394-395, 399-402, 404-406, 409, 412, 414-416, 418-420, 423-438, 491

Evidence-based curricula 7

Experiential laboratory situations 297

Experiential learning 135-136, 140

External accreditation 391, 393-394, 400

External curriculum evaluation 319-320, 324

External observers 423, 431

Faculty development plan 14, 21

Faculty evaluation 80, 87, 136, 321, 415, 423-426, 428, 430-432, 434-435, 437-438

Faculty politics 70-87

Faculty shortage 2-21, 83, 315, 478, 490

Fellowship grants 63

Friday File 473

Grant process 56, 61-62

Grant writing 55, 58, 60, 65, 69

Grantmaker 56, 59, 62-68

Grants 55-70, 81-82, 85, 88, 411

Grantseeker 55-65, 67-69

Grantsmanship 55-57

Health Education Systems, Inc. (HESI) 315, 318, 321, 325-331

Heideggerian thought 479

Hermeneutics 479

Host country 103-104, 108, 112-114, 119

Host site 465-467

Human dignity 283, 286, 289, 292, 349

Humanistic learning theory 126

Hybrid courses 18
Idea drawer 57-58
Immersion clinical experiences 115
Inclusion 210, 220, 225, 407
Inclusion-building activities 210
Individualized nursing education program 210, 216-217, 229, 232, 236
Individuals with Disabilities Education Act 216-217
Inspiration 90-99, 123, 363
Inspirational leader 95
Inspire 90, 93-96, 460
Inspired teaching 97
Interactive multimedia 130
Interactive teaching 448-449
Interpretive phenomenological approach 166, 176
Jigsaw 138-139
Joint Commission on Accreditation of Healthcare Organizations 338
Journal of Nursing Education 34, 38
Journal writing 57, 115
Laboratory simulation experiences 296-312
Laboratory simulations 300-301, 304
Learner-centered 149
Learning communities 139
Learning environments 126, 149, 297
Learning outcomes 27, 126, 137, 140, 283, 291, 304-305, 351
Liberal arts 25, 72, 102, 254, 265
List configuration 467-470
List owner 462-472, 474-475
List security 470
Listproc 455, 464-465, 475
Listserv 459, 464-465, 469, 475

L-Soft 465
Majordomo 464-465, 474
Manuscript 33-40, 42-53
Mentor 9-10, 12, 14, 16, 18, 20, 87, 228, 478, 484, 487-491
Mentoring 9, 105, 398, 478, 481-482, 484-485, 487-489, 491
Mentoring relationship 481, 484
Mind mapping 131
Mnemonic 129-130, 141
Narrative 46, 63, 67, 97, 134-135, 166-168, 171-173, 175-176, 180, 288, 401, 479
Narrative pedagogy 134-135, 166-167, 172, 175, 479
National Council Licensure Examination for Registered Nurses (NCLEX-RN) 237, 240-242, 245-246, 250-251, 253-257, 261, 274-275, 277-280, 315, 317-318, 320-322, 324-328, 330-331
National Council Licensure Examinations (NCLEX) 5, 15, 81, 90, 199, 217, 226, 236, 237-280, 314-315, 332, 432
National Council of State Boards of Nursing 15, 81, 237-238, 250, 253, 264, 274, 356
National League for Nursing (NLN) 3, 7, 10, 14, 17, 69, 146, 412, 425, 490
National League for Nursing Accrediting Commission (NLNAC) 146, 318, 336-337, 343, 352, 410, 411-421
NCLEX test plan 250-251, 273

NCLEX-PN 240, 243-245, 250-251, 264-267, 273-274

Nrsinged 459

Nurse Educator 3, 34, 38, 459, 473-474

Nursing research 6, 60

Nursing simulation laboratory 301, 303, 312

Office for Civil Rights 223, 229

Ongoing reflective practice 443

Online clinical discussion 146-162

Online course 59, 80, 152, 195, 203, 205, 356, 358, 363-365

Online discussion 146-147, 149, 151-154, 156-159, 290, 362-363, 459

Online discussion groups 146

Online discussion list 459

Online educators 150

Online instruction 18, 355-356, 358

Opposing opinion 136

Participation 74, 104, 138, 156, 158-159, 215, 228, 232, 294, 297, 303, 358, 363, 398, 420, 441, 443, 450, 452

Part-time faculty 19, 317, 425

Peer review 34-35, 48, 51, 411, 413, 423, 426-428, 433, 437, 488

People-first language 210-211

Personal reflection 91, 93, 133, 229, 442

Personal tutor system 194

Postclinical conferences 167

Post-tenure 434-435

Preceptor 10, 16, 78, 217

Problem solving 8, 26-27, 58, 94, 129, 131-132, 150, 167, 183, 243, 246,

255, 265, 267, 277, 296-298, 304, 311-312, 345, 368

Problem-based learning 15, 132-133, 362

Program grants 62

Promotion 33-34, 51, 80, 82, 87, 114, 122-123, 150, 160, 241-244, 254-257, 259, 265-266, 268, 270, 275-278, 356, 408, 425, 428

Proposal 56-57, 61, 63-69

Protégé 478, 484, 487-489, 491

Query letters 39, 63

Questioning 91, 133, 136, 358, 426, 444-445

Reasonable accommodations 210, 214, 216, 227, 229-230

Recursive reflection 442

Reflection 91, 93, 115, 133-134, 147-153, 166-168, 229, 286, 289, 362, 379, 400, 442, 446, 453-454, 478, 488

Reflective journaling 293

Reflective practice 386-388, 443

Reflective thought 133, 146-161

Rehabilitation Act of 1973 223, 229

Research grants 62

Responding 35, 48, 68, 156, 175-176, 265, 284-285, 292, 294, 377

Retention standards 210

Retirement 2-3, 16-17, 19-21, 83, 316-317

Revenue generation 55

Role play 104, 129, 136-137, 223, 286, 288-289, 292, 373, 446, 454

Scholarship 11, 34, 55, 63, 169, 320, 428

Search committee 71-72, 75

Service learning 128, 139-140

Short-term travel courses 101-124

Simulation 129, 131, 213, 225, 296-312

Skill performance scenarios 300

Socialization of nursing students 284, 293

Spam 462-464, 469-472

Standardized exams 317, 321-322, 324, 331

Standardized patients 131

Standardized testing 319, 331

Start-up grants 62

Storytelling 58, 67, 479

Student evaluation 29, 363, 423, 430-431, 433-434

Student-centered learning 126, 132

Students with disabilities 209-236

Synchronous 148, 153, 158, 201, 216, 358, 361-366

Teacher-focused 443

Tenure 6-7, 10, 16, 33-34, 51, 71, 79-80, 82, 84, 86-88, 323, 423, 425, 433-435, 437

Tenure-track appointment 79-80, 86

Terrorism 105, 111-112, 114, 434

Test plan 238-245, 250-251, 253-257, 262, 264-268, 273-280

Think aloud 127-128

Think-pair-share 138

Training grants 55, 63

Transformational leader 95

Transformational process 95

Triad of teaching 8

Triage 26-27

Tutor 18, 155, 193-208, 217, 232, 236, 245, 262, 273

Tutorials 196, 203, 245, 262, 273

Two-minute assessment 385-386

Universal instructional design 210, 215

Valuing 284-285, 289, 292-294, 299, 479

Virtual office hours 156

Virus 462-464, 469-471, 474

Web-based 14-15, 18-20, 29, 148, 150, 154, 194, 356

Web-enhanced discussions 148

Workload credit 72-75

Worksite host 466

Writing for Publication 32-53, 74

Tables

Table 3.1 - Online Directories of Nursing and Healthcare Journals   40

Table 3.2 - Sample Summary to Accompany Revised Manuscript   52

Table 8.1 - Explanation of Neuro-deficit Role Play   137

Table 9.1 - CMS Programs   154

Table 17.1 - Comparison of Academic Program Review   338
    and Accreditation Review

Table 20.1 - Sample Timeline for Accreditation Process   396-397

Table 22.1 - Methods of Evaluating Faculty Performance   436-437

Figures

Figure 1.1 - Grid for Grading a Term Paper   13

Figure 3.1 - Sample Query Letter   41

Figure 3.2 - Sample Cover Letter   49

Figure 3.3 - Sample Manuscript Review Form   50

Figure 7.1 - Sample Travel Course Syllabus   107

Figure 7.2 - Stages of Culture Shock   113

Figure 7.3 - Directions for Writing a Journal   116

Figure 8.1 - Illustration of Mnemonic for Auscultating Heart Sounds   130

Figure 10.1 - Postconference Phrases   169

Figure 11.1 - Modules in an Online Tutoring Program   196

Figure 11.2 - Content in an Online Tutoring Module   198

Figure 11.3 - Sample Test Questions Used in an Online Tutoring Module   200

Figure 11.4 - End-of-Term Survey   207

Figure 12.1 - Types of Accommodations   218

Figure 12.2 - Special Stethoscope   221

Figure 12.3 - Wheelchair-accessible ADA Exam Table   227

Figure 13.1 - The NCLEX Process   239

Figure 13.2 - Distribution of Content on the 2004 NCLEX-RN Test Plan   242

Figure 13.3 - Distribution Content on the NCLEX-PN Exam   244

Figure 13.4 - Multiple Response Item   247

Figure 13.5 - Fill-in-the-Blank Calculation Item   247

Figure 13.6 - Ordered-Response Item   248

Figure 13.7 - Hot-Spot Item   248

Figure 15.1 - Pediatric-Mental Health Scenario   307

Figure 15.2 - Adolescent Scenario   308

Figure 15.3 - Maternal Scenario   309

Figure 15.4 - Adult Medical-Surgical Scenario   310

Figure 15.5 - Older Adult Scenario   311

Figure 16.1 - NCLEX-RN Pass/Fail Rates by E_2 Scoring Intervals   326

Figure 16.2 - Progression Policies: Consequences of Benchmark Failure (N=35)   329

Figure 17.1 - Deming's 14 Points for Management   339

Figure 17.2 - Standard for Evaluating Program Reviews in   347-350
      Higher Education
Figure 19.1 - Sample Critical-Thinking Exercise   375
Figure 19.2 - Student Success Plan   376
Figure 19.3 - Chart Explorer   380
Figure 19.4 - Report Organizer   381
Figure 19.5 - Diagnostic Tests and Procedures   382
Figure 19.6 - IV Medication Administration and Monitoring   383
Figure 19.7 - Critical-Thinking Tool for the Client with   384
      Congestive Heart Failure
Figure 19.8 - Critical Thinking Tool for the Client with   385
      Renal Failure
Figure 19.9 - Two-Minute Assessment Tool   386
Figure 19.10 - Reflective Practice Tool   387
Figure 20.1 - Time-saving Strategies   403
Figure 25.1 - Mentoring, Empowering, and Role Modeling   485

Appendices

Appendix 7.1 - Student Health Promotion Teaching Project   122-124

Appendix 10.1 - Guidelines for Using Reflective Writing for   180-191
         Assessment and Dialogue

Appendix 12.1 - Example of an Individualized Nursing   232-236
         Education Program

Appendix 13.1 - NCLEX-RN Test Plan   253-263

Appendix 13.2 - NCLEX-PN Test Plan   264-273

Appendix 13.3 - NCLEX-RN Frequently Asked Questions   274-280